Glomerulopathies: Updated Reviews

Glomerulopathies: Updated Reviews

Edited by **Ida Waddell**

New Jersey

Published by Foster Academics,
61 Van Reypen Street,
Jersey City, NJ 07306, USA
www.fosteracademics.com

Glomerulopathies: Updated Reviews
Edited by Ida Waddell

International Standard Book Number: 978-1-63242-199-9 (Hardback)

Printed in the United States of America.

Contents

             Permissions

             List of Contributors

Preface

Kidney diseases can cause abnormalities in kidney functions. This book is a comprehensive overview of current developments in clinical features and therapeutic options in glomerulopathies physiology. The book has several chapters which discuss various topics regarding this subject. It deals with primary glomerulopathies and evaluates its complicating infectious circumstances. This book also discusses various disorders related to glomerulopathies. The objective of this book is to help students and experts in gaining more knowledge regarding this disease.

All of the data presented henceforth, was collaborated in the wake of recent advancements in the field. The aim of this book is to present the diversified developments from across the globe in a comprehensible manner. The opinions expressed in each chapter belong solely to the contributing authors. Their interpretations of the topics are the integral part of this book, which I have carefully compiled for a better understanding of the readers.

At the end, I would like to thank all those who dedicated their time and efforts for the successful completion of this book. I also wish to convey my gratitude towards my friends and family who supported me at every step.

Editor

Part 1

Primary Glomerulopathies

Membranous Nephropathy

Abdelaziz Elsanjak and Sharma S. Prabhakar
Department of Medicine, Texas Tech University Health Sciences Center
USA

1. Introduction

Membranous nephropathy (MN), a very common cause of nephrotic syndrome, is a glomerulopathy defined histopathologically by the presence of immune complexes on the extracapillary side of the glomerular basement membrane (GBM). Idiopathic membranous nephropathy (IMN) is an antibody-mediated glomerular disease with no defined etiology, histologically characterized by uniform thickening of glomerular basement membrane (GBM), caused by subepithelial immune complex deposits. Most cases of MN are idiopathic, for instance approximately 75% of the cases of MN in developed countries are idiopathic, or primary membranous nephropathy (IMN). MN can be secondary to a wide spectrum of infections, tumors, autoimmune diseases or exposure to drugs or toxic agents. Examples include systemic lupus erythematosus, hepatitis B antigenemia or other chronic infections, and historically graft vs. host disease, sickle cell anemia, a number of drugs and toxins such as therapeutic gold salts, penicillamine, tumors, and agents containing mercury

Idiopathic MN is a glomerulus-specific autoimmune disease and second only to focal glomerulosclerosis, is a leading primary cause of the nephrotic syndrome in adults. The name, '*membranous* nephropathy' reflects the pathological observation in light microscopy of thickening in the GBM between and around immune deposits that occur beneath the podocyte foot processes. The histological hallmarks of the disease were first described by Jones and Mellors and Ortega' over 60 years ago. These include "spikes," stained by methenamine silver, of normal GBM that extend between the immune deposits, a fine granular distribution of immunoglobulin (Ig) G and the complement component C3 in a capillary-loop pattern revealed by immunofluorescence, and the presence of electron-dense subepithelial immune deposits indicated by electron microscopy (EM). Idiopathic MN most commonly occurs in patients between the ages of 30 and 60 years, with men twice as likely to be affected as women. However, MN does occur in children as well as in the very elderly. Up to 70% of patients present with the nephrotic syndrome and the others garner clinical attention due to abnormalities in urine sediment such as proteinuria. Microscopic hematuria is observed in up to 50% of cases although red cell casts are rare. Hypertension and impaired renal function are uncommon at the outset of the disease and are more likely to occur with disease progression

2. Pathogenesis

Idiopathic membranous nephropathy (IMN) is an antibody-mediated glomerular disease that is histologically characterized by uniform thickening of glomerular basement membrane (GBM), caused by subepithelial immune complex deposits. The immune deposits consist of IgG, mainly IgG4 and IgG1 of antigens that have long escaped identification, and the membrane attack complex of complement C5b-9 (MAC). The formation of subepithelial immune deposits and complement activation are responsible for functional impairment of the glomerular capillary wall, causing proteinuria .Most data on the pathogenesis of MN comes from an animal model, the Heymann model of experimental MN in rats, which suggests that the podocyte is the target of injury. Studies show that there is in-situ binding of a circulating antibody to antigen in the subepithelial space. In the Heymann nephritis model, megalin was identified as the antigenic target. However, megalin, which is a member of the low-density lipoprotein receptor family and is expressed with clathrin at the base of podocyte foot processes (the site of immune complex formation) in rats, is an unlikely antigen for human MN.

In Heymann nephritis model of MN, rats are immunized against an antigenic fraction derived from rat proximal tubular brush border and develop subepithelial deposits virtually identical to those observed in human disease. The target antigen is a large transmembrane endocytic receptor known as megalin. In the rat (but not in human beings) megalin is additionally present on the foot processes of podocytes, allowing circulating antimegalin antibodies to cross the GBM, bind megalin at the podocyte cell surface, and ultimately form subepithelial immune deposits in situ. Complement, activated by the immune deposits, leads to insertion of the terminal complement components C5b-9 (the membrane attack complex) into the podocyte cell membrane, causing cell injury, effacement of the foot processes, and proteinuria.

In 2002, Debiec and Ronco identified neutral endopeptidase (NEP) as the responsible antigen in a rare subset of patients with alloimmune antenatal membranous nephropathy. This discovery supplied proof of concept that a human podocyte antigen could serve as a target for nephritogenic antibodies, as shown some 20 years earlier for the rat podocyte megalin in Heymann nephritis, the well established experimental model of membranous nephropathy.

Debiec and Ronco studied the development of neonatal MN in infants born of mothers genetically lacking neutral endopeptidase (NEP), a membrane-associated podocyte antigen that digests peptides. Because the fetus did not lack NEP, fetomaternal alloimmunization occurred and anti-NEP antibodies (often in very high titers) developed in the mothers. These antibodies (often of the IgG4 or IgG1 subclasses, similar to human idiopathic MN) crossed the placental barrier and interacted with the NEP, heavily expressed on the normal fetal podocyte. In situ immune complexes (containing both IgG1 and IgG4) developed in the newborn infant (or soon after birth) and typical MN ensued, along with proteinuria and nephrotic syndrome. The finding of the C5b-C9 membrane attack complex in the deposits, suggesting that this spontaneous human alloimmune disease also might be complement-dependent, was similar to what had been proposed for Heymann nephritis.

In 2009 Beck and et al identified circulating autoantibodies reactive with the transmembrane glycoprotein M-type phospholipase A2 receptor (PLA2R) in the majority of cases of adult IMN. This protein is expressed by the human podocyte, again suggesting a mechanism of disease that fits the paradigm established in Heymann nephritis. These anti-PLA2R autoantibodies were highly specific for IMN, and were not present in normal individuals, in patients with other causes of the nephrotic syndrome, or in cases of secondary MN. Levels of circulating anti- PLA2R antibodies parallel the course of clinical disease, declining or disappearing before a partial or complete remission of proteinuria, and reappearing with recurrence of nephrotic syndrome

T cells play a significant role in the pathogenesis. The presence of IgG4, which is a product of the type 2 response T helper cells (Th2) and an upregulation of cytokines, such as interleukins (IL) -4 and -10, suggest Th2 involvement. This CD4, T-cell dependent humoral response leads to subsequent Ig deposition and complement activation.

More recently Stanescu et al (2011) performed independent genome-wide association studies of single-nucleotide polymorphisms (SNPs) in patients with idiopathic membranous nephropathy from three populations of white ancestry (75 French, 146 Dutch, and 335 British patients). The patients were compared with racially matched control subjects; population stratification and quality controls were carried out according to standard criteria. In a joint analysis of data from the 556 patients studied (398 men), they identified significant alleles at two genomic loci associated with idiopathic membranous nephropathy. Chromosome 2q24 contains the gene encoding M-type phospholipase A_2 receptor (PLA$_2$R1) (SNP rs4664308, $P=8.6 \times 10^{-29}$), previously shown to be the target of an autoimmune response. Chromosome 6p21 contains the gene encoding HLA complex class II HLA-DQ alpha chain 1 (HLA-DQA1) (SNP rs2187668, $P=8.0 \times 10^{-93}$). The association with HLA-DQA1 was significant in all three populations ($P=1.8 \times 10^{-9}$, $P=5.6 \times 10^{-27}$, and $P=5.2 \times 10^{-36}$ in the French, Dutch, and British groups, respectively). The odds ratio for idiopathic membranous nephropathy with homozygosity for both risk alleles was 78.5 (95% confidence interval, 34.6 to 178.2). They concluded that an HLA-DQA1 allele on chromosome 6p21 is most closely associated with idiopathic membranous nephropathy in persons of white ancestry. This allele may facilitate an autoimmune response against targets such as variants of *PLA2R1*, findings which suggest a basis for understanding this disease and illuminate how adaptive immunity is regulated by HLA.

2.1 Natural history and prognosis of idiopathic MN

MN is a chronic disease, with spontaneous remission and relapses. In the United States and Europe, MN remains the second or third leading cause of ESRD among the primary glomerulonephritis types. Spontaneous remissions occur in up to 30% of cases and usually occur within the first 2 yrs after presentation. The percentage of patients going into spontaneous remission is much lower in patients with higher grades of proteinuria at presentation (*e.g.*, proteinuria >8 g/24 h). The remaining two thirds are divided into those with persistent proteinuria who maintain renal function long term, or who progress to renal failure. In white patients with NS, 10-yr kidney survival of 70% has been reported. Although the percentage of the IMGN population that progresses to end-stage renal failure remains relatively small, the absolute numbers are large. It affects people predominantly in their 30s and 40s, and has an enormous long-term impact on their quality of life and productivity. Because they have single-organ disease rather than multisystem organ failure (as is seen in diabetes), they survive longer on dialysis and after renal transplantation. However, even though these patients survive longer, they continue to function at a lower level in comparison with the age and gender matched normal population, and rarely returns to the same level of productivity or quality of life as their peers. Even in patients who do not progress to ESRD, complications often occur, including life-threatening thromboembolic phenomena and accelerated vascular disease. These may be due to an underlying specific defect in coagulation and/or tissue repair and/or the long-term sequelae of their prolonged nephrotic condition.

Today, once the diagnosis is made, the management of edema, BP, and hyperlipidemia is effective in almost all IMGN patients. The impact of the control of these factors alone on the natural history is expected to be positive but is currently unknown. This is partly due to the unusual phenomena of up to 30% of IMGN patients experiencing spontaneous remission. This wide variation in outcome is one of the factors that has led meta-analysis and systematic reviews of this disease to reach varying conclusions about the impact of immunosuppressive treatment on patient and renal survival and on proteinuria remission rates.

Female gender and low grade proteinuria is associated with good prognosis and associated with spontaneous remission. End-stage renal disease occurs at a 2-3:1 male:female ratio. Also, Asians with IMN appear to have a more favorable long-term prognosis than their non-Asian counterparts.

The Toronto Glomerulonephritis Registry created a model for identifying patients at risk for progression of renal insufficiency, taking into account the initial creatinine clearance (CrCl), the slope of the CrCl, and the lowest amount of proteinuria during a 6-month period. According to this model, patients who present with a normal CrCl (proteinuria <4 g/24 h), and stable renal function over 6 months are considered to be at low risk for progression. On the other hand, patients with persistent proteinuria (>8 g/24 h) have a 66−80% probability of progression to ESRD within 10 years, independent of the degree of renal dysfunction. Other factors associated with poor prognosis include older age, tubular interstitial changes on kidney biopsy and a high degree of glomerulosclerosis.

2.2 Clinical manifestations
MN affects patients of all ages and races, but is generally more common in men than women. It most commonly occurs in middle age, with peak incidence between the ages of 40-60. In contrast to primary MN, secondary forms of MN are most commonly encountered in young children and in individuals who are older than 60. At presentation, 60-70% of patients have nephrotic syndrome with the remaining 30-40% of patients presenting with subnephrotic range proteinuria (<3.5 g/24 h). 60 % of patients who present with subnephrotic range proteinuria will progress to full nephrotic syndrome in 1-2 years (Daniel Cattran 2006). Microscopic hematuria is common in MN (30 to 40%), but macroscopic hematuria and red cell casts are rare and should suggest other diagnoses .The majority of patients with MN are normotensive at presentation, however hypertension is present in 10-20 % of patients. Less than 20% present with renal insufficiency.

Serologic evaluation of all patients with MN should include anti-nuclear antibody HbsAg and hepatitis C virus antibody studies. Workup for malignancy is also warranted, to the extent that testing should be guided by the patient's age and whether there is a history of tobacco use.

2.3 Primary (idiopathic) vs. secondary forms of membraneous nephropathy
In developed countries, MN is primarily idiopathic, implying that known secondary causes have been effectively ruled out. Secondary forms of MN have been linked to multiple different agents and conditions. MN occurring post-hematopoietic stem cell transplantation (HSCT) may be a humoral manifestation of chronic graft-versus-host disease; it is the most common cause of post-HSCT nephrotic syndrome, and like idiopathic, post-HSCT MN disproportionately affects males. MN may recur in up to 42% of renal allografts with slowly progressive proteinuria; it is also possible for *de novo* MN to occur, perhaps as *an* alloimmune reactivation to minor histocompatibility antigens on the allograft podocytes.

Finally, MN may briefly occur early in infancy as a result of feto-maternal alloimmunization. Idiopathic MN must be distinguished from the various secondary causes, since treating or eliminating those underlying conditions are often sufficient to cause nephrotic syndrome remission.

The most common secondary form of MN in the United States (US) is membranous lupus nephritis (LN), designated class V LN by the International Society of Nephrology-Renal Pathology Society, and is seen in -10%-20% of LN cases (picture of LMN). The disease may occur in isolation and pre-date other symptoms or serological abnormalities suggestive of lupus. Thus, even in the absence of positive serological markers such as antinuclear antibodies (ANAs), membranous LN should remain a possibility in any young woman with a biopsy diagnosis of MN. Features that distinguish idiopathic MN from membranous LN and other secondary forms of MN include the glomerular location of the immune deposits, the predominance of a particular IgG subclass, and other pathological features. Clues to the diagnosis of membranous LN include the presence of subendothelial and mesangial deposits, in addition to the predominant subepithelial deposits, and a "full house" pattern of staining for IgG, IgA, IgM, C3, and Clq on immunofluorescence. In idiopathic MN the predominant IgG subclass found in the glomerular deposits is IgG4, whereas in many secondary forms, IgGl, IgG2, and IgG3 predorninate. Finally, an ultrastructural finding of tubuloreticular structures in the glomerular endothelium suggests lupus, although these structures can also be found in other non-idiopathic forms of MN.

Currently, renal biopsy is the sole means for diagnosis of MN and distinguishing it from other causes of nephrotic syndrome. The results of routine serological studies, including complement levels, are all normal in idiopathic MN. Possibly, antibodies to the human phospholipase A2 receptor (PLA2R) found in many patients with idiopathic MN may allow a serological diagnosis of MN, but this test is only available in research settings. Secondary causes of MN may be suggested by the presence of ANA, hepatitis B virus (HBV)-antigenemia, or concurrent infection with schistosomiasis or secondary syphilis. Hypocomplementemia may occur in lupus or HBV-associated MN, but normal complement levels do not rule out these diagnoses. Associations of MN with malignancy have been found in older individuals seemingly more frequent than chance. Therefore, in older individuals with newly diagnosed MN, tests to exclude malignancy is reasonable.

A number of secondary processes can also cause MN that are clinically and histologically similar to IMN. Worldwide, chronic infections such as hepatitis B, malaria, syphilis, and schistosomiasis are the most important causes of secondary MN. Systemic lupus erythematosus can give rise to a membranous form of glomerular disease, classified as class V lupus nephritis. Other autoimmune diseases such as rheumatoid arthritis, autoimmune thyroid diseases, and Sjogren's syndrome can all be associated with MN. Historically, certain medications used for the treatment of rheumatoid arthritis such as gold salts, penicillamine, and some NSAIDs were causally linked to MN. Solid tumors are associated with secondary MN more often than chance alone would predict, and on rare occasions remissions and relapses of the glomerular disease have been noted to occur with removal or relapse of the malignancy.

Finally, MN can occur de novo after renal transplantation or allogeneic hematopoietic stem cell transplantation, perhaps reflecting alloimmunization to a minor histocompatibility antigen expressed in the glomerulus. Secondary forms of MN often exhibit histopathological clues that distinguish them from IMN, although this is not always the case. As opposed to the exclusively subepithelial and intra-membranous deposits seen in IMN, secondary forms, especially membranous lupus nephritis, often have mesangial and subendothelial deposits. Tubuloreticular inclusions may also been seen within the glomerular endothelium on electron microscopy in lupus-associated MN. The IgG subclasses found within the glomerular deposits also differ. In contrast to the predominant IgG4 found in IMN, IgG2 and IgG3 are typically most abundant in secondary (lupus- and malignancy-associated) forms of MN. Finally, the nature of the electron dense material itself may herald a secondary cause. A form of MN characterized by spherular structures within the subepithelial deposits has been described that appears to be distinct from its idiopathic cousin.

Infectious
• Hepatitis B
• Hepatitis C
• Streptococcal Infections
• Malaria
• Schistosomiasis
• Syphilis
• Leprosy
• Tuberculosis
• Cytomegalovirus
Drugs
• Captopril
• Clopidogrel
• Mercury
• Penicillamine
• NSAIDs
• Gold
Autoimmune Diseases
• Systemic Lupus erythematosis
• Rheumatoid Arthritis
• Thyroiditis
• Sjogren's Disease
• Psoriasis
• Sarcoidosis
• Mixed Connective Tissue Disease
Neoplasms
• Carcinomas of the bladder, breast, pancreas, prostate, stomach cancer, lung cancer.
• Hematological malignancies: Lymphoma, Chronic Lymphoctic Leukemia
Others
• Sickle Cell
• Diabetes Mellitus
• Post-Transplant
• Hematopoietic Stem-cell transplant

Table 1. Secondary Causes of MN

2.4 Post-transplantation membranous glomerulopathy

Idiopathic MN recurs in 10–30% of patients after kidney transplantation. De novo MN, which is the most common de novo glomerulopathy in renal allografts, affects 2–9% of renal allografts. De novo MN occurs 2-3 years post-transplantation, while recurrent MN occurs after 1-2 years. The exact pathogenesis of de novo MN is unknown. Recurrence of membranous nephropathy is preceded by nephrotic range proteinuria. Recurrent membranous nephropathy usually presents sooner after transplantation (within 2 years) than *de novo* membranous nephropathy (after 2 years). Some data suggests that the actual risk of recurrence reaches 29% 3 years after transplantation. Half of the cases of recurrent membranous nephropathy progressed to end-stage renal disease within a decade. There is one case report in literature where the de novo MN was linked to antibody mediated rejection: the patient had donor specific antibody-DQ7. Remission of proteinuria was associated with a fall in the anti-DQ7 titer. This raised the possibility that *de novo* membranous nephropathy could be a particular manifestation of chronic antibody - mediated rejection (Menon, Shina et al 2010)

2.5 Histopathologic considerations of membranous nephropathy

The subtle nature of the light microscopic findings in some cases of Membranous Glomerulonephritis (MGN) and presence of basement membrane thickening in other glomerular diseases lead to the uncertainty in the diagnosis of MGN in its earlier days of evolution as a pathologic entity (Heptinstall R). Only after the development of electron microscopy and immunologic techniques MGN was distinguished with certainty from other causes of the nephrotic syndrome including minimal change disease and its variants and certain forms of chronic glomerulonephritis (Heptinstall).

3. Light microscopy

3.1 Glomeruli

The characteristic changes of MGN are seen in glomerular capillary walls. The other compartments may have secondary changes but are usually minor until the advanced stages of disease. The light microscopic appearance may be subtle, especially in early cases; however, in these cases immunopathology and electron microscopy can easily establish the diagnosis. Capillary loops may appear round and rigid in more advanced stages on hematoxylin and eosin stain (Fig.1).

The earliest sign by light microscopy is "moth-eaten" appearance of the GBM on silver stains (fig.2).

3.2 Immunopathology

The immunofluorescence characteristic of MGN is granular capillary wall staining for immunoglobulins and complement. IgG is present in almost all cases, and C3 staining is seen in approximately three quarter of cases (Fig. 3). The most important and invariable deposit is IgG, and even when other immunoglobulin or complement reactants are seen, they have a weaker staining and only segmental presence (Jenette JC 1983).

Mesangial deposits are usually not seen. The presence of prominent mesangial deposits or full house positivity with other immunoglobulins or complements should suggest MGN secondary to systemic lupus erythematosus.

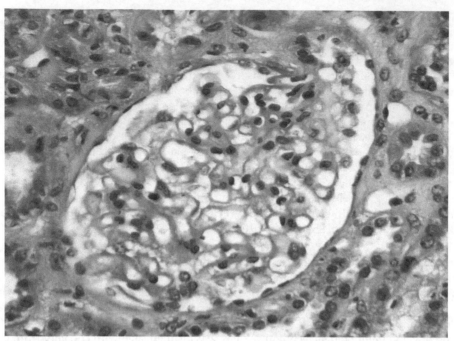

Fig. 1. Membranous glomerulonephropathy. Capillary loops may appear round and rigid in advanced cases. (H&E, 40X)

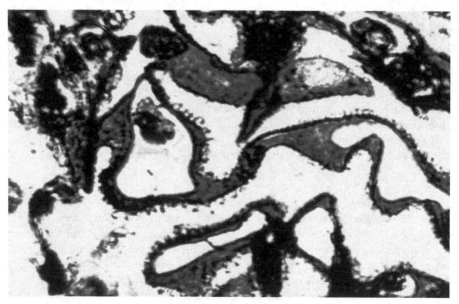

Fig. 2. Membranous glomerulonephropathy. Linear projections or "spikes" protrude from the outer surface of the GBM on silver stains (Periodic acid methenamine silver, 100X)

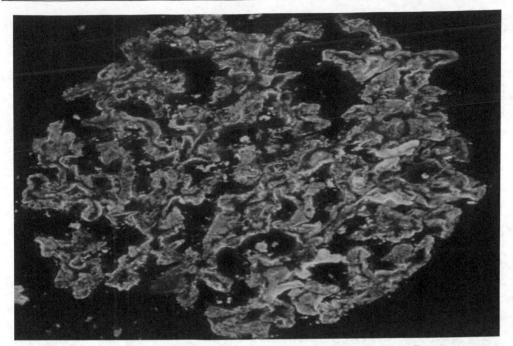

Fig.3. Membranous glomerulonephropathy. IgG is positive (2+) by immunofluorescence.

3.3 Electron microscopic findings
Electron microscopy findings helped define MGN by demonstrating the subepithelial and intramembranous (depending on the stage) location of electron-dense deposits (Gartner HV 1974). Electron-dense deposits are seen on the epithelial side of glomerular capillary loops (subepithelial). The location of electron-dense deposits at different levels in the GBM in the course of the disease led to the hypothesis that there is a sequence of changes in the GBM following initial subepithelial deposition (Ehrenreich T 1968).

3.4 Tubules
Tubular changes in MGN include progressive atrophy as the glomerular lesion progresses.

3.5 Interstitium
In uncomplicated cases, interstitial fibrosis may be seen without prominent inflammation or tubular atrophy. Development of interstitial fibrosis may reflect a progression of the glomerular lesion (Magill AB 1995).

3.6 Differential diagnosis
The light microscopic differential includes all glomerular diseases that have thickening of the glomerular basement membrane. In context of diseases associated with the nephrotic syndrome, the differential diagnosis includes minimal change disease, focal segmental glomerulosclerosis, membranoproliferative glomerulonephritis, diabetes mellitus and amyloidosis. In the past, before the development of electron microscopy and immunologic

techniques, many of these distinctions were made on clinical grounds or not at all. However, currently, characteristic histologic, immunopathologic, and ultrastructural findings can reliably distinguish it from other causes of nephrotic syndrome.

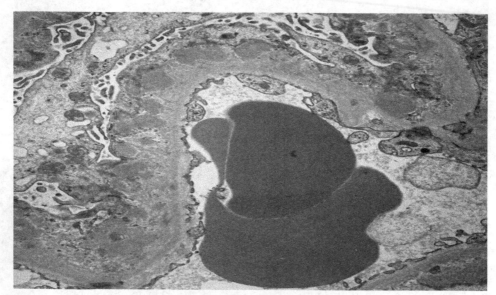

Fig. 4. Electron-dense deposits are present in subepithelial location.

3.7 Prognostic indicators

Ehrenreich and Churg (5) described the stages of membranous transformation as the morphologic representations of progression of the disease. Favorable outcomes are generally related to early stages (I and II) of membranous transformation. However, several later studies (Wahrmann 1989) did not find a relation between glomerular stage and outcome.

4. Natural history and prognosis of idiopathic MN

Although spontaneous remission of nephrotic syndrome occurs in about a third of patients, end-stage renal failure is observed in about 40% of patients after 10 years. Predicting the clinical course of a patient with MN at disease presentation is impossible given the variable and fluctuating disease course. A widely appreciated yet oversimplified view is that one-third of all patients will spontaneously remit without treatment, another third will remain proteinuric with preserved renal function and the final third will progress to end-stage renal disease (ESRD). Young females and those with subnephrotic levels of proteinuria are most likely to experience spontaneous remission, justifying several months of observation prior to any initiation of treatment in the absence of problematic clinical features. Baseline demographic differences in natural-history studies lead to a blurred prognostic picture. Several risk factors for MN progression have been proposed: older age at onset, male sex, nephrotic-range proteinuria (especially >8 g), and increased serum creatinine at presentation. As with most renal diseases, progression correlates with the amount of tubulointerstitial disease on renal biopsy, and a tubulointerstitial disease score has been included as a prognostic variable in several studies. Although the rate of renal decline may not differ in comparison with MN patients having preserved renal function, patients with a higher serum creatinine or increased interstitial disease at presentation will reach ESRD in a shorter time; therefore, it is advisable to consider early treatment in these patients. Asians with IMN appear to have a more favorable long-term prognosis than their non-Asian counterparts.

Achieving complete remission predicts an excellent long-term renal prognosis and those patients have nearly universal renal survival at 10 years, whereas the number falls to 90% with partial remission, and 45% with no remission. Cattran and his colleagues (Cattran 2005) proposed a prognostic model dividing patients with into low-, moderate-, and high-risk groups based on their degree of proteinuria and clinical course over 6 months of observation. Those with normal renal function and lower amounts of proteinuria <4 g daily) over 6 months constitute a group at low risk for developing progressive renal insufficiency from the disease. Intermediate levels of proteinuria (4-8 g daily) with stable renal function over 6 months define a group at moderate risk. The highest-risk patients are those with >8 g of daily proteinuria for 6 months, and/or reduced renal function at outset or deterioration of renal function over 6 months. The risk of further renal deterioration in this group is at least 75%.

A number of adult studies have allowed practitioners to characterize prognostic factors in adult patients with MN. Laluck et al. showed that low-grade, subnephrotic proteinuria and female gender were associated with spontaneous remission. Ideally, only patients unlikely to spontaneously remit and those at risk for significant renal deterioration should be treated. Male gender, age >50 years, persistent high-grade proteinuria, impaired renal function at onset, presence of segmental glomerular sclerosis, and tubulointerstitial damage on the kidney biopsy have been considered to be poor prognostic factors in adult idiopathic MN .

The Toronto Glomerulonephritis Registry created a model for identifying patients at risk for progression of renal insufficiency, taking into account the initial creatinine clearance (CrCl), the slope of the CrCl, and the lowest amount of proteinuria during a 6-month period. According to this model, patients who present with a normal CrCl, proteinuria <4 g/24 h, and stable renal function over 6 months are considered to be at low risk for progression. On the other hand, patients with persistent proteinuria (>8 g/24 h) have a 66–80% probability of progression to ESRD within10 years, independent of the degree of renal dysfunction

5. Treatment of idiopathic membranous nephropathy

5.1 General outlines

Treatment goals in IMN are to prevent loss of renal function and to prevent the complications of the nephrotic syndrome (eg, hyperlipidemia, volume overload hypertension, and thrombophilia). Opinions vary on how best to obtain the desired results, and the literature concerning the treatment of IMN is still unclear. The relatively low incidence of MN hampers recruitment into clinical trials, and the variable natural history of the disease adds further treatment complications. In addition, substantial risks for treatment are associated with established immunosuppressive agents and newer, potentially less toxic agents (eg, mycophenolate or rituximab) have been introduced for the treatment of MN without the benefit of long-term clinical trials. A meta-analysis on 1025 patients with MN from 18 randomized clinical trials concluded that immunosuppressive treatment had no benefits in patient or renal survival; however some data suggest that the treatment is warranted. Because of the high rate of spontaneous remission in MN, newly diagnosed patients with nephritic syndrome and normal renal function should initially receive conservative therapy with an ACE inhibitor or ARB, diuretics, salt restriction, and statins. If a patient remains proteinuric with normal renal function, such conservative treatment can be continued, but those patients who remain frankly nephrotic after 6 months or who initially present with (or develop) renal dysfunction should be treated with an immunosuppressive agent.

The treatment of MN depends on patient presentation and disease progression after diagnosis is made by biopsy. The two leading immunomodulatory therapies used are alkylating agents (cyclophosphamide or chlorambucil) and calcineurin inhibitors (cyclosporine or tacrolimus), both typically given orally or intravenous with corticosteroids . Given the limited efficacy, high rate of relapse, and toxicities of alkylating agents, calcineurin inhibitors, and corticosteroids, other therapies for MN are needed. Recently, rituximab has surfaced as a potential treatment option for MN. This monoclonal antibody directed against the B cell antigen CD20 may be beneficial in MN on the basis of experimental evidence that B cell activation is a key step in the pathogenesis of MN. Furthermore, rituximab is generally well tolerated with a limited short-term toxicity profile. A significant amount of literature is emerging on the benefits of rituximab in MN as primary treatment and as treatment for IMN refractory to other immunosuppressant regimens.

The treatment of membranous nephropathy in patients with normal renal function remains controversial. However in patients with deteriorating renal function, a combination therapy with steroids and cytotoxic agents is considered beneficial . It remains unclear if therapy is effective in more advanced renal failure since there is no published data on such cases. There are some cases reported in literature   with near end-stage renal failure in whom treatment resulted in clinical improvement. Thus therapy is effective in patients with primary membranous nephropathy and advanced azotemia especially in those who had never been treated.((Prabhakar S et al 1996)

5.2 Alkylating agents

Corticosteroids as monotherapy for treatment of IMN is not effective, instead, typical immunosuppressive regimens for idiopathic MN combine corticosteroids with alkylating agents for 6-12 months. Treatment with cyclophosphamide or chlorambucil in conjunction with corticosteroids is supported by randomized controlled trials (RCTs) cumulative data suggest that 30%-40% of those treated will achieve complete remission, with 30%-50% attaining partial remission and only 10% developing progressive renal disease," Relapse occurs in approximately 25%- 30% within 5 years of discontinuing the alkylating agent, but often responds to a repeat course of immunosuppressive therapy arm. A 6-month regimen consisting of alternating months of corticosteroids and alkylating agents has both short-term and long-term beneficial effects on proteinuria and renal survival. Ponticelli and colleagues found that this regimen increased remission rates at the final follow-up visit from 36% in untreated patients to 76%, and improved 10-year renal survival from 60% to 92%. The long-term outcomes of a randomized, controlled trial from India (Jha et al) found the same result. Some studies indicated that a delay in therapy did not lead to differences in efficacy. Studies showed immunosuppressive therapy markedly lessened the decline in renal function.

Despite the favorable results of alkylating agents in IMN, many physicians are reluctant to use these drugs, because of increased risk of infection and myelosuppression, particularly those with reduced GFR. Cancer risk is increased when alkylating agents are used for a long time. There are some reports of increased risk of wegener granulomatosis with cyclophosphamide when the dose is more than 36 gmr (equivalent to 100 mg daily for one year) were associated with a 9.5-fold increased risk of bladder cancer. Use of cyclophosphamide for long time have also been associated with an increased risk of lympho-proliferative disorders. Relapses occur in 25–30% of patients within 5 years of discontinuation of therapy with alkylating agents. While this rate of relapse is lower than that observed after discontinuation of cyclosporine, it is still disconcerting since relapses generally necessitate increased immunosuppression. Despite reduction in proteinuria, these agents failed to show beneficial effects on overall mortality or risk of ESRD.

5.3 The calcineurin inhibitors (CNIs): Cyclosporine and tacrolimus

Cyclosporine is an alternative, clinically validated immunosuppressive agent used in the treatment of IMN. In one randomized clinical trial (RCT), 51 patients with steroid-resistant IMN, treatment with cyclosporine plus steroids for 6 months with tapering over 4 weeks resulted in a 75% complete or partial remission rate, versus only 22% in the placebo (steroids alone) group. Typically, many patients in cyclosporine based treatment regimens achieved partial remissions, and many relapsed after discontinuing treatment. Another similarly-sized trial compared 12 months of cyclosporine and corticosteroids to cyclosporine alone." Although both groups achieved -80% remission rates at 12 months, the relapse rate was lower in the group receiving adjunctive corticosteroids from the beginning. Longer courses of cyclosporine (1-2 years) with a slow taper may be necessary to avoid a high rate of relapse. Other investigators demonstrated that treatment with tacrolimus in heavily nephrotic patients resulted in higher remission rates compared with conservative treatment alone; however, nearly half of these patients had a nephritic relapse within several months of tapering tacrolimus. Cyclosporine reduces proteinuria and the rate of decline in renal function in patients with IMN. These effects have been demonstrated in patients with preserved renal function, in those with declining or impaired renal function and also in patients resistant to other immunosuppressants. In some studies almost 50% of patients who had achieved remission relapsed within 1 year of cyclosporine withdrawal, especially in the first 6 months. In high-risk patients with declining renal function a 12 month treatment of cyclosporine led to a 50% reduction in proteinuria in half of the patients, and slowed the rate of renal deterioration compared with placebo. Notably, no prospective, randomized, head-to-head comparisons of cyclosporine and alkylating agents have been conducted in IMN.

On the basis of the available data, extended therapy seems to enhance the likelihood of remission. In one analysis, the majority of complete remissions occurred after at least 6 months of therapy, and the number increased as treatment continued for more than 12 months. Thereafter, the combination of low-dose cyclosporine (1.4–1.5 mg/kg per day; trough levels >100 ng/ml) and prednisolone (0.1 mg/kg per day) might be more beneficial than cyclosporin monotherapy for maintaining remission and preventing relapse.

Several investigators have evaluated whether tacrolimus could provide similar efficacy to cyclosporine in IMN. Tacrolimus is considered to be more potent than cyclosporine, has a more favorable cardiovascular risk profile and leads to better long-term renal function after renal transplantation. Studies showed the overall remission rate achieved with tacrolimus is similar to that reported with cyclosporine but the rate of complete remission is higher with tacrolimus. This difference might be, in part, related to the long duration of therapy used in these studies (18 months, compared with 26 weeks in the study of cyclosporine by Cattran et al). The nephrotoxic effects of calcineurin inhibitors are of concern, particularly if long-term treatment is required as a result of relapses. Managing the use of these agents in patients with reduced GFR can be difficult. Due to this issue, Ponticelli and Villa recommend alternative agents in patients with impaired renal function (creatinine clearance <60 ml/min), severe hypertension or severe interstitial fibrosis and tubular atrophy. Finally, the extent to which calcineurin inhibitors affect the underlying immune process rather than merely modifying disease expression is unclear. In view of the broad range of toxic effects and the high rates of relapse associated with the use of steroids, alkylating agents and calcineurin inhibitors, alternative treatments have been investigated

6. Antimetabolites

6.1 Mycophenolate mofetil

Mycophenolate is another agent used for MN treatment with varying results. Initial studies suggested that mycophenolate could reduce proteinuria in patients with MN resistant to other conventional therapies. However, a recent RCT detected no effect of mycophenolate monotherapy in patients with normal renal function and nephrotic levels of proteinuria, when compared to conservative antiproteinuric therapy. Corticosteroid treatment with mycophenolate therapy achieved a 1-year cumulative remission rate of 66% in a group of MN patients with moderate renal dysfunction, but was inferior to alkalating agents and steroids in a historically treated control group and demonstrated a relapse rate of nearly 40%. However, a small RCT revealed similar effects from 6 months of mycophenolate and steroids compared with chlorambucil and steroids at 15 months of follow-up. Given these small studies and lack of consistently demonstrated superior efficacy, mycophenolate is not a first-line agent for the treatment of MN, but may be considered with adjunctive corticosteroids, if standard therapies are not effective or cannot be tolerated.

Clinical efficacy studies of mycophenolate mofetil (MMF) in IMN have produced mixed results in a multicenter study (Chan *et al.*) randomized 20 newly diagnosed patients with persistent proteinuria ≥3 g per day to undergo 6 months of treatment with either MMF plus prednisolone or with a regimen of chlorambucil alternating monthly with corticosteroids. The groups achieved similar remission rates (65%) and experienced few relapses, which suggests that MMF in conjunction with steroids has similar efficacy to a modified Ponticelli regimen. An open-label trial in the Netherlands evaluated the efficacy of MMF in patients considered to be at high risk of disease progression. The outcomes of 32 patients treated for 1 year with MMF 2 g per day and steroids were compared with those of historic matched controls treated with oral cyclophosphamide plus corticosteroids for 1 year. Patients in both groups had reduced GFR at baseline (median approximately 40 ml/min) and median proteinuria was >8 g/g creatinine. The two groups achieved similar remission rates (approximately 70%), but the relapse was higher in the MMF group such that by the end of follow-up, patients in the MMF arm were less likely to be in remission than those in the cyclophosphamide . Both treatments resulted in stabilization or improvement of renal function in the majority of patients, and infections and hospitalization occurred at a similar frequency in the two groups. Although the investigators concluded that MMF did not seem to be as effective as, or any better tolerated than cyclophosphamide, this study does suggest that a prolonged course of MMF might be of benefit even in patients with unfavorable baseline characteristics.

In contrast to the above-mentioned studies, responses to MMF in other multicenter randomized controlled trials the have been poor. Firm recommendations regarding the use of this agent as initial therapy are difficult to make. MMF might be a reasonable option when the toxic effects of alkylating agents and high-dose steroids are of particular concern or when severe azotemia prohibits use of calcineurin inhibitors. Studies in large numbers of patients with prolonged follow-up are needed to determine the long-term effectiveness of MMF for maintenance of remission and preservation of renal function. Additional information is also needed to fully evaluate the adverse effect profile of MMF. MMF is also associated with pregnancy loss and congenital malformations and it can also increase the risk of lymphoma and infection. Cases of JC-virus-associated progressive multifocal leukoencephalopathy in patients with systemic lupus erythematosus receiving MMF have elicited concern. All these considerations must be weighed in the decision to use MMF in IMN,

6.2 Azathioprine

Before the use of MMF became widespread, azathioprine was tested as a treatment for IMN in several small studies, with mixed results. A combination of azathioprine and corticosteroids was reported to be beneficial in high-risk patients with declining renal function. Some patients experienced reduction in proteinuria and stabilization or improvement of renal function. However, these studies were case series with no control groups and the combined number of patients analyzed was small. In contrast to these favorable findings, a recent retrospective review indicated that azathioprine had no long-term benefit in IMN. Due to the conflicting evidence regarding the efficacy of azathioprine in IMN and the popularity of MMF, azathioprine is unlikely to be tested in future randomized trials in this setting.

7. Alternative agents

Due to the often severe adverse or nephrotoxic effects associated with cyclophosphamide and cyclosporine, several newer and potentially less toxic agents are under evaluation for the treatment of MN. Several small studies indicate the potential efficacy of rituximab, mycophenolate, or synthetic adrenocorticotrophic hormone (ACTH) in MN; unfortunately, none are large RCTs nor do they provide long-term follow-up data

7.1 Rituximab

Rituximab is a monoclonal anti-CD20 antibody that depletes B cells, Its rationale for use is provided by the suggested pathophysiological basis for MN of autoantibodies targeting a suspected glomerular antigen. Rituximab has been used in treatment of non-Hodgkin Lymphoma and others diseases. Although Rituximab appears to induce remission with an initial efficacy comparable to alkylating agents and corticosteroids, long-term data on dialysis-free survival have not been reported. In an open label trial of rituximab with a group of 15 high-risk idiopathic MN patients, there were 2 complete and 6 partial remissions at final follow-up. Others reported the effects of treatment with 4 weekly doses of rituximab on 50 consecutive patients with persistent nephrotic levels of proteinuria despite 6 months of conservative therapy," Ten patients achieved a full remission after treatment; however, they were more likely female and with lower baseline serum creatinine values, which is a population of high spontaneous remission. Recently, a small RCT study conducted in Spain demonstrated that rituximab was of benefit in 13 Spanish patients with idiopathic MN and CNI dependence, allowing successful weaning of the nephrotoxic CN. A review of the published literature about rituximab describing the use of rituximab in MN highlights that, while promising, the existing literature consists of too few patients, heterogeneous populations, and insufficient follow-up to recommend the use of rituximab outside the research setting.

There may be potentially fatal mucocutaneous reactions, such as stevens–Johnson syndrome and toxic epidermal necrolysis, can occur following rituximab exposure. Severe infections are infrequent, occurring in only 1–2% of patients. Of great concern, rare cases of progressive multifocal leukoencephalopathy have been reported with rituximab use, particularly as part of a multidrug immunosuppressive regimen. Physicians and patients need to be aware of the presenting features of this devastating demyelinating disease of the central nervous system, which include altered mental status, visual symptoms, motor deficits and ataxia. The preliminary results of rituximab treatment are encouraging, but concerns remain before this agent can be recommended for routine use in IMN. So far, no randomized, controlled trials have been conducted to clarify the role of rituximab in the treatment of IMN. Adequately powered, randomized, controlled trials with prolonged follow-up are needed to determine the long-term course of the disease following B-cell reconstitution; rates of relapse; subsequent redosing regimens; and effects on renal survival. Further studies must clarify whether rituximab should be used as monotherapy or in combination with other immunosuppressive drugs to achieve maximum anti proteinuric effect and durable remission. The preliminary small, uncontrolled study suggests that the addition of rituximab to tacrolimus can induce sustained remission of the nephrotic syndrome, allowing early tacrolimus withdrawal and thereby overcoming the issue of tacrolimus dependence.

7.2 Adrenocorticotrophic hormone (ACTH)

Several small, uncontrolled trials have reported beneficial effects of synthetic adrenocorticotropic hormone ACTH in patients with IMN. One small, randomized, controlled trial by Ponticelli et al. compared treatment with ACTH for 1 year to a 6-month regimen of methylprednisolone alternating monthly with a cytotoxic agent in 32 (mostly medium-risk) patients with IMN. The probability of complete or partial remission did not differ substantially between the groups (87% versus 93%), and the number of remissions, mean time to response and number of relapses were also comparable between the groups. The results suggest that prolonged ACTH treatment could be equivalent to the combined use of cytotoxic drugs and steroids. The side effects of ACTH include glucose intolerance, fluid retention, hypertension, diarrhea, bronze discoloration of the skin, dizziness and fatigue, all of which resolve after discontinuation of treatment. Extensive studies with long follow-up are needed to confirm the preliminary data on the use of ACTH in IMN. Further investigation is also required to find the mechanisms by which ACTH seems to decrease proteinuria and alter apolipoprotein metabolism. These effects are probably not entirely attributable to an increase in endogenous cortisol synthesis, since steroid monotherapy has not been shown to be effective in IMN. ACTH therapy can be effective in patients who are unresponsive to steroids. On the other hand, the endogenous cortisol liberated by the actions of exogenous ACTH might act differently and perhaps more effectively than orally administered steroid

7.3 Sirolimus

The role of sirolimus in IMN has been evaluated in two small pilot studies, with unfavorable results. No remissions occurred during therapy, but one patient achieved a partial remission after cessation of therapy. Severe adverse events, including pneumonitis, infection, persistent proteinuria and azotemia, necessitated discontinuation of the drug in the majority of cases. These trials were prematurely terminated owing to the unfavorable risk–benefit ratio. An open-label trial of sirolimus in 11 patients with a variety of chronic glomerulopathies and declining renal function, including three with membranous nephropathy, was associated with acute kidney injury in more than half of the patients; this event generally occurred within weeks of starting sirolimus. Thus, sirolimus does not seem to have a role in the treatment of IMN

7.4 Eculizumab

Eculizumab is a fully humanized monoclonal antibody directed against the complement protein C5, approved for the treatment of Paroxysmal Nocturnal Hematuria. Ecluzimab inhibit C5a and C5 b thus preventing complement activation. Treatment with eculizumab improves the quality of life and reduces the need of transfusions and the risk of thrombosis in patients with PNH. However, eculizumab can increase the risk of meningococcal infections perhaps due to the reduction in the levels of C5 activity. Patients should therefore be vaccinated or revaccinated with a meningococcal vaccine at least 2 weeks before receiving the first dose of eculizumab. Other side effects include headache, nasopharingitis, back pain and cough; nausea may occur in the period following injection. The mechanism of action of eculizumab renders this monoclonal antibody potentially attractive for treating patients with IMN, as the terminal components of the complement C5b--C9 play a prominent role in mediating the inflammation and the damage of podocytes and glomerular basement membrane. However, a RCT conducted in IMN failed to show any advantage over placebo of eculizumab 8 mg/kg every other week or every 4 weeks. Further trials are needed to establish whether a different dosage or more prolonged treatment may obtain therapeutic results in IMN

8. Intravenous high-dose immunoglobulins [IVIG]

IVIG have been used in high dose in treatment of IMN. IVIG interferes with complement-mediated immune damage by binding to C3b and C4b, by this mechanism preventing glomerular injury. This mechanism may be involved in IMN, as suggested by a study in passive Heymann nephritis, in which treatment with systemic immunoglobulin obtained a decrease in proteinuria, associated with a decreased glomerular deposition of C3c and C5b--9, without changes in the amount, size or distribution of the subepithelial immune complexes . A few anecdotal uncontrolled studies suggested a possible benefit of IVIG therapy in IMN.

8.1 Anticoagulation

Use of anticoagulation in nephrotic syndrome is controversial issue. Nephrotic syndrome (NS) is associated with high risk of for thromboembolic complications, including deep venous thrombosis, renal vein thrombosis, and pulmonary embolism; this risk seems to be greater for IMN especially in patient with low albumin and previous history of thrombo-embolic disease. Analyses showed that in patients with IMN the benefits of oral anticoagulation outweigh the risks. However, before prescribing anticoagulants the physician should take into account the severity of the NS (as assessed by serum albumin concentration), pre-existing thrombotic states, and the overall likelihood of serious bleeding events consequent to oral anticoagulation The optimal duration of prophylactic anticoagulation is unknown but should probably last for as long as NS persists (Ponticelli C et al 2010).

IMGN TREATMENT ALGORITHM

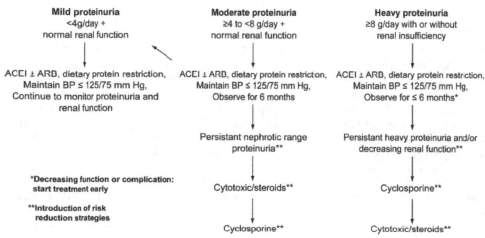

[Cattran et al 2010].

9. Future directions

If anti-PLA2R or other MN-specific autoantibodies can be demonstrated to be tightly associated with immunological disease activity in idiopathic MN, a serologic immunoassay would have several potential applications. it could use the anti- PLA2R as an initial assay for the diagnosis of idiopathic MN without kidney biopsy. Serial assays for the presence and titer of anti-PLA2R prior to therapeutic intervention in clinical trials could help reduce uncertainty as to whether rapid responders represent a true therapeutic effect or a spontaneous remission. Anti-PLA2R could also be followed during treatment to assess the efficacy of immunosuppressive therapy and to determine the length of treatment. It could also be useful in partial remission, when residual proteinuria could be caused either by ongoing but attenuated immune activity or by structural glomerular changes without immune activity.

10. Summary

Membranous Nephropathy is a common cause of nephrotic syndrome in adults of all races and ethnicities. Its molecular pathogenesis is increasingly well understood, and identification of PLA2R as a target antigen may allow better diagnosis, better following of the disease course, and improved decision-making regarding necessity and duration of treatment. Treatment should be provided to those at high risk of progression to ESRD, including patients with persistent severe proteinuria or a documented loss of renal function. At present, alkylating agents and cyclosporine are the only clinically validated treatments with sufficient follow-up data; however, as the roles of tacrolimus, rituximab, mycophenolate, and ACTH grow, these agents may become the new treatments of choice for idiopathic MN.

11. Acknowledgements

We sincerely thank Dr. Irfan Warraich, Department of Pathology, Texas Tech University Medical Center for providing the photomicrographs from biopsies in subjects with membranous nephropathy for inclusion in this chapter.

12. References

Ahmed M, Wong C .Rituximab and nephrotic syndrome: a new therapeutic hope? Nephrol Dial Transplant (2008) 23: 11–17

Alexopoulos1 E, Papagianni1 A, Tsamelashvili M.Induction and long-term treatment with cyclosporine in membranous nephropathy with the nephrotic syndrome Nephrol Dial Transplant (2006) 21: 3127-3132

Beck L, Salant D.Membranous nephropathy:recent travels and new roads ahead Kidney International (2010) 77, 765–770

Beck L. Membranous Nephropathy and Malignancy,Seminars in Nephrology, Vol 30, No 6, November 2010, pp 635-644

Bomback A , Derebail V, McGregor JG, Kshirsagar AJ, FalkRJ ,PatrickH. Rituximab Therapy for Membranous Nephropathy:A Systematic Review Clin J Am Soc Nephrol 4: 734–744, 2009. doi:10.2215/CJN.05231008

BrantenA, du Buf-Vereijken PW. Mycophenolate Mofetil in Idiopathic Membranous Nephropathy: AClinical Trial With Comparison to a Historic Control Group Treated With Cyclophosphamide .Clin J Am Soc Nephrol 2: 932-937, 2007

Cattran D, Management of Membranous Nephropathy: When and What for Treatment: J Am Soc Nephrol 16: 1188–1194,2005

Cattran DC . Idiopathic membranous glomerulonephritis Kidney International, Vol. 59 (2001), pp. 1983–1994

Chan T M ,Lin AW,Tang SC, Prospective controlled study on mycophenolate mofetil and prednisolone in the treatment of membranous nephropathy with nephrotic syndrome.Nephrology 2007; 12, 576–581

Chen A, Frank R, VentoS, Crosby V, Chandra M,Gauthier B, Valderrama E and Trachtman H Idiopathic membranous nephropathy in pediatric patients: presentation, response to therapy, and long-term outcome. BMC Nephrology 2007, 8:11

Chen,M, Li H, MD, Li XY, Lu FM, Ni Z,Xu FF.Tacrolimus Combined With Corticosteroids in Treatment of Nephrotic Idiopathic Membranous Nephropathy: A Multicenter Randomized Controlled Trial.The American Journal of the Medical Sciences • Volume 339, Number 3, March 2010

Cravedi P, Ruggenenti P,Sghirlanzoni MC.Titrating Rituximab to Circulating B Cells to Optimize Lymphocytolytic Therapy in Idiopathic Membranous Nephropathy.Clin J Am Soc Nephrol 2: 932-937, 2007

Deegens J, Wetzels JF .Membranous Nephropathy in the Older Adult Epidemiology, Diagnosis and Management.Drugs Aging 2007; 24 (9): 717-732

Du Buf-Vereijken P.W .G , Branten AJ, Wetzels JF. Idiopathic Membranous Nephropathy: Outline and Rationaleof a Treatment Strategy. American Journal of Kidney Diseases, Vol 46, No 6 (December), 2005: pp 1012-1029.

Dusso B, Morange S, Burtey S. Mycophenolate Mofetil Monotherapy in Membranous Nephropathy:A 1-Year Randomized Controlled Trial.American Journal of Kidney Diseases, Vol 52, No 4 (October), 2008: pp 699-705

Ehrenreich T, Churg J. Pathology of membranous nephropathy. Pathol Ann 1968;3:145.

Ehrenreich T, Churg J. Pathology of membranous nephropathy. Pathol Ann 1968;3:145.

Fervenza FC, Sethi S and Specks U, Idiopathic Membranous Nephropathy: Diagnosis and Treatment .Clin J Am Soc Nephrol 3: 905-919, 2008

Fervenza1 FC,Cosio1FG , Erickson SB1, U Specks2, AM Herzenberg.Rituximab treatment of idiopathic membranous nephropathy.Kidney International (2008) 73, 117–125

Floccari VF,Cosentini M. Giacobbe G. Coppolino S,Campo D, Bolignano A. Case-by-Case Protocol of Membranous Nephropathy Treatment with Endovenous Infusion of High Doses of Human Immunoglobulins

Gartner HV, Fischbach H, Wehner H, et al. Comparison of clinical and morphological features of peri(epi-extra) membranous glomerulonephritis. Nephron 1974;13:288

Glassock R.The Pathogenesis of Idiopathic Membranous Nephropathy:A 50-Year Odyssey American Journal of Kidney Diseases, Vol 56, No 1 (July), 2010: pp 157-167-

Hepinstall's Pathology of the Kidney, 6th Edition Lippincott Williams & WilkinsHeptinstall RH, Idiopathic membranous, membranoproliferative, and lobular glomerulonephritis. In: Heptinstall RH, ed. The Pathology of the Kidney. Boston: Little, Brown and Company, 1974:393

Hofstra J,Wetzels JF.Alkylating agents in membranous nephropathy: efficacy proven beyond doubt:Nephrol Dial Transplant (2010) 25: 1760-1766

Hofstra1 J, Branten AJ, WirtzJJ, Noordzij TC,du Buf-Vereijken PW WetzelsJF.Early versus late start of immunosuppressive therapy in idiopathic membranous nephropathy: a randomized controlled trial.Nephrol Dial Transplant (2010) 25: 129-136

Idasiak-Piechocka I,Katarzyna AO, Łochyńska B,Skrobańska B. Efficacy and Safety of Low-Dose Chlorambucil in Nephrotic Patients with Idiopathic Membranous Nephropathy:Kidney Blood Press Res 2009;32:263–267

Ivanyi A.A primer on recurrent and de novo glomerulonephritis in renal allografts. nature clinical practice nephrology ,august 2008 vol 4 no 8

Jennette JC, Iskandar SS, Dalldorf FG. Pathologic differentiation between lupus and nonlupus membranous glomerulopathy. Kidney Int 1983;24:377.

Jha V,GanguliA, Saha TA .Randomized, Controlled Trial of Steroids and Cyclophosphamide in Adults with Nephrotic Syndrome Caused by IdiopathicMembranous Nephropathy-journal

Kosmadakis G, Filiopoulos V, Smirloglou D,Skarlas P,Georgoulias C,MichailS.Comparison of immunosuppressive therapeutic regimens in patientswith nephrotic syndrome due to idiopathic membranous nephropathy. Renal Failure, 32, 566–571, 2010

Laluck BJ Jr, Cattran DC. Prognosis after a complete remission in adult patients with idiopathic membranous nephropathy. Am J Kidney Dis. ;33(6):1026-32. 1999.

Lefaucheur C, Stengel B,NochyD, Martel P ,Hill GS, Jacquot C and Rosser J for the GN-PROGRESS Study Group.Membranous nephropathy and cancer: Epidemiologic evidence and determinants of high-risk cancer association .Kidney International (2006) 70, 1510–1517

Lionaki1 S,Siamopoulos K, Theodorou I. Inhibition of tumour necrosis factor alpha in idiopathic membranous nephropathy: a pilot study Nephrol Dial Transplant (2009) 24: 2144–2150

Magil AB. Tubulointerstitial lesions in human membranous glomerulonephritis: Relationship to proteinuria. Am J Kidney Dis 1995;25:375.

Menon S,Valentini RP.Membranous nephropathy in children: clinical presentation and therapeutic approach.Pediatric Nephrology (2010) 25:1419–1428 DOI 10.1007/00467-009-1324-5

Mok CC:Membranous nephropathy in systemic lupus erythematosus: a therapeutic enigma: Nat. Rev. Nephrol. 5, 212–22(2009)doi:10.1038/nrneph.2009.14

Mok1 CC,Ying KY, Yim CW, Ng WL ,Wong WS.Very long-term outcome of pure lupus membranous nephropathy treated with glucocorticoid and azathioprine.Lupus (2009) 18, 1091–1095

Nayagam L,Ganguli SA. Mycophenolate mofetil or standard therapy for membranous nephropathy and focal segmental glomerulosclerosis: a pilot study Nephrol Dial Transplant (2008) 23: 1926–1930

Pantelista K. Koutroulia E. Sotsiou F. Vlachiojannis JG., Oumenos DS: Benefit and cost from the long-term use of cyclosporine-A in idiopathic membranous nephropathy Nephrology 15 (2010) 762–767 Expert Opin. Pharmacothery. (2010) 11(13):2163-2175

Polanco N, Gutierrez E: Spontaneous Remission of Nephrotic Syndrome in Idiopathic Membranous Nephropathy.J Am Soc Nephrol 21: 697–704, 2010.

Ponticelli C,Passerini P. Can prognostic factors assist therapeutic decisions in idiopathic membranous nephropathy.J Nephrology 2010 ; 23 (02): 156-163

Ponticelli C. Membranous nephropathy J. Nephrol 2007 May-Jun;20(3):268-87

Prabhakar Kahn. Therapy of membranous nephropathy with severe azotemia. Clinical NephroLogy, v.45 .No.6 - 1996

Praga M,Passerini P.Management of idiopathic membranous nephropathyExpert Opin. Pharmacotherapy. (2010) 11(13):2163-2175 M

Praga1 M, Barrio V,Fernandez J G ,J Lun .Tacrolimus monotherapy in membranous nephropathy: A randomized controlled trial .Kidney International (2007) 71, 924–930

Ronco P, Debiec H.Target antigens and nephritogenic antibodies in membranous nephropathy: of rats and men: Semin Immunopathol (2007) 29:445–458 DOI 10.1007/s00281-007-0091-2

Roncoa P , Debieca H.Membranous glomerulopathy: the evolving story Curr Opin Nephrol Hypertens 2010, 19:254–25919:254–259

Ruggenenti P, Cravedi P,Remuzzi G .Rituximab for membranous nephropathy and immune disease: less might be enough: Piero nature clinical practice Nephrology february 2009 vol 5 no 2

Ruggenenti P,Cravedi P.Effects of Rituximab on Morphofunctional Abnormalities of Membranous Glomerulopathy, Clin J Am Soc Nephrol 3: 1652–1659, 2008.

Salant D.In Search of the Elusive Membranous Nephropathy Antigen Nephron Physiol 2009;112:p11–p12

Segara A ,Praga M,Ramos N.Successful treatment of membranous glomerulonephritis with rituximab in calcineurin inhibitor-dependent patients Clin J Am Soc Nephrol. 2009 Jun;4(6):1083-8. Epub 2009 May 28

Sepe1 V, Libetta1C, GiulianoMG, Adamo G, Canton AD.Mycophenolate mofetil in primary glomerulopathies .Kidney International (2008) 73, 154–162

Stanescu HC, Arcos-Burgos M, Medlar A, et al. Risk HLADQA1 and PLA2R1 alleles in idiopathic membranous nephropathy. N Engl J Med 2011;364:616-26.

Troyanov S,Wall CA, Miller JA. Scholey JW, Cattran DC, Idiopathic membranous nephropathy: Definition and relevance of a partial remission. Kidney International, Vol. 66 (2004), pp. 1199–1205

Waldman M,Austin HA.Controversies in the treatment of idiopathic membranous nephropathy Nat. Rev. Nephrol. 5, 469–479 (2009); published online 7 July 2009

Wehrmann M, Bohle A, Bogenschutz O, et al. Long-term prognosis of chronic idiopathic membranous glomerulonephritis: An analysis of 334 cases with particular regard to tubulointerstitial changes. Clin Nephrol 1989;3:67.

Membranoproliferative Glomerulonephritis

Matthew C. Pickering[1] and Joshua M. Thurman[2]
[1]Centre for Complement & Inflammation Research (CCIR), Imperial College, London,
[2]Division of Nephrology and Hypertension,
University of Colorado Denver School of Medicine, Colorado
[1]United Kingdom
[2]United States of America

1. Introduction

Membranoproliferative glomerulonephritis (MPGN) refers to glomerular pathology in which there is thickening of the capillary wall together with mesangial expansion. In this article we firstly review the pathological features of MPGN and discuss how advances in our understanding of the association between abnormalities in the regulation of complement and MPGN have revealed limitations in the historical pathological sub-division of MPGN. Secondly we review the clinical presentation of MPGN, its prognosis and therapeutic considerations.

2. Pathological features of MPGN

The name 'membranoproliferative glomerulonephritis' derives from the light microscopic glomerular histologic pattern. MPGN is synonymous with 'mesangiocapillary glomerulonephritis'. The glomeruli are large and hypercellular. The hypercellularity is typically uniform though-out the glomeruli. Mesangial hypercellularity and expansion of the mesangial matrix can accentuate the appearance of discrete lobules within the glomeruli. In some cases the hypercellularity includes infiltration of the glomerulus with neutrophils [1] and in severe cases monocytes have been detected in the glomerulus [2]. The degree of leukocyte infiltration shows some correlation with the degree of C3d deposition, possibly due to the chemotactic effects of complement split products. In patients who have undergone two biopsies, for example, when the abundance of C3d decreased in the second biopsy fewer leukocytes were observed [3]. The basement membranes of glomerular capillaries in MPGN are thickened. A characteristic change in the capillary wall is splitting of the glomerular basement membrane (GBM), termed 'tram-tracking' or 'double-contours'. This is due to the inter-position of the proliferated mesangial cells between the endothelial cells and the GBM. The inter-positioned mesangial cells generate new basement membrane material between the endothelial and mesangial cells, a process that is readily identifiable on electron microscopy.

Immunofluorescence studies of glomerular immunoglobulin and C3 in MPGN typically demonstrated granular deposition of these immune factors along the capillary loops. Staining for IgG is often fainter than it is for complement C3 and is sometimes absent [4 5].

An early study described three immunofluorescence patterns in MPGN: glomerular deposition of both immunoglobulin and C3 (66%), predominant deposition of C3 (21%) and deposition of C3 only (13%) [4]. The finding of immunoglobulin and complement is characteristic of immune complex-mediated glomerular inflammation and suggests that the MPGN is secondary to systemic disorders in which there is a propensity for immune-complexes to deposit or form within the kidney. The known conditions include diseases such as autoimmune disorders (e.g. systemic lupus erythematosus), malignancies and chronic infections. Hepatitis C, for example, is now recognized as a major cause of mixed cryoglobulinemia and MPGN [6]. Where a systemic disorder is identifiable the MPGN is referred to as secondary MPGN. In the absence of a clear aetiology MPGN is appropriately termed 'idiopathic or primary MPGN'.

The finding of glomerular complement deposition alone suggests activation of the complement system in the absence of immunoglobulin. This most commonly is a consequence of activation of the complement alternative pathway. Perhaps not surprisingly we now know that inherited and acquired disorders of the alternative pathway are associated with MPGN in which the histological features are characterized by predominant or isolated glomerular C3 deposition. The prototypic example of this is dense deposit disease. In the 1960s it was recognized that ribbon-like electron dense deposits are detectable within the lamina densa of the glomerular basement membrane in some patients with glomerulonephritis [7]. These intra-membranous deposits are the histological defining feature of dense deposit disease and this, rather than mesangial inter-positioning, produces thickening of the GBM. Dense deposit disease is rare: of children whose biopsies demonstrate an MPGN pattern by light microscopy, less than 20% have dense deposit disease [8 9]. Prominent C3 deposits are virtually always present in the glomeruli of patients with dense deposit disease. Granular C3 deposits are almost always present within the mesangium, although different patterns have also been observed [8], e.g. "ring-like" pattern of mesangial C3 staining. Glomerular C1q and/or immunoglobulins may be seen [10]. Our current understanding of dense deposit disease has recently been reviewed [11].

Since the MPGN in dense deposit disease was associated with distinct immunofluorescence studies (predominant or isolated glomerular C3 deposition) and GBM ultrastructural appearances (striking linear electron dense transformation of the lamina densa) an MPGN classification emerged which sub-divided MPGN initially into two groups: MPGN type I and MPGN type II. MPGN type I was characterized by immunoglobulin and C3 deposition and sub-endothelial electron dense GBM deposits [5]. MPGN type I contained both primary and secondary types. MPGN type II was used to describe dense deposit disease. Hence in the literature dense deposit disease was renamed MPGN type II. A further group, MPGN type III was subsequently added to describe MPGN where there were prominent subepithelial GBM deposits, possibly caused by immune-complexes similar to those found in membranous disease [12]. As in membranous disease, the deposits are associated with spikes along the GBM that can be detected by silver stain. A further MPGN type III variant was characterized by the presence of basement membrane ruptures on electron microscopy [13]. C3 deposition is invariably present in the glomeruli of patients with MPGN type III whilst immunoglobulin deposition is variable [13]. The traditional classification of MPGN is depicted in figure 1.

Subsequent studies have revealed limitations in this MPGN classification. Firstly, it is now recognized that patients with the dense deposit disease may present with many different patterns of glomerular injury by light microscopy. These patterns, in addition to MPGN, include mesangial proliferative and crescentic lesions [10]. In fact more than half of the dense deposit disease biopsies did not show MPGN. The emerging consensus is that dense deposit disease is a distinct pathologic entity and should not be thought of as an MPGN variant [10 14]. Secondly, we now know that defects in complement regulation are strongly associated with glomerular inflammation in which there is isolated glomerular C3 deposition irrespective of whether the glomerular lesion is MPGN. We discuss the intimate association between complement and MPGN next.

MEMBRANOPROLIFERATIVE GLOMERULONEPHRITIS

	type I	type II	type III
Immunofluorescence:	complement C3 and IgG	complement C3	complement C3 variable IgG
GBM deposits:	sub-endothelial	intra-membranous	sub-endothelial & sub-epithelial

Fig. 1. The traditional classification of MPGN. Dense deposit disease was renamed MPGN type II in this classification. Immunofluorescence refers to glomerular staining for complement C3 and IgG. GBM – glomerular basement membrane.

3. Complement and MPGN

The complement system is an integral component of immunity. Its principal role is concerned with host defence against pathogens and it forms an important component of innate immunity. Complement also acts as natural adjuvant enhancing the B cell response to antigen and more recent data implicates an important role for complement in T cell responses [15]. To understand the relationship between MPGN and complement it is important to understand how complement is activated. Binding of antibody to antigen forms an immune complex and immune complexes are the triggers of the complement classical pathway. In immune-complex associated MPGN the classical pathway is activated and contributes to glomerular inflammation. The complement alternative pathway is continuously activated i.e. requires no specific activating trigger. Unlike the classical pathway, the alternative pathway is antibody-independent and, through this pathway, the key effector molecules of the pathway (C3 and C5) can be deposited on surfaces in the absence of immunoglobulin. The key negative regulator of the alternative pathway is an abundant plasma protein called complement factor H (CFH). Early investigators studying MPGN hypothesized that MPGN lesions in which complement components such as C3 were present in the absence of immunoglobulin, were mediated by alternative pathway activation. We now know that both inherited and acquired causes of alternative pathway regulation are associated with this type of MPGN. Dense deposit disease, in which glomerular C3 deposition is typically seen with little or no immunoglobulin, is associated with genetic and acquired factors that enhance alternative pathway activation (reviewed in [11]). C3 nephritic factor was associated with dense deposit disease decades ago [14] and the 'factor' is now known to be an immunoglobulin which targets an enzyme complex within the alternative pathway. This autoantibody stabilizes the enzyme complex and enhances alternative pathway activation. Hence C3 nephritic factor is associated with over-activation of the alternative pathway. Consequently, through consumption, plasma C3 levels are typically low in individuals with C3 nephritic factor. Genetic factors include genetic deficiency of the alternative pathway regulatory protein, CFH (reviewed in [16]) and 'gain of function' mutations in the alternative pathway activation protein, complement C3 [17]. Genetic deficiency of CFH in pigs and gene-targeted CFH-deficient mice also results in spontaneous MPGN [18 19]. Acquired dysregulation of the alternative pathway due to neutralizing autoantibodies against CFH [20] has also been described. Recently, an autoantibody to factor B, an activation protein within the alternative pathway, has also been associated with MPGN [21]. In summary factors that increase alternative pathway activation have been associated with MPGN in which there is glomerular C3 with little or no immunoglobulin. It is clearly important to distinguish MPGN driven by these factors from MPGN associated with systemic immune complex disease or MPGN due to other aetiologies. Consequently, there has been much discussion on how to develop our current classification of MPGN.

4. C3 glomerulopathy – moving away from the traditional classification of MPGN

In order to identify individuals with inherited or acquired defects in complement regulation we proposed a classification called C3 glomerulopathy (Figure 2) [22]. C3 glomerulopathy defines glomerular pathology characterized by isolated or predominant glomerular C3 deposition in the absence of immunoglobulin irrespective of both the glomerular light microscopic appearances and the ultrastructural appearance of the GBM [22]. Whilst many patients with isolated glomerular C3 deposition and complement abnormalities develop MPGN some do not [23 24]. For example, Servais and colleagues described 19 cases of primary glomerulonephritis cases with isolated deposition of C3 in the absence of morphological GBM changes of dense deposit disease [24]. Thirteen cases had an MPGN pattern by light microscopy whilst the remaining 6 did not [24]. They used the term 'C3 glomerulonephritis'. Recently a familial C3 glomerulopathy associated with a mutation in a complement protein called complement factor H-related protein 5 (CFHR5) was characterised [23]. Affected individuals have renal biopsies consistent with C3 glomerulonephritis. Biopsies show mesangial C3 deposition and variable degrees of mesangial hypercellularity. Mesangial and sub-endothelial GBM electron dense deposits are typical and some develop MPGN. These patients were identified and specifically investigated for complement disorders because renal biopsies demonstrated glomerular C3 deposition in the absence of immunoglobulin. The discovery of CFHR5 nephropathy is fascinating and we direct the interested reader to [25]. The impetus to propose the term C3 glomerulopathy was to enable the rapid identification of patients with glomerular disease who ought to be investigated for complement abnormalities and who may benefit from complement modulating therapeutic strategies. The relationship between C3 glomerulopathy and MPGN is discussed in detail in reference [26].

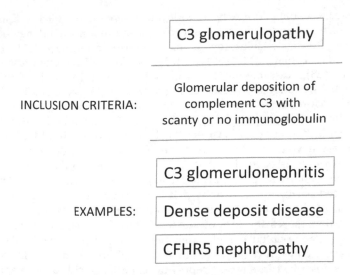

Fig. 2. Definition and examples of C3 glomerulopathy

In summary the traditional MPGN classification has become outdated due to advances in our understanding of complement-mediated glomerular inflammation and our knowledge of the histopathological spectrum of dense deposit disease. Nevertheless, in reviewing historical studies the use of the traditional MPGN sub-groups is unavoidable. In the next sections we have used the traditional sub-groups acknowledging that the reader will now be aware of the limitations of this classification. The recent descriptions of C3 glomerulonephritis and CFHR5 nephropathy are discussed separately.

5. Clinical features of MPGN

MPGN commonly presents with the nephritic syndrome (microscopic hematuria, non-nephrotic proteinuria, and renal insufficiency). However, up to one third of the patients present with relatively preserved renal function and the nephrotic syndrome [27]. The spectrum of clinical findings is generally the same for all of the subgroups considered in this review, but some differences exist and are discussed under individual headings below.

MPGN type I

MPGN type I may be more common in children than in adults [28]. It typically presents as a renal limited disease, although many patients have hypertension at the time of diagnosis [29]. Hypertension may be less common in children [29], particularly when the disease is detected early through screening of asymptomatic individuals. The majority of patients have microscopic hematuria, and some have macroscopic haematuria [29]. Cameron reported that 75% of their patients with MPGN type I had normal C3 levels at the time of disease onset [29]. In an analysis of 9 patients with MPGN type I, however, Ooi and colleagues reported depressed C3 levels for all of the patients on at least one occasion [30]. Approximately 30% of patients have a C3 nephritic factor [29 30]. C4 levels were low for some of the patients.

MPGN type II/Dense deposit disease

Dense deposit disease usually presents in children between the ages of 5 and 15 [14], although a recent series included more patients diagnosed in adulthood than in childhood (12). There appears to be a slight female to male preponderance [31]. The clinical presentation is similar to that of MPGN type I. MPGN type II usually presents with the nephritic syndrome [28], but proteinuria is usually present and is in the nephrotic range in approximately 50% of patients [31]. Interestingly, the renal disease is often preceded by an infection [31]. More than 80% of patients with dense deposit disease have hypocomplementemia at some point [29], and 100% of children with the disease had depressed C3 levels in the report of Nasr et al. [31]. Approximately 80% of patients with dense deposit disease have detectable C3 nephritic factor [32]. As described above, dense deposit disease is strongly associated with defects in regulation of the alternative pathway of complement. This underlying defect probably explains the association of dense deposit disease with acquired partial lipodystrophy [33] and with retinal drusen (deposits within Bruch's membrane of the retina) [34]. In acquired partial lipodystrophy, uncontrolled complement activation causes the loss of subcutaneous fat. The drusen resemble those seen in patients with age related macular degeneration and presumably also form as a result of defective complement regulation. However, only one patient with each of these co-morbidities was described in a recent report of 32 patients with dense deposit disease [31].

MPGN type III

MPGN type III usually presents with similar clinical findings to those seen in MPGN type I. The proportion of patients with hypocomplementaemia was comparable to that of MPGN type I [35].

C3 glomerulonephritis

C3 glomerulonephritis is a recently described entity so the full spectrum of its clinical manifestations is not yet known. Servais et al. reported a series of 19 patients [24]. Men and women were represented nearly equally, and the patients ranged in age from 7 years old to 70. Sethi et al. recently reported three more cases of C3 glomerulopathy [36], all of whom were adult males (aged 38-73). Approximately 30% of the patients in the two reports had a creatinine clearance below 60 ml/min. Most of the patients had proteinuria (eight of the 22 patients described had nephrotic range proteinuria) and 15 patients had hematuria [24 36]. A comprehensive evaluation of the complement system was performed in both reports. Nine of the 22 total patients had depressed C3 levels. Six patients in the first series had C3 nephritic factor, and one of the patients reported by Sethi et al. had C3 nephritic factor. Mutations in complement regulatory proteins were identified in six of the patients reported by Servais et al. [24]. The three patients reported by Sethi et al. all carried the Tyr402His allele of CFH which has been identified as a risk allele for dense deposit disease [36].

CFHR5 nephropathy

CFHR5 nephropathy is a familial form of C3 glomerulopathy that has to date only been described among individuals with Cypriot ancestry. It was characterized only recently [23 25]. Affected individuals all carry a mutation in CFHR5 and to date only heterozygous affected individuals have been identified. The biological role of CFHR5 is unknown although there is evidence that it interacts with complement deposited within the glomeruli in many different glomerular pathologies [37 38]. The mutation in CFHR5 nephropathy is an internal duplication in exons 2 and 3 of the *CFHR5* gene. This results in a secreted abnormally large CFHR5 protein. The clinical course of CFHR5 nephropathy has been described in a comprehensive review of 91 patients from 16 pedigrees [39]. Affected patients have continuous microscopic haematuria and often develop macroscopic haematuria during periods of infection. Hypertension, proteinuria and end-stage renal failure are more common in men. In this report of affected individuals aged over 50 years, 80% of affected men developed chronic renal failure whilst 21% of affected women developed chronic renal failure [39]. The condition recurs in the transplanted kidney [40].

6. Prognostic considerations in MPGN

As highlighted in the above discussion, many of the patients who were previously identified simply as having MPGN are now recognized as having distinct disease processes. Consequently, older data regarding the prognosis of MPGN may have combined patients who would now be categorized differently. For example, early studies of MPGN may well have included patients with dense deposit disease due to defective complement regulation or patients with secondary MPGN caused by hepatitis C associated cryoglobulinemia.

MPGN type I

Studies of patients with MPGN type I have reported fairly wide variation in the long-term prognosis of the disease. The 10-year renal survival for children has been reported to be 60-80% [41 42]. The patients included in these studies were treated with corticosteroids and other immunosuppression. The prognosis may be improved by early detection, such as that afforded by screening of school children [43]. This improvement could be due to lead-time bias, however. Adverse prognostic features include nephrotic syndrome [32 44], an elevated creatinine at presentation or within the first year, and structural injury on the renal biopsy [44].

MPGN type II/Dense deposit disease

The prognosis of dense deposit disease may be worse than that for MPGN type I [8 9 29], although the small numbers of patients with each disease make it difficult to control for other variables. Spontaneous remissions of dense deposit disease are rare, and approximately 50% of patients will reach end-stage renal disease within 10 years [29]. Of the 27 patients in the report by Nasr *et al.* for whom follow-up was known, 25.9% had a complete response to therapy. There was no response in the remaining patients and 25.9% progressed to end-stage renal disease (duration of follow-up 2 months to 24 years) [31]. Age and the serum creatinine at biopsy were predictive of progression to end-stage renal disease. Only 7.1% of the adults had a complete response to therapy. Although uncontrolled complement activation is believed to be pathogenic in this disease, perturbations in C3 levels do not appear to correlate with clinical outcomes [29 31]. Recurrence in renal allografts is common [31 45].

C3 glomerulonephritis

During the period of follow-up (ranging from 0.4 – 34 years) in the series reported by Servais *et al.* [24], most of the patients had a decline in renal function. Three patients reached end stage renal disease, and another two patients had creatinine clearances below 15 mL/min. The patients described by Sethi et al. did not show a decline in renal function during the short period of follow-up (6 months to 3 years) [36].

CFHR5 nephropathy

As mentioned above the course of this condition is more severe in males. In affected individuals aged over 50 years the incidence of end-stage renal failure was 78% in men and 22% in women [39].

7. Therapeutic approaches to MPGN

Given the distinct mechanisms of glomerular injury between immune-complex-mediated MPGN and the primary complement-mediated MPGN groups, evidence of treatment efficacy in one group may not be applicable to the other. However, for both groups non-specific therapies may be beneficial at slowing the progression of renal disease. The blood pressure should be rigorously controlled, and ACE inhibitors or angiotensin receptor blockers are probably agents of choice [46]. Complications of the nephrotic syndrome, such as hyperlipidemia, should be treated.

MPGN type I

As this is a disease of immune-complex deposition, there is a rationale for treating this disease with immunosuppression. Unfortunately, there is not conclusive evidence that any of the common treatments are effective. Perhaps the best study to date was a randomized controlled trial of alternate day prednisone that included 41 children with MPGN type I [47]. The patients had high-grade proteinuria or renal impairment, and renal survival was better in the group that received steroids. Although this difference did not reach significance (P = 0.07), the authors concluded that this was due to the small number of patients. Other uncontrolled studies further support the finding that long-term treatment with corticosteroids may be effective at inducing disease remission [9 48 49]. One of these studies included patients with diffuse lesions on their biopsies, but who were detected early through school-based screening [49]. These patients were treated with alternate day steroids, and all of the patients but one was treated for at least four years. Of 19 patients evaluated, four patients had persistent mild proteinuria but only one patient had a disease relapse (successfully treated with a second course of steroids). Other case series have not shown improved outcomes in patients who received steroids. In one such study, however, the authors determined that patients who received steroids were more likely to have had the nephrotic syndrome [44]. They concluded, therefore, that steroids may, in fact, have been beneficial. After analyzing the available data, Levin concluded that corticosteroids are indicated for children with nephrotic syndrome or with renal insufficiency [50], but the optimal criteria by which patients should be stratified for treatment are still under debate [44].

Similarly, some studies have suggested a benefit of treatment with anti-platelet agents [51 52]. A randomized, controlled trial of aspirin and dipyridamole, for example, indicated that treatment with these agents was effective at preserving renal function [51]. However, a long-term follow-up study that examined renal survival in these patients from the time of diagnosis (not from the start of treatment) did not see a sustained benefit [53]. Another randomized trial of patients demonstrated that aspirin plus dipyridamole was effective at reducing proteinuria at 36 months [54]. The serum creatinines in both groups were unchanged, however, so the effect of this treatment on the progression of renal disease remains uncertain.

Several case series and case reports have described patients treated with other immunosuppressive agents, such as cyclophosphamide or calcineurin inhibitors [29 44 55 56].

The patients treated with these agents are probably selected because they have concerning prognostic factors. Thus, it is difficult to determine the efficacy of these agents. Case reports have also described patients with steroid-resistant MPGN type I who responded to mycophenolate mofetil [57 58]. Certainly more data is needed, but given the relative safety of this medication it is a reasonable choice for patients who do not respond to steroids.

Approximately 30-60% of patients with MPGN type I who undergo renal transplantation have a recurrence of the disease, and disease recurrence adversely affects graft survival [59 60]. Although there are anecdotal reports that increasing immunosuppression may be beneficial, there is no well established therapy for recurrent disease [60].

MPGN type II/Dense deposit disease

No clinical trials have been conducted in patients with dense deposit disease. Based upon what is known about the pathophysiology of the disease, the complement inhibitor eculizumab may be beneficial, and a clinical trial of this agent in dense deposit disease is currently underway. Eculizumab is a monoclonal antibody that blocks C5 activation and is currently licensed for treatment of anemia in paroxysmal nocturnal haemoglobinuria. It has been used successfully to treat atypical haemolytic uraemic syndrome and is likely to be licensed for this indication soon.

Plasma exchange may be effective at removing autoantibodies or dysfunctional complement components, while also enhancing CFH function through the infusion of plasma. Plasma exchange was reported to be effective in two affected sisters who had a factor H mutation and C3 nephritic factor [61].

The role of immunosuppressive agents in dense deposit disease is uncertain. Theoretically, immunosuppressive drugs may be beneficial in patients with evidence of autoantibodies, yet corticosteroids are not of clear benefit in this disease [14]. The patients reported by Nasr et al. included 18 patients who received immunosuppression [31]. The immunosuppression regimens included steroids in all patients. Two patients were also treated with mycophenolate mofetil and three received calcineurin inhibitors. A trend towards a benefit was seen in patients treated with immunosuppression but this did not reach significance. The greatest benefit was seen in those who received immunosuppression and a renin-angiotensin system inhibitor. Recently, a patient with fulminant disease was treated with high-dose corticosteroids, plasma exchange, and cyclophosphamide, and apparently responded to treatment [62]. This patient had a low C3 level, but did not have C3 nephritic factor or a complement mutation, so the mechanism by which the treatment benefited the patient is difficult to infer.

Based on existing data, the optimal treatment of patients with dense deposit disease is uncertain. A treatment algorithm incorporating complement testing and the above treatment options has been proposed [63]. Treatment may need to be initiated before genetic testing can be performed, however, and the presence or absence of C3 nephritic factor is probably not sufficiently accurate to guide therapy. Thus, the decision to use plasma exchange, standard immunosuppressive drugs, and/or eculizumab must ultimately be made based on the clinical severity of the disease.

Recurrence of MPGN type II is very common in patients who receive renal transplants, and some estimate the recurrence rate is 100% [60]. Graft survival at 5 years is approximately 50%, and the most common cause of graft loss is recurrent disease [64]. The impact of more aggressive (e.g. peri-transplant plasma exchange) or newer therapies (e.g eculizumab) remain unknown.

MPGN type III

Patients with MPGN type III do not seem to respond as well to corticosteroids as do those with type I disease as assessed by disease relapse and estimated GFR [35]. Thus, other than non-specfic therapies there is scant evidence to guide the treatment of these patients.

C3 glomerulonephritis

In the series by Servais et al., five of the patients were treated with steroids [24]. The authors reported that there was no clear effect of treatment on the disease outcomes. The patients reported by Sethi et al. were treated conservatively (no patients received immunosuppression), and no deterioration in renal function was seen during the period of follow-up [36]. Thus, based upon the available data there is little evidence to support immunosuppression in these patients.

CFHR5 nephropathy

The optimum treatment for CFHR5 nephropathy presently remains unknown. There are theoretical grounds to investigate the utility of eculizumab in this condition e.g. during disease flares. The relationship between renal decline and infective episodes in CFHR5 nephropathy implies that immunosuppressive strategies may be a potentially harmful approach.

8. Conclusions

MPGN is a fascinating glomerular pathology. We have made significant progress in understanding the role of complement in MPGN. There are limitations to the traditional histological classification. Dense deposit disease should not be referred to as MPGN type II since many patients with dense deposit disease do not have MPGN. C3 glomerulopathy is a new term which encompasses glomerular pathologies in which there is isolated or predominant deposition of glomerular C3. C3 glomerulopathy includes dense deposit disease and C3 glomerulonephritis. The most recent addition is CFHR5 nephropathy. Individuals with C3 glomerulopathy should be investigated for complement dysregulation and represent logical patient populations in which to explore the efficacy of complement modulating therapies.

9. References

[1] Jones DB. Membranoproliferative glomerulonephritis. One of many diseases? Arch Pathol Lab Med 1977; 101:457-461.

[2] Laohapand T, Cattell V, Gabriel JR. Monocyte infiltration in human glomerulonephritis: alpha-1-antitrypsin as a marker for mononuclear phagocytes in renal biopsies. Clin Nephrol 1983; 19:309-316.

[3] Soma J, Saito T, Sato H, *et al*. Intraglomerular immune cell infiltration and complement 3 deposits in membranoproliferative glomerulonephritis type I: a serial-biopsy study of 25 cases. Am J Kidney Dis 1994; 23:365-373.

[4] Belgiojoso GB, Tarantino A, Bazzi C, *et al*. Immunofluorescence patterns in chronic membranoproliferative glomerulonephritis (MPGN). Clin Nephrol 1976; 6:303-310.

[5] Zhou XJ, Silva FG. *Membranoproliferative Glomerulonephritis*. Philadelphia: Lippincott Williams & Wilkins, 2007.

[6] Alpers CE, Smith KD. Cryoglobulinemia and renal disease. Curr Opin Nephrol Hypertens 2008; 17:243-249.

[7] Berger J, Galle P. [Dense Deposits within the Basal Membranes of the Kidney. Optical and Electron Microscopic Study]. Presse Med 1963; 71:2351-2354.

[8] Habib R, Gubler MC, Loirat C, et al. Dense deposit disease: a variant of membranoproliferative glomerulonephritis. Kidney Int 1975; 7:204-215.

[9] Habib R, Kleinknecht C, Gubler MC, et al. Idiopathic membranoproliferative glomerulonephritis in children. Report of 105 cases. Clin Nephrol 1973; 1:194-214.

[10] Walker PD, Ferrario F, Joh K, et al. Dense deposit disease is not a membranoproliferative glomerulonephritis. Mod Pathol 2007; 20:605-616.

[11] Smith RJ, Harris CL, Pickering MC. Dense deposit disease. Mol Immunol 2011.

[12] Burkholder PM, Marchand A, Krueger RP. Mixed membranous and proliferative glomerulonephritis. A correlative light, immunofluorescence, and electron microscopic study. Lab Invest 1970; 23:459-479.

[13] Strife CF, McEnery PT, McAdams AJ, et al. Membranoproliferative glomerulonephritis with disruption of the glomerular basement membrane. Clin Nephrol 1977; 7:65-72.

[14] Appel GB, Cook HT, Hageman G, et al. Membranoproliferative glomerulonephritis type II (dense deposit disease): an update. J Am Soc Nephrol 2005; 16:1392-1403.

[15] Kemper C, Atkinson JP. T-cell regulation: with complements from innate immunity. Nat Rev Immunol 2007; 7:9-18.

[16] Pickering MC, Cook HT. Translational mini-review series on complement factor H: renal diseases associated with complement factor H: novel insights from humans and animals. Clin Exp Immunol 2008; 151:210-230.

[17] Martinez-Barricarte R, Heurich M, Valdes-Canedo F, et al. Human C3 mutation reveals a mechanism of dense deposit disease pathogenesis and provides insights into complement activation and regulation. J Clin Invest 2010; 120:3702-3712.

[18] Hogasen K, Jansen JH, Mollnes TE, et al. Hereditary porcine membranoproliferative glomerulonephritis type II is caused by factor H deficiency. J Clin Invest 1995; 95:1054-1061.

[19] Pickering MC, Cook HT, Warren J, et al. Uncontrolled C3 activation causes membranoproliferative glomerulonephritis in mice deficient in complement factor H. Nat Genet 2002; 31:424-428.

[20] Meri S, Koistinen V, Miettinen A, et al. Activation of the alternative pathway of complement by monoclonal lambda light chains in membranoproliferative glomerulonephritis. J Exp Med 1992; 175:939-950.

[21] Strobel S, Zimmering M, Papp K, et al. Anti-factor B autoantibody in dense deposit disease. Mol Immunol 2010; 47:1476-1483.

[22] Fakhouri F, Fremeaux-Bacchi V, Noel LH, et al. C3 glomerulopathy: a new classification. Nat Rev Nephrol 2010; 6:494-499.

[23] Gale DP, de Jorge EG, Cook HT, et al. Identification of a mutation in complement factor H-related protein 5 in patients of Cypriot origin with glomerulonephritis. Lancet 2010; 376:794-801.

[24] Servais A, Fremeaux-Bacchi V, Lequintrec M, et al. Primary glomerulonephritis with isolated C3 deposits: a new entity which shares common genetic risk factors with haemolytic uraemic syndrome. J Med Genet 2007; 44:193-199.

[25] Gale DP. The identification of CFHR5 nephropathy. J R Soc Med 2011; 104:186-190.

[26] Pickering M, Cook HT. Complement and glomerular disease: new insights. Curr Opin Nephrol Hypertens 2011; 20:271-277.

[27] Watson AR, Poucell S, Thorner P, et al. Membranoproliferative glomerulonephritis type I in children: correlation of clinical features with pathologic subtypes. Am J Kidney Dis 1984; 4:141-146.

[28] Magil AB, Price JD, Bower G, et al. Membranoproliferative glomerulonephritis type 1: comparison of natural history in children and adults. Clin Nephrol 1979; 11:239-244.

[29] Cameron JS, Turner DR, Heaton J, et al. Idiopathic mesangiocapillary glomerulonephritis. Comparison of types I and II in children and adults and long-term prognosis. Am J Med 1983; 74:175-192.

[30] Ooi YM, Vallota EH, West CD. Classical complement pathway activation in membranoproliferative glomerulonephritis. Kidney Int 1976; 9:46-53.

[31] Nasr SH, Valeri AM, Appel GB, et al. Dense deposit disease: clinicopathologic study of 32 pediatric and adult patients. Clin J Am Soc Nephrol 2009; 4:22-32.

[32] Schwertz R, Rother U, Anders D, et al. Complement analysis in children with idiopathic membranoproliferative glomerulonephritis: a long-term follow-up. Pediatr Allergy Immunol 2001; 12:166-172.

[33] Eisinger AJ, Shortland JR, Moorhead PJ. Renal disease in partial lipodystrophy. Q J Med 1972; 41:343-354.

[34] Duvall-Young J, Short CD, Raines MF, et al. Fundus changes in mesangiocapillary glomerulonephritis type II: clinical and fluorescein angiographic findings. Br J Ophthalmol 1989; 73:900-906.

[35] Braun MC, West CD, Strife CF. Differences between membranoproliferative glomerulonephritis types I and III in long-term response to an alternate-day prednisone regimen. Am J Kidney Dis 1999; 34:1022-1032.

[36] Sethi S, Fervenza FC, Zhang Y, et al. Proliferative glomerulonephritis secondary to dysfunction of the alternative pathway of complement. Clin J Am Soc Nephrol 2011; 6:1009-1017.

[37] McRae JL, Cowan PJ, Power DA, et al. Human factor H-related protein 5 (FHR-5). A new complement-associated protein. J Biol Chem 2001; 276:6747-6754.

[38] McRae JL, Duthy TG, Griggs KM, et al. Human factor H-related protein 5 has cofactor activity, inhibits C3 convertase activity, binds heparin and C-reactive protein, and associates with lipoprotein. J Immunol 2005; 174:6250-6256.

[39] Athanasiou Y, Voskarides K, Gale DP, et al. Familial C3 Glomerulopathy Associated with CFHR5 Mutations: Clinical Characteristics of 91 Patients in 16 Pedigrees. Clin J Am Soc Nephrol 2011; 6:1436-1446.

[40] Vernon KA, Gale DP, de Jorge EG, et al. Recurrence of complement factor H-related protein 5 nephropathy in a renal transplant. Am J Transplant 2011; 11:152-155.

[41] Arslan S, Saatci U, Ozen S, et al. Membranoproliferative glomerulonephritis in childhood: factors affecting prognosis. Int Urol Nephrol 1997; 29:711-716.

[42] McEnery PT. Membranoproliferative glomerulonephritis: the Cincinnati experience--cumulative renal survival from 1957 to 1989. J Pediatr 1990; 116:S109-114.

[43] Kawasaki Y, Suzuki J, Nozawa R, et al. Efficacy of school urinary screening for membranoproliferative glomerulonephritis type 1. Arch Dis Child 2002; 86:21-25.

[44] Cansick JC, Lennon R, Cummins CL, et al. Prognosis, treatment and outcome of childhood mesangiocapillary (membranoproliferative) glomerulonephritis. Nephrol Dial Transplant 2004; 19:2769-2777.

[45] Bennett WM, Fassett RG, Walker RG, et al. Mesangiocapillary glomerulonephritis type II (dense-deposit disease): clinical features of progressive disease. Am J Kidney Dis 1989; 13:469-476.

[46] Kent DM, Jafar TH, Hayward RA, et al. Progression risk, urinary protein excretion, and treatment effects of angiotensin-converting enzyme inhibitors in nondiabetic kidney disease. J Am Soc Nephrol 2007; 18:1959-1965.

[47] Tarshish P, Bernstein J, Tobin JN, et al. Treatment of mesangiocapillary glomerulonephritis with alternate-day prednisone--a report of the International Study of Kidney Disease in Children. Pediatr Nephrol 1992; 6:123-130.

[48] Ford DM, Briscoe DM, Shanley PF, et al. Childhood membranoproliferative glomerulonephritis type I: limited steroid therapy. Kidney Int 1992; 41:1606-1612.

[49] Yanagihara T, Hayakawa M, Yoshida J, et al. Long-term follow-up of diffuse membranoproliferative glomerulonephritis type I. Pediatr Nephrol 2005; 20:585-590.

[50] Levin A. Management of membranoproliferative glomerulonephritis: evidence-based recommendations. Kidney Int Suppl 1999; 70:S41-46.

[51] Donadio JV, Jr., Anderson CF, Mitchell JC, 3rd, et al. Membranoproliferative glomerulonephritis. A prospective clinical trial of platelet-inhibitor therapy. N Engl J Med 1984; 310:1421-1426.

[52] Zimmerman SW, Moorthy AV, Dreher WH, et al. Prospective trial of warfarin and dipyridamole in patients with membranoproliferative glomerulonephritis. Am J Med 1983; 75:920-927.

[53] Donadio JV, Jr., Offord KP. Reassessment of treatment results in membranoproliferative glomerulonephritis, with emphasis on life-table analysis. Am J Kidney Dis 1989; 14:445-451.

[54] Zauner I, Bohler J, Braun N, et al. Effect of aspirin and dipyridamole on proteinuria in idiopathic membranoproliferative glomerulonephritis: a multicentre prospective clinical trial. Collaborative Glomerulonephritis Therapy Study Group (CGTS). Nephrol Dial Transplant 1994; 9:619-622.

[55] Cattran DC, Cardella CJ, Roscoe JM, et al. Results of a controlled drug trial in membranoproliferative glomerulonephritis. Kidney Int 1985; 27:436-441.

[56] Haddad M, Lau K, Butani L. Remission of membranoproliferative glomerulonephritis type I with the use of tacrolimus. Pediatr Nephrol 2007; 22:1787-1791.

[57] De S, Al-Nabhani D, Thorner P, et al. Remission of resistant MPGN type I with mycophenolate mofetil and steroids. Pediatr Nephrol 2009; 24:597-600.

[58] Ito S, Tsutsumi A, Inaba A, et al. Efficacy of mycophenolate mofetil for steroid and cyclosporine resistant membranoproliferative glomerulonephritis type I. Pediatr Nephrol 2009; 24:1593-1594.

[59] Andresdottir MB, Assmann KJ, Hoitsma AJ, et al. Recurrence of type I membranoproliferative glomerulonephritis after renal transplantation: analysis of the incidence, risk factors, and impact on graft survival. Transplantation 1997; 63:1628-1633.

[60] Ponticelli C, Glassock RJ. Posttransplant recurrence of primary glomerulonephritis. Clin J Am Soc Nephrol 2010; 5:2363-2372.

[61] Licht C, Heinen S, Jozsi M, *et al.* Deletion of Lys224 in regulatory domain 4 of Factor H reveals a novel pathomechanism for dense deposit disease (MPGN II). Kidney Int 2006; 70:42-50.

[62] Krmar RT, Holtback U, Linne T, *et al.* Acute renal failure in dense deposit disease: complete recovery after combination therapy with immunosuppressant and plasma exchange. Clin Nephrol 2011; 75 Suppl 1:4-10.

[63] Smith RJ, Alexander J, Barlow PN, *et al.* New approaches to the treatment of dense deposit disease. J Am Soc Nephrol 2007; 18:2447-2456.

[64] Braun MC, Stablein DM, Hamiwka LA, *et al.* Recurrence of membranoproliferative glomerulonephritis type II in renal allografts: The North American Pediatric Renal Transplant Cooperative Study experience. J Am Soc Nephrol 2005; 16:2225-2233.

3

Focal Segmental Glomerulosclerosis

Dawinder S. Sohal and Sharma S. Prabhakar

Department of Medicine, Texas Tech University Health Sciences Center
USA

1. Introduction

Focal segmental glomerulosclerosis (FSGS) as the name implies is a histopathological pattern of lesions, where the "focal" refers to, involving minority of glomeruli and the "segmental" refers to, involving a portion of the glomerular capillary tuft caused by injury to podocytes (Fig 1A). Clinically it manifests proteinuria which can progress to nephrotic syndrome and eventually to end stage renal failure.

1.1 Historical aspects

Karl T. Fahr, a German pathologist, described "Progressive lipoid nephrosis" in 1925 which is currently recognized as FSGS. Arnold Rich (1957) was the first to report segmental sclerosis in juxtamedullary glomeruli in autopsy cases of children with nephrosis and uremia. In this report, he hypothesized that the progression to end stage renal disease (ESRD) in a subset of children with idiopathic nephrotic syndrome was because of the development of glomerular sclerosis. Churg et al published histopathological classification of nephrotic syndrome in children for the International Study of Kidney Disease in Children (ISKDC) in 1970, and the disease entity of FSGS was emphasized as a clinicopathological entity separate from minimal change disease (MCD) by its marked resistance to steroids and progression to ESRD. Habib (1973) described clinical and histopathological features of this entity as a separate disease entity using the term 'focal glomerular scleroses'.

Brown et al (1978) reported the malignant form of FSGS, which is characterized by FSGS with rapid decline in renal function. Howie et al. (1984) described the glomerular tip lesion in FSGS, as glomeruli with segmental lesions at the outer 25% with adhesion or prominence of podocytes at the tubular neck. Patients with the glomerular tip lesion often develop nephrotic syndrome and have excellent response to steroids, favorable outcome, and their clinical course is similar to that of patients with MCD. Schwartz et al. (1985) reported another form of FSGS-related cellular lesion characterized by glomerular extracapillary epithelial hypercellularity and endocapillary hypercellularity with foam cells and infiltrating leukocytes, and this was considered to represent an early stage in the development of FSGS. Soon after a collapsing form of FSGS as a new clinic-pathological entity was described by Weiss et al. (1986), which is characterized by nephrotic syndrome with progressive irreversible ESRD and by glomerular collapse with epithelial hypercellularity. Subsequently, many cases of renal disease associated with HIV infection, (Rao TK et al 1984) termed as HIV-associated nephropathies, were reported with features similar to the collapsing form of FSGS.

Between 1980–2000, secondary FSGS (Rennke HG et al. 1989 & D'Agati V. 1994) was established as FSGS with recognized etiologic associations, including genetic mutations in podocyte-associated proteins, virus, drug toxicities, and structural–functional adaptations. Finally in 2004, the Columbia classification was proposed by D' Agati, Fogo, Bruijn, and Jenette, as a working classification for FSGS as given in table 2. Lately some celebrity figures like Sean Elliott and Alonzo Mourning (National Basketball Association) have been diagnosed with FSGS which has further enhanced awareness of this disease in public.

1.2 Epidemiology

Focal segmental glomerulosclerosis (FSGS) currently is the leading cause of nephrotic syndrome in adults and children, particularly in the United States, Australia, Brazil, Canada, Kuwait, India and many other countries. (reference from: http://eng.hi138.com/?i295373_The-epidemiology-of-focal-segmental-glomerulosclerosis). Renal biopsy survey for idiopathic nephrotic syndrome in adults in United States between 1995 to 1997, has revealed that FSGS is the most common cause of nephrotic syndrome, responsible for 35 percent of all cases and more than 50 percent of cases among black population, (67 percent of such cases in black adults were younger than 45 years of age). Idiopathic FSGS is now the most common cause of end stage renal disease (ESRD) caused by primary glomerular disease in the United States in both the black and white populations. The proportion of ESRD attributed to FSGS has increased 11-fold, from 0.2% in 1980 to 2.3% in 2000 (excluding patients with HIV). As per Kitiyakara C. et al (2004) the peak decade for FSGS ESRD incidence is 40 to 49 years among black patients as compared to, 70 to 79 years among white and Asian patients. Males have 1.5- to 2-fold greater risk than females. Recent incidence of end stage renal disease secondary to FSGS is five cases per million population in Caucasian US population and 30-40 cases per million population for African-American population (Hogg R. et al 2007).

2. Etio-pathogenesis

While majority of FSGS cases are still considered idiopathic, the etiologies and mechanisms involved in FSGS development continue to be elucidated. FSGS can be divided into primary or idiopathic and secondary depending upon if the etiology is unknown vs. known respectively. For FSGS to produce nephrotic range or non-nephrotic range proteinuria, alterations of normal glomerular structure and function has to occur. Normal glomerular function requires, that the three major components of glomerular filter, namely *endothelial cells, podocytes, and glomerular basement membrane (GBM)*, be intact and are able to provide a permselective filtration barrier. Specialized tight junctions between podocyte foot processes create a slit diaphragm (SD) which is integral in preventing the loss of protein into Bowman's space (Kimberly et al. 2007 & Asanma et al 2003) . Even though the clinical presentation of FSGS is often heterogeneous, a cardinal feature of the disease is proteinuria, which implies loss of this permselective barrier (Schnaper HW, 2003 & Fogo AB, 2003). Electron microscopic picture clearly reveals distortion of normal architecture (or effacement) of the foot processes of podocytes in FSGS
(Fig 1B).
A key factor in the pathogenesis of FSGS is damage and loss of podocytes. Asanuma K. et al. (2003) described that based on recent insights into the molecular pathology of podocyte injury, at least four major causes have been identified that lead to the uniform reaction of

pododcyte foot processes effacement and proteinuria: (1) interference with the slit diaphragm complex and its lipid rafts (2) direct interference with the actin cytoskeleton (3) interference with the GBM or with podocyte-GBM interaction, and (4) interference with negative surface charge of podocytes. Damage to podocytes triggers apoptosis and the detachment of podocytes from the glomerular basement membrane. The resulting reduction in podocyte number (podocytopenia) leaves the glomerular basement membrane to be exposed, (Fogo AB 2003) which leads to development of maladaptive interactions between the glomerular basement membrane and epithelial cells. This is followed by proliferation of epithelial, endothelial and mesangial cells. The combined reaction of cell proliferation and leakage of proteins into Bowman's space results in deposition of the collagen. Eventually the capillary loop collapses and endothelial cells are lost and the affected part of the glomerular tuft heals by scarring causing a characteristic lesion of FSGS. Thus the lesions initially are limited to a few segments in the glomerulus (segmental) and in a few regions of the kidney (focal) but the disease ultimately progresses to involve the entire kidney leading to end stage renal disease (ESRD).

The precise initial insult that leads to the above cascade of events is still unknown. A 'circulating permeability factor' which leads to glomerular basement membrane injury has been proposed in the pathogenesis of FSGS (Shalhoub RJ, 1974). The following information favors the hypothesis of 'circulating Permeability factor' (1) frequent recurrence of proteinuria after renal transplant [Ingulli E. et al. 1991] (2) the efficacy of extracorporeal techniques such as plasmapheresis in reducing the post renal transplant proteinuria [Artero M. et al 1992 and 1994]. (3) the results of *in vitro* bioassay which detects permeability changes induced by FSGS serum on isolated glomeruli [Savin VJ et al in 1992 and 1996].

(4)Rea et al (2001) demonstrated that the main clinical feature of FSGS i.e. proteinuria, disappeared within one year after transplantation in two recipients of kidneys from a patient with FSGS. Not taking into account ethical and legal implications, good outcome of the FSGS allograft kidneys into non FSGS recipients is another good evidence for humoral genesis/circulating permeability factor, as a cause of the FSGS. (5) Kemper M. et al (2001) demonstrated transmission of glomerular permeability factor from the mother affected by FSGS to her infant during gestation. After birth, proteinuria in the child decreased and then disappeared, suggesting a strong correlation with some circulating factor transmitted from the mother to the child.

At the molecular level, cytokines and vasoactive factors are believed to play a major role in the progression of FSGS. The overexpression of transforming growth factor β (TGFβ) or its downstream proteins, the 'Smads' lead to glomerulosclerosis in animal models. Activation of the renin-angiotensin system upregulates TGFβ, which is considered to cause further progression of the disease (Harris RC et al. 2006). Angiogenic factors, like platelet-derived growth factor (PDGF) and vascular endothelial growth factor (VEGF) seem to play a role in disease progression. This is based upon the rat remnant kidney model (RK model) experimental studies of progressive glomerulosclerosis. In this model, VEGF upregulation soon after the renal injury and later loss of VEGF expression correlates well with progression of the glomerulosclerosis (Kang DH et al. 2001).

Mechanical stress is also believed to play a role in the progression of FSGS. (Hostetter TH. 2003 & Kwoh C. et al 2006) The hyperfiltration due to the defects of the filtration barrier results in increased single nephron glomerular filtration rate (SNGFR), which results in hypertrophy of glomeruli. The hypertrophy exacerbates the mismatch between the glomerular basement membrane and the decreased numbers of podocytes, propagating the injury further. Another factor in the progression of FSGS is tubulointerstitial injury. Clinically, tubulointerstitial injury is a predictor of the loss of renal function in FSGS (D'Agati VD 2003 & Rodriguez-Iturbe B et al. 2005). The nonspecific entry of proteins into the tubular lumen is one potential source of damage to the tubulointerstitlum. Indeed, persistence of nephrotic-range proteinuria is a negative prognostic factor for the progression of FSGS to ESRD (Walls J. 2001). Cytokines (such as TGFβ), when present in the tubules, will recruit monocytes, macrophage, and T-cells. This stimulates other cytokines, including interleukin-1, tumor necrosis factor alpha, and other chemokines. This inflammatory infiltrate leads to mesangial matrix deposition, promoting the collapse of glomeruli. The cellular infiltrate and cytokines also damage tubular epithelial cells, and some tubular epithelial cells may undergo transformation to mesenchymal cells. These mesenchymal cells, as well as recruited and stimulated fibroblasts, result in collagen matrix deposition and tubulointerstitial fibrosis

(Harris RC et al. 2006).

Regardless of the cause of podocyte injury, when the podocytes start dying, leakage of protein across the GBM leading to proteinuria and hypoalbuminemia ensues. At this time cholesterol levels start rising due to increased synthesis of cholesterol by the liver and loss of lipid regulating proteins in the urine, the underlying mechanism of these effects is not completely known yet. The beneficial effects of blocking the renin-angiotensin system may not be limited to their antiproteinuric or antihypertensive effects. As noted earlier, angiotensin stimulates TGFβ, in turn contributing to fibrosis. In addition, angiotensin affects intracellular calcium concentrations and the podocyte cytoskeleton (Harris RC et al. 2006). Inhibition of angiotensin may slow progression by these local mechanisms (Korbert SM, 2003).

With increasing incidence of FSGS, these pathways of podocyte injury and disease progression provide important targets for future intervention. Trials have already been initiated to antagonize cytokines, such as TGFβ (as discussed later in this chapter in treatment section).

Genetic mutations seen in congenital forms of nephrotic syndrome and FSGS enabled researchers to identify specific gene mutations involved in podocyte damage (Tryggvason K. et al. 2006). Mutations of the nephrin gene, a podocyte-specific transmembrane component of the slit diaphragm, are found in congenital Finnish-type nephrotic syndrome, and may lead to loss of normal caliber slit diaphragms. (Kestila M. et al. 1998, Tryggvason K. et al. 2006, Kwoh et al. 2006). In mouse models, mutations of nephrin-like transmembrane genes (NEPH-1) which also localize to the slit diaphragm result in proteinuria and early death. Other proteins which are part of the slit diaphragm complex include: podocin, CD2-associated protein (CD2AP), FAT, P-cadherin,ZO-1, LAP (leucine rich repeat and PDZ domain) protein. (Asanuma K et al 2003, Tryggvason K. et al. 2006). Mutations in podocin (a transmembrane protein that interacts with nephrin, NEPH-1 and CD2AP) have been identified in familial FSGS. Recently, mutations in CD2AP, an immunoglobulin-like protein that is involved in nephrin integration with podocyte cytoskeleton, have also been linked to genetic forms of FSGS (Shih NY. et al. 1999, Kim JM et al 2003, Tyggvason K. et al 2006). In mouse models, the loss of FAT1 and FAT2 (transmembrane proteins with cadherin-like repeats) results in the absence of slit diaphragms, proteinuria, and early death. Alpha-actinin-4, an important structural component of the podocyte cytoskeleton, is mutated in some autosomal dominant forms of FSGS (Kaplan JM et al 2000, Yao J et al. 2004). In addition to the abnormal structural proteins mutations, some other mutations have been identified in association with FSGS like TRPC6 (Transient receptor potential cation chanel, subfamily C, member 6) which is a cation-selective, ion-channel protein that mediates calcium signals (Winn MP et al. 2005). The role of the other components of the slit diaphragm in the pathophysiology of FSGS is not yet clear.

In summary, these data suggest that mutations in the cytoskeleton and membrane proteins specific to podocytes are responsible for most inherited forms of disease. The frequency of spontaneous mutations in the general population who develop nephrotic syndromes or FSGS still needs to be assessed as it has diagnostic, prognostic and therapeutic implications in case of FSGS. For example, patients who possess genetically defective podocytes should be unresponsive to conventional steroid treatment. Similarly, these patients should not have recurrent FSGS when transplanted with a structurally normal kidney allograft. Furthermore, family members who are potential living donors could be genetically screened for mutations associated with the development of kidney disease and excluded as candidate donors.

3. Secondary FSGS

Secondary FSGS can be seen in a variety of conditions such as renal agenesis, obesity, or sickle cell disease etc where hyperfiltration is a characteristic abnormality. Glomerulomegaly is common in situations with hyperfiltration. Obesity-associated FSGS needs a definitive diagnosis with a renal biopsy to exclude the presence of concurrent early diabetic nephropathy. Secondary FSGS may also result from intravenous drug abuse and reflux disease. It has been reported that toxins, including lithium and pamidronate, and sirolimus are associated with the development of FSGS lesions. Among the viral infections, HIV is the most common cause. Rarer viral causes of secondary FSGS include persistent parvovirus B19, simian virus 40, and cytomegalovirus infection.

4. Clinical presentation

Primary FSGS more likely presents with sudden-onset nephrotic syndrome, whereas secondary FSGS presents more insidiously with subnephrotic range proteinuria and renal insufficiency. But the secondary FSGS from pamidronate toxicity though typically presents with full nephrotic syndrome and acute or subacute renal failure, with collapsing FSGS lesions on biopsy. Physical exam reveals elevated blood pressure and edema. Urine may be foamy and may have hematuria. The relative frequencies of these findings at presentation or biopsy based diagnosis in published series (Rydell JJ et al. 1995 & Chun MJ et al 2004) are as follows. Primary FSGS can present with nephrotic range proteinuria (60 to 75%), microscopic hematuria with variable degrees of proteinuria (30 to 50%), hypertension (45 to 65 %), renal insufficiency (25 to 50 %) and with overlapping of these presentations. Children tend to present with more proteinuria whereas hypertension is more common in adults. A case of FSGS should be considered idiopathic only when other etiologies are thoroughly excluded. Uncommonly Muehrcke's lines (white banding on the nails due to hypoalbuminaemia), xanthelasma and xanthomata (cholesterol deposits in skin) are associated with FSGS as well. Following risk factors need to be considered when doing history and physical examination on such patients: male gender, black race, positive family history, heroin abuse, use of known causative medications, chronic viral infection, a solitary kidney, and obesity.

Primary or idiopathic FSGS: Refer to Table 2

Secondary FSGS:
1. Virus assoiated
    a. HIV associated nephropathy (HIVAN)
    b. Parvovirus B19
    c. SV40
    d. CMV
2. Drug toxicity
    a. Pamidronate
    b. Lithium
    c. Interferon –alpha
    d. Heroin
    e. Sirolimus
3. Secondary FSGS mediated by adaptive structural-functional responses
    a. Reduced renal mass
        Unilateral renal agenesis
        Oligomeganephronia
        Renal dysplasia
        Reflux nephropathy
        Sequela to cortical necrosis
        Surgical renal ablation
        Chronic allograft nephropathy
        Any advanced renal disease with reduction in functioning nephrons
    b. Initially normal renal mass
        Obesity
        Hypertension
        Atheroembolic or other acute vaso-occlusive processes
        Cyanotic congenital heart disease
        Sickle cell anemia
        Anabolic steroids
4. Familial FSGS
    a. Autosomal recessive :
        mutations in genes NPHS1 (coding for nephrin) ,NPHS2 (coding for podocin) and
        PLCE1 (coding for PLC epsilon1)
        LAMB2 (coding for Laminin beta 2 chain)
    b. Autosomal dominant
        Mutations in genes ACTN1 (coding for alpha actinin4), TRPC6 (coding for TRPC6),
        INF2 (coding for INF2)
        WT1 (coding for WT1)

Table 1. Etiologic Classification of Focal Segmental Glomerulosclerosis

Differences in clinical manifestations correlate with differences in pathologic phenotypes. Collapsing variant of FSGS often has more severe proteinuria and renal insufficiency but less hypertension than typical variant. Patients with collapsing FSGS frequently have extrarenal manifestations of the disease, a few weeks before the onset of the nephrosis e.g. episodes of upper respiratory infections, diarrhea that are usually ascribed to the viral or other infectious processes. However, the symptoms of fever, anorexia, aches and pains are present only in 20% of patients at the time of onset of nephrosis. Glomerular tip lesion variant (Fig 4) often presents with rapid onset of edema similar to minimal change disease. Glomerular tip lesion patients may develop reversible acute renal failure, at the times of initial presentation when the degree of proteinuria, edema, hypoalbuminemia are at their peak. This behaves like minimal change disease and this rarely happens in any other forms of FSGS. Patients with glomerular tip lesion FSGS tend to be older white males in comparison to younger black males predominance in collapsing variant FSGS.

Distinguishing between primary and secondary FSGS is important, since secondary FSGS should not respond to immunosuppressive therapy. Instead, the inciting condition or toxin should be alleviated or stopped in secondary form FSGS if possible. Unfortunately, distinguishing between primary vs. secondary FSGS can be challenging, since focal sclerosis lesions may be present in a diverse assortment of glomerular, vascular, and tubular injuries, just as global sclerosis represents a common endpoint lesion for the end-stage renal disease.

5. Laboratory findings

Urine analysis may have wide range of findings starting from fatty casts to dysmorphic red blood cells and red blood cell casts. Proteinuria varies from less than 1 gm to 30g/day. Hypoproteinemia is common in patients with FSGS, with total serum protein reduced to varying extents. Hypoalbuminemia may drop as low as below 2 g/dL, especially in patients with the collapsing and glomerular tip variants of FSGS. Cholesterol levels are increased. Serum complement components are typically in normal range in FSGS. CD4 cell count and HIV test is essential in all patients with FSGS, especially those with the collapsing pattern. DNA/PCR for Parvo B19 and CMV test is an essential part of work up to rule out the rare forms of secondary FSGS. Finally renal biopsy is the final step to make the diagnosis of FSGS.

6. Histopathology

The diagnosis of FSGS is not an easy one to make, because the morphologic features of FSGS are nonspecific and can occur in a variety of other conditions or superimposed on other glomerular disease processes. Additionally, because the defining glomerular lesion is focal, it may not be adequately sampled in small needle biopsies. The diagnosis of FSGS is further complicated by the existence of a primary (or idiopathic) form and many secondary forms (Table 1). Before a diagnosis of primary FSGS can be made, secondary forms must be excluded. Idiopathic FSGS must be distinguished from human immunodeficiency virus (HIV) -associated nephropathy, heroin nephropathy and other large group of secondary FSGS caused by structural-functional adaptations mediated by intrarenal vasodilatation, and increased glomerular capillary pressures, (as listed in Table 1). The morphological types are not used to guide treatment but to provide useful prognostic information. Electron microscopy can be used to distinguish primary and secondary FSGS. In primary FSGS, foot process fusion is diffuse and occurs throughout the glomeruli. In secondary FSGS, foot process fusion is mostly limited to the sclerotic areas.

Five main light microscopic patterns of FSGS have been defined, as given below:

Variant	Positive Criteria	Negative Criteria
FSGS NOS	At least one glomerulus with segmental increase in matrix obliterating the capillary lumina. There may be segmental glomerular basement membrane collapse without podocyte hyperplasia.	Exclude perihilar,cellular,tip and collapsing variant.
Perihillar Variant	Perihillar sclerosis and hyalinosis involving >50% of segmentally sclerotic glomeruli.	Exclude cellular,tip and collapsing variant.
Cellular Variant	At least one glomerulus with segmental endocapillary hypercelllularity occluding lumina, with or without foam cells with karyorrhexis.	Exclude tip and collapsing variant.
Tip variant	At least one segmental lesion involving the tip domain (outer 25% of tuft next to origin of the proximal tubule) The tubular pole must be identified in the defining lesion. The lesion must have either an adhesion or confluence of podocyte with parietal or tubular cells at the tubular lumen or neck. The tip lesion may be sclerosing or cellular.	Exclude callasping variant . Exclude any perihilar sclerosis.
Collapsing variant	At least one glomerulus with segmental or global collapse Podocyte hypertrophy/hyperplasia	none

Classified based upon the 'Working Columbia Classification 2004'.

Table 2. Morphological variants of FSGS

Although appearance of the glomerular tuft differs in these forms, all share the common feature of podocyte alterations at the ultrastructural level. At present, it is unclear if these morphologic variants reflect pathogenetic differences or they are the consequence of different severities of podocyte injury or histopathologic evolution. Future studies are needed to address these questions.

Classic Focal Segmental Glomerulosclerosis (Focal Segmental Glomerulosclerosis Not Otherwise Specified) : also called FSGS NOS, or typical FSGS. FSGS NOS requires exclusion of the other more specific subtypes described in the table 2. Light Micrscopic examination reveals accumulation of extracellular matrix which occlude glomerular capillaries, forming discrete segmental solidifications involving affected portion of the glomerular tuft. Also seen is plasmatic insudation of amorphous glassy material beneath the GBM, endocapillary foam cells, and wrinkling of the GBM. Adhesions to Bowman's capsule are common, and overlying visceral epithelial cells often appear swollen over the sclerosing segment. Non sclerotic glomerular lobules appear normal by light microscopy except for mild podocyte swelling.

Immunofluorescence: focal and segmental granular deposition of IgM, and C3 is seen often, but C1 in the distribution of segmental glomerular sclerosis may also be seen. Nonsclerotic glomeruli may have weak mesangial staining for IgM and C3. By electron microscopic examination, segmental sclerotic lesions exhibit increased matrix, wrinkling and retraction of GBM. Accumulation of inframembranous hyaline material but *no immune complex* electron-dense deposits are seen. Overlying the segmental sclerosis, there is usually effacement of foot processes (Fig 1.B)and podocyte hypertrophy. The adjacent nonsclerotic glomerular capillaries show only foot process effacement.

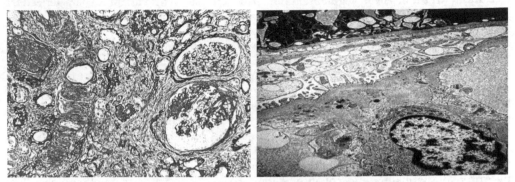

Fig. 1. (A-left) Focal segmental distribution of glomerular lesions. The glomerulus at the top right of the picture is normal. The glomerulus at the bottom shows dense segmental scars with adhesion to Bowman's capsule. (Periodic acid methenamine silver, 20X). (B-Right) Patchy effacement of foot processes is present. No immune complex-type deposits are seen along the GBM. (Electron Microscopy).

Perihilar Variant of Focal Segmental Glomerulosclerosis : This variant is defined as perihilar hyalinosis and sclerosis (Fig 2. A & B) which involves more than 50% of glomeruli with segmental lesions. This category requires that the cellular, tip, and collapsing variants be excluded. Podocyte hyperplasia is uncommon.

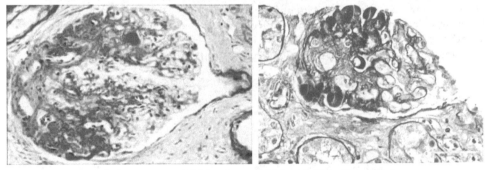

Fig. 2. (A-left): Perihillar variant FSGS (B): Glomerulus with "Hyalinosis": homogeneous, eosinophilic material may be present at the periphery of sclerotic foci, or within the capillary subendothelial space (PAS, 40X). (Fig 2A-obtained from http://www.unckidneycenter.org/kidneyhealthlibrary/fsgs.html#causes)

Immunofluorescence (IF) reveals segmental deposits of IgM and C3 in areas of sclerosis and hyalinosis.

Electron microscopy (EM) demonstrates variable foot process effacement. The perihilar variant may occur in primary or secondary FSGS. It is more common in secondary forms of FSGS mediated by adaptive structural-functional responses, in which it is typically accompanied by glomerular hypertrophy. In this setting, the greater filtration pressures at the proximal end of the glomerular capillary bed may favor the development of lesions at the vascular pole.

Cellular Variant of Focal Segmental Glomerulosclerosis : This variant is characterized by focal and segmental endocapillary hypercellularity that may mimic a form of focal proliferative glomerulonephritis. Glomerular capillaries are segmentally occluded by endocapillary hypercellularity, including foam cells, infiltrating leukocytes, karyorrhectic debris, and hyaline. There is often hyperplasia of the visceral epithelial cells, which may appear swollen and crowded, sometimes forming pseudocrescents. This variant requires that tip lesions and collapsing lesions be excluded.

IF shows focal and segmental glomerular positivity for IgM and C3 and EM reveals severe foot process effacement.

Collapsing Variant of Focal Segmental Glomerulosclerosis: This variant is defined by at least one glomerulus with segmental or global collapse (Fig 3) and overlying hypertrophy and hyperplasia of visceral epithelial cells. There is occlusion of glomerular capillary lumina by implosive wrinkling and collapse of the GBMs. This lesion is more often global than segmental. Overlying podocytes display striking hypertrophy, hyperplasia and express proliferation markers. Podocytes often contain prominent intracytoplasmic protein resorption droplets and may fill Bowman's space, forming pseudocrescents . Although podocyte hyperplasia is found in both the collapsing and cellular variants of FSGS, collapsing glomerulopathy is distinguished by the absence of endocapillary hypercellularity. In collapsing FSGS, there is prominent tubulointerstitial disease, including tubular atrophy, interstitial fibrosis, interstitial edema, and inflammation. A distinctive feature is the presence of dilated tubules forming microcysts that contain loose proteinaceous casts. This pattern can occur both in primary FSGS and also in secondary FSGS due to HIV,parvovirus B12,pamidronate toxicity and interferon therapy. Endothelial tubuloreticular inclusions are identified in over 90% of patients with HIVinfection collapsing glomerulopathy and interferon therapy, whereas only in 10% cases with idiopathic collapsing glomerulopathy. Besides these conditions endothelial tubuloreticular inclusions are seen commonly in systemic lupus erythematosus nephritis.

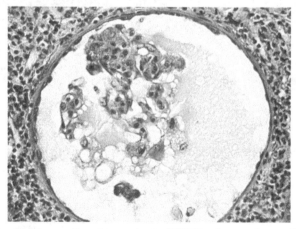

Fig. 3. A glomerulus displays collapsing variant of FSGS , glomerular capillaries show collapse with absent lumen (H&E, 40X).

IF microscopy of collapsing lesions often is positive for IgM and C3. EM reveals severe foot process effacement affecting both collapsed and noncollapsed glomeruli

Tip Variant of Focal Segmental Glomerulosclerosis :

This variant is defined by the presence of at least one segmental lesion involving the tip domain (i.e., the outer 25% of the tuft next to the origin of the proximal tubule). There is either adhesion (Fig 4) between the tuft and Bowman's capsule or confluence of swollen podocytes with parietal or tubular epithelial cells at the tubular lumen or neck. In some cases, the affected segment appears to herniate into the tubular lumen. The segmental lesions may be cellular or sclerosing type. Although initially peripherally located, these lesions may progress more centrally. The presence of perihilar sclerosis or collapsing sclerosis rules out the tip variant.

IF microscopy reveals involved tip area positive for IgM and C3 and EM findings demonstrate foot process effacement.

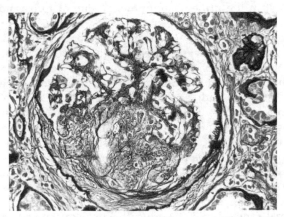

Fig. 4. Sclerotic glomerular segment with a small adhesion; "Glomerular tip lesion" (Periodic acid methenamine silver, 40X)

7. Treatment

Typically the goals of treatment in FSGS include-(1) to reduce, eliminate or at least suppress the proteinuria and (2) to avoid or at least retard the progression to ESRD. Treatment of the FSGS can be arbitrarily divided into (1) **Nonspecific; nutritional management** (2)**Non immunosuppressive therapy**: diuretics and RAS interference. (3) **Immunosuppressive treatment: which includes the use of** steroids, steroid sparing medications like cyclophosphamide, cyclosporine A, tacrolimus and mycophenolic mofetil. **(4)-Antifibrotic drugs:Pirfenidone, Rosiglitazone (FONT Phase 1 trial completed and now FONT phase II trial is ongoing) (5)-Monoclonal/polyclonal Antibodies: Adalimumab, Rituximab, Fresolmumab (6)-Plasmapheresis**

Nonspecific treatment: Nonspecific treatment goals in FSGS are like any other glomerulopathy associated with nephrotic syndrome, which include maintenance of adequate nutrition, minimization or elimination of proteinuria, and prevention of complications resulting from edema. The mainstay of treatment is reduction in daily salt intake to 2 g of sodium. A high level of protein intake may further aggravate proteinuria, adversely affecting renal function. Current recommendations call for an intake of 1to1.3 g of high biologic value protein per kilogram of body weight and a reduction of fat intake. Lipid lowering is necessary to reduce cardiovascular risk and to possibly delay the progression of renal disease.

7.1 Non-immunosuppressive drug treatment

Symptomatic relief of edema helps the patient feel better. In most patients, loop diuretics are needed to promote diuresis. Patients with massive edema with impaired oral absorption may require intravenous administration of loop diuretics. In patients with refractory conditions, addition of other diuretics (eg, metolazone) and potassium-sparing agents (eg, spironolactone, triamterene) facilitates diuresis and prevents hypokalemia. Rarely, some patients (especially children) with intractable edema may need intravenous albumin and diuretics in a hospital setting to initiate diuresis. Protracted use of intravenous albumin should be discouraged; the regimen is expensive and ineffective, because most of the infused albumin is lost in the urine. Continuous IV drip of furosemide is preferred over large boluses of IV push to avoid side effects.

Control of hypertension is one of the most important aspects of overall management in FSGS, like any other glomerular disease. Angiotensin-converting enzyme inhibitors (ACEIs) and angiotensin receptor blockers (ARBs) are nonspecific agents that reduce proteinuria because of their antihypertensive and intrarenal hemodynamic effects of reducing glomerular capillary pressure and resistance. ACEIs and ARBs are effective in reducing protein loss even in normotensive patients. These agents do have an effect in slowing down of the disease progression by downregulating the TGFβ by interfering with renin angiotensin system, regardless of any antihypertensive effects.These agents do not abolish proteinuria completely or reverse the primary glomerular disease process per se.

As hypertension develops in most patients with FSGS which further causes deterioration of renal function, the control of blood pressure is an important part of the treatment of FSGS. Many patients, may require combination antihypertensive therapy to maintain blood pressure in the normal range. Lipid lowering therapy like statins is warranted to correct hyperlipidemia to reduce the risk of cardiovascular disease in this subset of patient population.

7.2 Immunosuppressive treatment

Idiopathic FSGS is a difficult disease to treat because of its highly variable clinical course. The specific treatment approach is still empirical, and no consensus has evolved because of a lack of prospective controlled trials. Current evidence is, mostly derived from retrospective analyses, and favors prolonged steroid therapy (6 months or longer) to induce remission in patients with idiopathic FSGS.

Criteria for remission: (1) complete remission is considered when urinary protein excretion of less than 200-300 mg/day, and (2) partial response is considered when urinary protein excretion of 200-3500 mg/day, or a greater than 50% reduction in baseline proteinuria.

Since long-term steroid therapy is not without serious toxicity, the patient counselling regarding the goals of the therapy, possible potential side affects and expected outcomes, is essential before starting such treatment. The current consensus is to initiate therapy with prednisone in a dose of 1 mg/kg (60-80 mg/d) for 2-6 months or longer, depending on patient's response as assessed by presence or absence of edema, 24-hour urine protein excretions, creatinine clearance, serum creatinine, serum albumin, and lipid levels. Literature reveals that 30-60% of patients may undergo complete or partial remission with this treatment regimen, and relapses are frequent when steroids are discontinued. Blacks and patients with collapsing FSGS are generally refractory to treatment and progress to renal failure. In steroid responsive patients, the goal is to titrate prednisone to the lowest dose needed to stop proteinuria and to prevent relapses. Use of steroids on alternate days can also reduce toxicity. The optimal duration of treatment is uncertain; some authorities recommend use of steroids indefinitely. If no remission after 4 months of corticosteroid treatment, disease is defined as being corticosteroid-resistant (Meyrier A.,2009).

In patients who are refractory to 2-3 months of prednisone therapy, the recommendation is to reduce the steroid dose and to add cyclophosphamide (2.5 mg/kg [150-200 mg/day]), monitor patients for bone marrow suppression, and encourage adequate fluid intake to prevent hemorrhagic cystitis. Prolonged use of cyclophosphamide may lead to gonadal toxicity; therefore, persisting with cyclophosphamide beyond 3 months in patients who do not respond is unwise. Cyclosporine (3.5mg/kg/day) can induce remission and preserve renal function, although relapse occurs in 60% of patients when cyclosporine alone is used (Ponticelli C. et al. 1993 & Cattran DC et al. 1999). Continuing treatment with cyclosporine for 1 year after remission followed by a slow tapering of the dose results in a longer remission (Meyrier A 1994). Low-dose cyclosporine in combination with low-dose prednisone (0.15mg/kg/day) in corticosteroid-resistant patients is more effective than cyclosporine alone (Cattaran DC. Et al 1999 & Meyrier A 2009). Rates of complete (Niaudet P. 1994 & Braun N et al 2008) and partial remission achieved with cyclosporine are greater if low-dose prednisone is given at the same time. Continuous use of cyclosporine for >12 months is associated with a significant increase in tubulointerstitial fibrosis. Its use should, therefore, be limited to patients with creatinine clearance >60 ml/min/1.73 m^2

Isolated reports have suggested that patients who are refractory to steroids and cyclophosphamide, treatment with other immunosuppressive agents, such as tacrolimus and sirolimus, may be beneficial in inducing remission. However, studies using these agents were uncontrolled investigations that were limited to a few patients.

7.3 Tacrolimus

Few studies have reported the use of tacrolimus for Idiopathic FSGS. In the largest study, 25 patients with nephrotic syndrome due to primary FSGS and known resistance to or dependence on cyclosporine (cyclosporine) were given tacrolimus plus prednisolone (prednisone) for 6 months. Seventeen patients had a reduced proteinuria to <3 g/day, and 12 had complete or partial remission. Thirteen patients relapsed after discontinuing tacrolimus; reinstitution of therapy for 1 year resulted in complete remission (5 patients) and partial remission (4 patients). [Segarra A et al 2002].

7.4 Mycophenolate mofetil

Mycophenolate mofetil (MMF) is a reversible inhibitor of inosine monophosphate dehydrogenase (IMPDH) in purine biosynthesis. MMF is selective for the de novo pathway critical to lymphocytic proliferation and activation. Because of favorable results in other glomerular diseases, mycophenolate mofetil has also been evaluated in FSGS. Although the experience is limited, the suggested dose is 750-1000 mg twice daily in patients who are refractory to corticosteroids and in whom calcineurin inhibitors may not be appropriate. However, adequate randomized studies supporting this approach are lacking (Cattran DC et al. 2004). If mycophenolate is being considered, cyclosporine should not be used concurrently. Mycophenolate can be either used alone or in combination with corticosteroids.

7.5 Monoclonal antibody treatment

Rituximab: Rituximab is an anti CD20 chimeric monoclonal antibody. Case reports have suggested rituximab may be effective in treating patients with minimal change nephropathy and FSGS. (Peters HP et al 2008). Four patients with nephrotic syndrome due to minimal change nephropathy or FSGS were treated with rituximab because of failure of or intolerance to the standard immunosuppressive therapy. Other cases of FSGS reported in the literature (6 pediatric patients) that were successfully treated with rituximab were also included. Complete remission was reported within 1 month for a 7-year-old boy with FSGS during treatment with rituximab and concurrent treatment with mycophenolate, low-dose prednisolone (prednisone), and tacrolimus. Controlled trials are needed to further evaluate the efficacy of rituximab in FSGS.

Fresolimumab: Recently a phase one trial (Trachtman H. et al 2011) has been completed which evaluated the safety and pharmacokinetics of single-dose infusions of fresolimumab, a human monoclonal antibody that inactivates all forms of transforming growth factor-beta (TGF-β), in a phase I open-label, dose-ranging study. Patients with biopsy-confirmed, treatment-resistant, primary FSGS with a minimum estimated glomerular filtration rate (eGFR) of 25 ml/min per 1.73m2, and a urine protein to creatinine ratio over 1.8mg/mg were enrolled. All 16 patients completed the study in which each received one of four single-dose levels of fresolimumab (up to 4mg/kg) and was followed for 112 days. Fresolimumab was well tolerated with pustular rash, the only adverse event, developing in two patients. Single-dose fresolimumab was well tolerated in patients with primary resistant FSGS. Additional evaluation in a larger dose-ranging study is necessary.

7.6 Antifibrotic agents

Pirfenidone has been shown to have therapeutic potential in fibrotic diseases, although the mechanism of action is not well understood. It has been shown to reduce transforming growth factor-β 1 production, antagonize TNF-α signaling, and scavenge reactive oxygen species. It also reduces fibrosis and prevents loss of glomerular filtration in animal models of renal disease. An open-label trial evaluated the safety and efficacy of pirfenidone in patients with idiopathic and post adaptive FSGS. Pirfenidone had no effect on BP or proteinuria but it did preserve renal function. Controlled trials are needed to further evaluate the efficacy of pirfenidone in FSGS (Cho ME. et al 2007).

Rosiglitazone: Renal mesangial cells express peroxisome proliferator-activated receptor (PPAR –gamma). PPAR-gamma activation, can exhibit anti-inflammatory effects. Weissgarten et al (2006) demonstrated that PPAR-gamma activation by rosiglitazone resulted in decreased manifestation of inflammatory hallmarks, including inhibition of mesangial cell proliferation, downregulation of apoptosis and blunted responsiveness to angiotensin II in animal models. FONT-I (a phase 1 clinical trial) showed that this agent was safe and well tolerated in 11 patients with biopsy-demonstrated FSGS. The results of further studies are awaited.

Despite all attempts, some patients continue to deteriorate and progress to ESRD. Patients and their families should be counselled in detail regarding the treatment options for ESRD so that they can choose appropriate treatment tailored to their life style among maintenance hemodialysis, continuous ambulatory peritoneal dialysis, or renal transplantation. FSGS may recur in the transplanted kidney, but most centers do not consider this a contraindication for renal transplantation.

Secondary FSGS treatment management is directed toward the etiology or associated disorder. For example, discontinuing pamidronate in pamidronate induced FSGS, and in HIV-associated FSGS, HAART is associated with remission of proteinuria and preservation of renal function. In heroin-associated FSGS, discontinuation of the drug may result in remission of proteinuria and improvement in renal function.

8. Prognosis

Prognosis of idiopathic FSGS is variable. Important prognostic factors are, the amount of proteinuria, the level of plasma creatinine, the morphological subtype, and the response to therapy as listed in table 3. Korbet SM (1999) described that nephrotic patients with FSGS, particularly those with massive proteinuria, have a significantly poorer prognosis than non-nephrotic patients, with 50% progressing to end-stage renal disease (ESRD) over 3-8 years as compared with a 10-year survival of >80%, respectively. In addition, the recurrence rate of this lesion is high in transplanted patients with primary FSGS. When clinical and histological features at presentation have been evaluated by multivariate analysis, the significant positive predictors of progression to ESRD have consistently been the serum creatinine (>1.3 mg/dl), amount of proteinuria and the presence of interstitial fibrosis (> or =20%). The one factor which is a significant negative predictor of progression to ESRD is the achievement of a remission in proteinuria. Unfortunately, spontaneous remissions are rare in FSGS, occurring in < or =6% of patients only.

1. Clinical features at the time of biopsy
   a. Nephrotic range proteinuria or massive proteinuria
   b. Elevated serum creatinine
   c. Black race
2. Histopathologic features at the time of biopsy
   a. Collapsing variant
   b. Tubulointerstitial fibrosis
3. Clinical features during the course of the FSGS
   a. Failure to achieve partial or complete remission.

Table 3. Risk factors for progressive loss of renal function in FSGS

Thomas DB et al. (2006) described that the morphological subtype identified on renal biopsy also provided useful prognostic information. The collapsing variant, the main variant seen in HIV-induced FSGS, is associated with a worse prognosis than the other forms. The tip variant has a better prognosis than the other forms.

9. Summary

Focal segmental glomerulosclerosis is still largely an idiopathic disease but in the recent past, more genetic mutations and secondary causes have been described. As more and more pathogenetic mechanisms involved in idiopathic FSGS are coming into light and more secondary causes of FSGS are described, the occurrence of true idiopathic FSGS diagnosis is decreasing and thus the frequency of the latter is often overstated. Other than the genetic and secondary causes of FSGS, the treatment strategies are still not based upon multiple large randomized controlled trials, and in fact are based upon predominantly anecdotal experiences. Still there are more questions than the answers for the pathogenesis, classification, treatment and prognosis of this an almost a century old disease. This clincopathologic entity still remains a challenge for the nephrologists and transplant physicians.

10. Acknowledgements

We acknowledge and thank Irfan Warraich, MD (Dept. of pathology, Texas Tech University Health Science Center Lubbock, Texas) for his generous contribution by providing us with histopathology figures used in this chapter.

11. References

Asanuma K, Mundel P (2003) The role of podocytes in glomerular pathobiology. Clin. Exp. Nephrol 7(4):255–259

Bahiense-Oliveira M, Saldanha LB, Mota EL, et al. Primary glomerular diseases in Brazil (1979-1999): is the frequency of focal and segmental glomerulosclerosis increasing? Clin Nephrol 2004; 61:90.

Barisoni L, Kriz W, Mundel P, D'Agati V (1999) The dysregulated podocyte phenotype: a novel concept in the pathogenesis of collapsing idiopathic focal segmental glomerulosclerosis and HIV-associated nephropathy. J Am Soc Nephrol 10 (1):51–61

Braden GL, Mulhern JG, O'Shea MH, et al. Changing incidence of glomerular diseases in adults. Am J Kidney Dis 2000; 35:878.

Braun N, Schmutzler F, Lange C, et al. Immunosuppressive treatment for focal segmental glomerulosclerosis in adults. Cochrane Database Syst Rev. 2008;(3):CD003233.

Brown CB, Cameron JS, Turner DR et al. Focal segmental glomerulosclerosis with rapid decline in renal function ("malignant FSGS"). Clin Nephrol 1978: 10: 51

Cattran DC, Appel GB, Herbert LA, et al. A randomized trial of cyclosporine in patients with steroid-resistant focal segmental glomerulosclerosis. Kidney Int. 1999;56:2220-2226.

Cattran DC, Wang MM, Appel G, et al. Mycophenolate mofetil in the treatment of focal segmental glomerulosclerosis. Clin Nephrol. 2004;62:405-411.

Cho ME, Smith DC, Branton MH, et al. Pirfenidone slows renal function decline in patients with focal segmental glomerulosclerosis. Clin J Am Soc Nephrol. 2007;2:906-913.

Chun MJ, Korbet SM, Schwartz MM, Lewis EJ. Focal segmental glomerulosclerosis in nephrotic adults: presentation, prognosis, and response to therapy of the histologic variants. J Am Soc Nephrol 2004; 15:2169.

Churg J, Habib R, White RH. Pathology of the nephrotic syndrome in children: a report for the International Study of Kidney Disease in Children. Lancet 1970: 760: 1299.

D'Agati V. The many masks of focal segmental glomerulosclerosis. Kidney Int 1994: 46: 1223.

D'Agati VD, Fogo AB, Bruijn JA, Jennette JC. Pathologic classification of focal segmental glomerulosclerosis: a working proposal. Am J Kidney Dis 2004: 43: 368.

D'Agati VD (2003) Pathologic classification of focal segmental glomerulosclerosis. Semin Nephrol 23(2):117–134

Daskalakis N, Winn MP (2006) Focal and segmental glomerulosclerosis: varying biologic mechanisms underlie a final histopathologic end point. Semin Nephrol 26(2):89–94

Dijkman H, Smeets B, van der Laak J, Steenbergen E, Wetzels J (2005) The parietal epithelial cell is crucially involved in human idiopathic focal segmental glomerulosclerosis. Kidney Int 68 (4):1562–1572

Fahr T. Pathologische anatomie des morbus brightii. In: Henke F, Lubarsch O, eds.

Handbuch der Speziellen Pathologischen Anatomie und Histologie (Vol. 6) ; | Springer, Berlin: 1925; 156

Filler G, Young E, Geier P, Carpenter B, Drukker A, Feber J (2003) Is there really an increase in non-minimal change nephrotic syndrome in children? Am J Kidney Dis 2003: 42(6):1107– 1113

Fogo AB (2003) Animal models of FSGS: lessons for pathogenesis and treatment. Semin Nephrol 23(2):161–171

Ghiggeri GM, Artero M, Carraro M, Perfumo F (2001) Permeability plasma factors in nephrotic syndrome: more than one factor, more than one inhibitor. Nephrol Dial Transplant 16 (5):882–885

Haas M, Meehan SM, Karrison TG, Spargo BH. Changing etiologies of unexplained adult nephrotic syndrome: a comparison of renal biopsy findings from 1976-1979 and 1995-1997. Am J Kidney Dis 1997; 30:621.

Habib R. Focal glomerular sclerosis. Kidney Int 1973: 4: 355.

Harris RC, Neilson EG (2006) Toward a unified theory of renal progression. Annu Rev Med 57:365–380

Hogg R, Middleton J, Vehaskari VM. Focal segmental glomerulosclerosis: epidemiology aspects in children and adults. Pediatr Nephrol. 2007;22:183-186.

Hostetter TH (2003) Hyperfiltration and glomerulosclerosis.Semin Nephrol 23(2):194–199

Howie AJ, Brewer DB. The glomerular tip lesion: a previously undescribed type of segmental glomerular abnormality. J Pathol 1984: 142: 205.

http://eng.hi138.com/?i295373_The-epidemiology-of-focal-segmental-glomerulosclerosis

Johnson RJ (2001) Impaired angiogenesis in the remnant kidney model: I. Potential role of vascular endothelial growth factor and thrombospondin-1. J Am Soc Nephrol 12(7):1434–1447 26.

Kang DH, Joly AH, Oh S-W, Hugo C, Kerjaschki D, Gordon KL, Mazzali M, Jefferson JA, Hughes J, Madsen KM, Schreiner GF,

Kaplan JM, Kim SH, North KN, Rennke H, Correia LA, Tong HQ, Mathis BJ, Rodriguez-Perez JC, Allen PG, Beggs AH, Pollak MR (2000) Mutations in ACTN4, encoding alpha-actinin-4, cause familial focal segmental glomerulosclerosis. Nat Genet 24 (3):251–256

Karle SM, Uetz B, Ronner V, Glaeser L, Hildebrandt F, Fuchshuber A (2002) Novel mutations in NPHS2 detected in both familial and sporadic steroid-resistant nephrotic syndrome. J Am Soc Nephrol 13(2):388–393

Kestila M, Lenkkeri U, Mannikko M, Lamerdin J, McCready P, Putaala H, Ruotsalainen V, Morita T, Nissinen M, Herva R,

Kashtan C, Peltonen L, Holmberg C, Olsen A, Tryggvason K (1998) Positionally cloned gene for a novel glomerular protein—nephrin—is mutated in congenital nephrotic syndrome. Mol Cell 1(4):575–582

Kim JM, Wu H, Green G, Winkler CA, Kopp JB, Miner JH, Unanue ER, Shaw AS (2003) CD2-associated protein haploinsufficiency is linked to glomerular disease susceptibility. Science 300(5623):1298–1300

Kimberly Reidy & Frederick J. Kaskel. Pathophysiology of focal segmental glomerulosclerosis Pediatr Nephrol (2007) 22:350–354

Kitiyakara C, Eggers P, Kopp JB. Twenty-one-year trend in ESRD due to focal segmental glomerulosclerosis in the United States. Am J Kidney Dis 2004; 44:815.

Korbet SM. Clinical picture and outcome of primary focal segmental glomerulosclerosis. Nephrol Dial Transplant. 1999;14(suppl 3):68S-73S.

Korbet SM (2003) Angiotensin antagonists and steroids in the treatment of focal segmental glomerulosclerosis. Semin Nephrol 23(2):219–228

Kwoh C, Shannon MB, Miner JH, Shaw A (2006) Pathogenesis of nonimmune glomerulopathies. Annu Rev Pathol Mech Dis 1:349–374

Meyrier A, Noel LH, Auriche P, et al. Long-term renal tolerance of cyclosporin A treatment in adult idiopathic nephrotic syndrome. Collaborative Group of the Societe de Nephrologie. Kidney Int. 1994;45:1446-1456.

Meyrier A (2003) E pluribus unum: the riddle of focal segmental glomerulosclerosis. Semin Nephrol 23(2):135–140

Meyrier A. An update on the treatment options for focal segmental glomerulosclerosis. Expert Opin. Pharmacother. 2009;10:615-628.

Niaudet P. Treatment of childhood steroid-resistant idiopathic nephrosis with a combination of cyclosporine and prednisone. J Pediatr. 1994;125:981-986.

Peters HP, van de Kar NC, Wetzels JF. Rituximab in minimal change nephropathy and focal segmental glomerulosclerosis: report of four cases and review of the literature. Neth J Med. 2008;66:408-415.

Ponticelli C, Rizzoni G, Edefonti A, et al. A randomized trial of cyclosporine in steroid-resistant idiopathic nephrotic syndrome. Kidney Int. 1993;43:1377-1384.

Rao TK, Fillippone EJ, Nicastri AD et al. Associated focal and segmental glomerulosclerosis in the acquired immunodeficiency syndrome. N Engl J Med 1984: 310: 669.

Rennke HG, Klein PS. Pathogenesis and significance of nonprimary focal and segmental glomerulosclerosis. Am J Kidney Dis 1989: 13: 443.

Rich A. A hitherto undescribed vulnerability of the juxtamedullary glomeruli in lipoid nephrosis. Bull Johns Hopkins Hosp 1957;100: 173–186

Rodriguez-Iturbe B, Johnson RJ, Herrera-Acosta J (2005) Tubulointerstitial damage and progression of renal failure. Kidney Int 68(Supp 99):S82–S86

Rydel JJ, Korbet SM, Borok RZ, Schwartz MM. Focal segmental glomerular sclerosis in adults: presentation, course, and response to treatment. Am J Kidney Dis 1995; 25:534.

Savin VJ, McCarthy ET, Sharma M (2003) Permeability factors in focal segmental glomerulosclerosis. Semin Nephrol 23(2):147–160

Schnaper HW (2003) Idiopathic focal segmental glomerulosclerosis. Semin Nephrol 23(2):183–193

Schwartz MM, Lewis EJ. Focal segmental glomerular sclerosis: the cellular lesion. Kidney Int 1985: 28: 968.

Schwimmer JA, Markowitz GS, Valeri A, Appel GB (2003) Collapsing glomerulopathy. Semin Nephrol 23(2):209–218

Segarra A, Vila J, Pou L, et al. Combined therapy of tacrolimus and corticosteroids in cyclosporin-resistant or -dependent idiopathic focal glomerulosclerosis: a preliminary uncontrolled study with prospective follow-up. Nephrol Dial Transplant. 2002;17:655-662.

Shih NY, Li J, Karpitskii V, Nguyen A, Dustin ML, Kanagawa O, Miner JH, Shaw AS (1999) Congenital nephrotic syndrome in mice lacking CD2-associated protein. Science 286(5438):312–315

Shimizu A, Higo S, Fujita E, Mii A, Kaneko T. Focal segmental glomerulosclerosis after renal transplantation. Clin Transplant 2011: 25 (Suppl. 23): 6–14.

Thomas DB, Franceschini N, Hogan SL, et al. Clinical and pathologic characteristics of focal segmental glomerulosclerosis pathologic variants. Kidney Int. 2006;69:920-926

Trachtman H. et al; A phase 1, single-dose study of fresolimumab, an anti-TGF-beta antibody, in treatment-resistant primary focal segmental glomerulosclerosis. Kidney International (2011) 79, 1236–1243

Tryggvason K, Patrakka J, Wartiovaara J (2006) Hereditary proteinuria syndromes and mechanisms of proteinuria. N Engl J Med 354(13):1387–1401

Weiss MA, Daquioag E, Margolin EG, Pollak VE. Nephrotic syndrome, progressive irreversible renal failure, and glomerular "collapse": a new clinicopathologic entity? Am J Kidney Dis 1986: 7: 20.

Weissgarten J, Berman S, Efrati S, et al. Apoptosis and proliferation of cultured mesangial cells isolated from kidneys of rosiglitazone-treated pregnant diabetic rats. Nephrol Dial Transplant. 2006;21:1198-1204

Winn MP. Approach to the evaluation of heritable diseases and update on familial focal segmental glomerulosclerosis: Nephrol Dial Transplant 2003 Aug;18 Suppl 6:vi14-20.

Winn MP, Conlon PJ, Lynn KL, Farrington MK, Creazzo T, Hawkins AF, Daskalakis N, Kwan SY, Ebersviller S, Burchette

JL, Pericak-Vance MA, Howell DN, Vance JM, Rosenberg PB (2005) A mutation in the TRPC6 cation channel causes familial focal segmental glomerulosclerosis. Science 17(5729):1801– 1804

Walls J (2001) Relationship between proteinuria and progressive renal disease. Am J Kidney Dis 37(1 Supp 2):S13–S16

Weiss MA, Daquioag E, Margolin EG, Pollak VE. Nephrotic syndrome, progressive irreversible renal failure, and glomerular "collapse": a new clinicopathologic entity? Am J Kidney Dis 1986: 7: 20.

Yao J, Le TC, Kos CH, Henderson JM, Allen PG, Denker BM, Pollak MR (2004) Alpha-actinin-4-mediated FSGS: an inherited kidney disease caused by an aggregated and rapidly degraded cytoskeletal protein. PLoS Biol 2(6):787–794

4

Primary IgA Nephropathy: An Update in 2011

Francois Berthoux[1] and Amir Kamal Aziz[2]
[1]*Dialysis and Renal Transplantation Department, University Hospital of Saint-Etienne,*
Medical Faculty of Saint-Etienne, Saint-Etienne Cedex 2
[2]*Nephrology and Dialysis Department, Louis Pasteur Hospital, Dole*
France

1. Introduction

IgA Nephropathy (IGAN) is also called mesangial IgA glomerulonephritis and was first described by Jean Berger, a French general pathologist, in 1968 in the journal d'Urologie-Néphrologie [1, 2]. Many reviews have been written on the subject [3, 4, 5].

2. Definition [3, 4, 5]

The definition is histopathologic with the characteristical **deposition** of the **immunoglobulin A** in the renal **mesangium**: these deposits are **predominant** (or codominant with other immunoglobulins, IgG and/or IgM), **granular, coarse** (with the "en mottes" aspect), **generalized** in the glomerulus and **diffuse** to all glomeruli. These deposits are evidenced usually by the technique of direct immunofluorescence on a semi-quantitative scale: traces (+/-), 1+, 2+, and ≥ 3+. There is a general agreement to accept **at least 1+ IgA deposits** for the definition.

By contrast, the lesions observed by light microscopy are often segmental and focal. The main lesions concern the mesangium with increased matrix and hypercellularity with in addition endocapillary proliferation. The most severe lesions are represented by obsolescent glomeruli ("pains à cacheter"), focal and segmental glomerulosclerosis (FSGS) with capsular adhesions, and extracapillary proliferation with the formation of cellular/hyalinized crescents.

3. The IgA nephritides [3, 4, 5]

The deposition of mesangial IgA has been observed in different types of glomerulonephritis leading to the classification of **Primary IgA nephropathy** (Berger's disease) versus the **Secondary IgA nephropathies**: associated to Schönlein-Henoch Purpura, to patent Alcoholic Liver Cirrhosis, to Systemic lupus Erythematosus, or to Ankylosing Spondylarthritis. Primary disease represents at least 80 % of the cases.

4. Epidemiology [3, 4, 5]

Primary IGAN is worldwide the most frequent glomerulonephritis; it accounts for about a quarter of the percutaneous renal biopsies performed on native kidneys. In France, the **incidence** is about 30 new cases per million inhabitants (pmp) and its **prevalence** is closed to 1000 pmp according to the disease duration from onset to dialysis or to last follow-up (from few months to more than 5O years). All these numbers are of course dependent of the "politic" of renal biopsy: liberal indication or restricted to the most severe cases with already proteinuria over 1g/day or already some degree of renal insufficiency (Glomerular Filtration Rate <60 ml/mn/1.73 m² body surface area).

The disease is more frequent in men than in women, about 70% males, in most continents except in Asia. Age at onset ranges from 5 years to 75 with a peak frequency in adolescents and young adults.

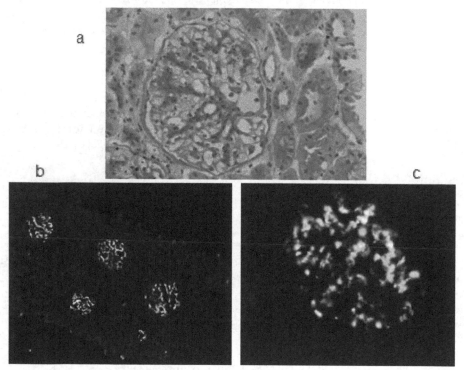

Fig. 1. HistoPathology of IgA Nephropathy:
(a) Light microscopy showing one glomerulus with segmental increased in mesangial matrix and mild hypercellularity.
(b) Immunofluorescent microscopy showing diffuse IgA deposits in all glomeruli.
(c) Immunofluorescent microscopy showing generalized mesangial IgA deposits within all the glomerulus surface/volume.

5. Mode of onset/initial presentation [3, 4, 5]

The onset of the disease can be **acute/subacute** in about 30 to 35 % of the patients with the classical **intra-infectious gross haematuria**: at time of an infectious episode of various origin (pharyngitis, bronchitis, or even intestinal or urinary infection), the patient is urinating blood with colored urine, more brown than red with a color of coffee or coca-cola; this is a total haematuria (sometimes with loin pain) which lasts from few hours to few days; there is no clot and the characteristics of this gross haematuria is nephrological with the presence on urine cytology of typical red blood cell casts. After such an episode, the patient is usually presenting microscopic haematuria or could be in total remission until the next episode.

The discovery can be **chance proteinuria** or **chance microscopic haematuria** at time of systemic urine control for medical check-up at school, at different institutions or at work; the time of onset is therefore imprecise and we should refer to the last negative control if any.

The disease can be diagnosed later on with arterial hypertension (HT) and/or oedema and/or chronic kidney disease stage 3 or up (CKD-3+).

6. Progression of the disease [6-12]

Overall, IGAN is a **progressive disease** both clinically and pathologically. The **clinical progression** starts with urine abnormalities, followed by occurrence of HT, sometimes oedema related to massive proteinuria or nephrotic syndrome, and later on occurrence of CKD-3 through CKD-5 and ultimately renal death necessitating chronic dialysis. The progression is also **pathological** and this was demonstrated by repeated renal biopsies 5 years later [6, 13]: it was shown that the global optical score (GOS) progressed in the majority of the patients with increased glomerular but also vascular and tubular/interstitial indices.

We are taking as example our prospective cohort of primary IGAN patients [12] whose diagnostic biopsy was performed between January 1st 1990 and December 31st 1999 at our institution with loco-regional patients coming from the Saint-Etienne area, the IGAN-STET-CO. This cohort is composed of 332 patients (237 men, 71.4 %) with a mean age of 35.9 at onset, 41.4 at diagnosis and 48.8 years at dialysis/death or at last follow-up visit. The total exposure time was about 13 years. Overall, 32 patients needed dialysis, 13 died before reaching dialysis, and 45 (13.6 %) reached the primary composite outcome while 99 (29.8 %) presented the secondary outcome (CKD-3+).

7. Predictive risk factors and the absolute renal risk of dialysis/death: A new concept [12]

One very important goal was to sort out the major and independent risk factors (RF), present at diagnosis, able to predict accurately the ultimate final prognosis (dialysis or death as primary end-point). From the literature, we already know that the amount of proteinuria (g per day), the occurrence/presence of HT, and the severity of renal lesions on the initial biopsy were associated with progression [6-11]. Many other risk factors were also described such as gender, overweight/obesity [14], metabolic syndrome, age at onset [15], hypertriglyceridemia/hyperuricemia [16], and also different immunogenetic markers (HLA antigens, different cytokines polymorphisms [17, 18],...) but they were not consistent or controversial in different published cohorts. We recently confirmed [12] that these 3 major risk factors were sufficient to cover the whole prediction in our cohort. These risk factors were simplified, dichotomized for easier use and shown to be independent predictors in a multivariate model of Cox regression: - the most important is the **presence of HT (Yes or No)** defined according to WHO (≥ 140/90); - the next is the **presence of Proteinuria ≥ 1g/d (Yes or No);** and - the last is the scoring of the renal lesions; we have used our own **global**

optical score (GOS) developed 20 years ago and integrating all elementary lesions (glomerular from 0 to 6, vascular from 0 to 5, tubular from 0 to 4, and interstitial from 0 to 5) with a GOS up to 20. We set up by ROC analysis that the best cut-off for predicting dialysis was the **presence of GOS ≥ 8 (Yes or No).** These 3 RF turned out to have a similar weight in the prediction of dialysis/death by the different accuracy parameters and also by the Cox regression (β/SE ratio of the same magnitude).

In analogy to the absolute cardio-vascular risk (ACVR) of death or major CV events at 10 years [19, 20], we proposed the **Absolute Renal Risk of Dialysis/Death;** this ARR is calculated at diagnosis and is very simply the number of these RF present: 0, 1, 2 or 3. By Kaplan-Meier survival curves, we could calculate the cumulative rate of primary event at 10 and 20 years after onset (time zero); it was respectively 2 and 4 % for ARR=0; 2 and 9 % for ARR=1; 7 and 18 % for ARR=2; and 29 and 64% for ARR=3.

In addition, this ARR integrates gender (less RF for women), age at diagnosis (more RF for older patients), and also body mass index (more RF in overweight/obese patients). We could also use it as prospective with time zero set-up at diagnosis and not at onset; the cumulative incidence of dialysis/death 10 years after diagnosis is 4% for ARR=0, 8% for ARR=1, 18% for ARR=2, and 68% for ARR=3. It is remarkable to underline the similarity of the values obtained 20 y after onset and 10y after diagnosis.

Distribution of these Risk Factors at time of Diagnosis and at last follow-up (LFU): HT was present in 120 patients (36.1%) at diagnosis and in 164 (49.4%) at LFU; Proteinuria ≥1g/d was present in 100 patients (30.1%) at diagnosis and in only 61 (18.4%) at LFU; and GOS ≥ 8 was present in 120 patients (36.1%) at time of diagnosis. The distribution of the ARR was as follows at time of diagnosis: 151 patients (45.5%) with ARR=0, 69 (20.8%) with ARR=1, 65 (19.6%) with ARR=2, and 47 patients (14.1%) with ARR=3.

It should be stressed that this cohort is an adequately treated cohort with all RF targeted as soon as they were identified: perfect control of blood pressure (target <130/80) with all antihypertensive agents; persistent reduction of proteinuria with ACEI and ARBs; and prednisolone for severe renal lesions.

8. Pathological classification of IgA nephropathy

We have developed our own classification in 1990 [6, 13] with the Global Optical Score already described. During the past decades, the classifications of Haas [21] or Hass modified by Lee [22] were frequently used. The international Oxford classification was published in 2009 [23, 24] and retained only 4 parameters with significant clinical prediction: - mesangial hypercellularity (M score= 0 or 1); - endocapillary hypercellurarity (E score= 0 or 1); - segmental glomerulosclerosis (S score= 0 or 1); and - tubular atrophy/interstitial fibrosis (T score= 0 or 1 or 2). Overall, the MEST score ranges from 0 to 5. One limitation is that patients were only included if proteinuria was ≥ 1g/d in adults and there was no patients with ARR=0 who are in fact the majority of the patients; in addition patients with extracapillary GN (≥ 50% crescents) were also excluded; the two tails of the IGAN cohorts were therefore lacking!

9. Principles of treatment in IGAN

The treatment should in fact target all major risk factors when present: hypertension, proteinuria, and severe renal lesions.

The permanent control of HT is a major step; the goal is to lower BP ≤ 130/80. Sodium chloride restriction is recommended with 24 h urinary sodium below 100 mmol/d corresponding to a maximum of 6 g daily sodium chloride. All antihypertensive agents can be used: diuretics, beta blockers, calcium blockers, central-acting, ACE inhibitors, angiotensin-2-receptor blockers (ARBs), and more recently renin inhibitors. However two classes have demonstrated a better protection and should be used alone or in association: ACEI and ARBs [25, 26]. In our prospective cohort [12], we have demonstrated that survival without dialysis/death improved in patients with adequately controlled BP on long term [27].

The significant reduction of proteinuria is another major step [28]; the reduction can be obtained with the use of ACEI and ARBs which have a significant antiproteinuric effect. It is recommended to start with either one of these drugs, to titrate the dose to the effect, and to use the association in case of resistant proteinuria; the goal is to bring proteinuria ≤ 1g/d or ideally < 0.30 g/d. We have also demonstrated [12] that the permanent reduction of proteinuria is associated with a better survival on long-term.

The **treatment of severe renal lesions** on the biopsy; this could be achieved by Prednisone or Prednisolone treatment [29-31] which should be in theory able to reduce hypercellularity and cellular infiltration within the glomeruli; however in the trial, there was no repeated biopsies at the end of the steroid therapy. For the most severe cases with extracapillary GN (>50 % crescents), the association of high dose steroids and immunosuppressive agents as already proposed might be a good option.

The use of Fish Oil was limited with controversial results [32, 33].

We are still in the need of large randomized controlled trials with a long duration (5 years seems optimal) to draw definite conclusions on the treatment of IGAN.

10. Pathogenesis and patho-physiology of primary IgA nephropathy

Very significant progress has been made during the last decades. The key protein in this disease is the immunoglobulin A and more precisely the subgroup 1; in fact IgA1 is deposited in the mesangium but not IgA2 [34]. The major difference between IgA1 and IgA2 is the presence of an hinge region in IgA1 composed of 23 aminoacids with usually five sugar side chains linked to threonin or serin. There is now a consensus [35-39] about the fact that the main difference between IgA1 in Controls and in IGAN patients is the hypo-galactosylation of these glycosylated side chains. The normal complete sugar chain is O-linked to threonine or serin and composed of one molecule of N-acetyl galactosamine (GalNac) and one molecule of Galactose; in addition a molecule of sialic acid can be bound in terminal to Galactose or in lateral to GalNac. In IGAN, more side chains are truncated with loss of terminal Galactose with its terminal sialic acid and is referred to the Galactose-deficient IgA1 (deGal-IgA1). This deGal-IgA1 represents the specific autoantigen in this disease and is present in the serum, within the circulating immune complexes and in the mesangial deposits [40]. This loss in terminal galactose is associated with a down-regulation of the gene controlling the linkage of galactose to GalNac, C1GALT1 [41] and the description of specific polymorphism [42] raising the possibility of genetic predisposition [43].

The loss of terminal galactose unusually exposed the GalNac molecules, which become antigenic with elicitation of a specific antibody response [44, 45]: IgG and/or IgA anti O-GalNac, the specific auto-antibodies. It is now possible to measure the amount of circulating autoantigen and autoantibodies in patients sera and to discriminate between Controls and IGAN patients [46, 47].

The mesangial deposition of deGal-IgA1 is dependent on physical characteristics of this molecule (more sticky) and the presence of transferrin receptor (CD71) which is able to bind IgA1 variants [48]. After binding, the deGal-IgA1 and the deposited immune complexes are able to activate the different mediators of inflammation both cellular [49] and in fluid phase. There is also the CD89 system [50] that we personally consider as an amplification loop. This is a specific receptor for IgA1 variants, FcαRI, present on circulating monocytes but not in the mesangium; this receptor is able to bind immune complexes with further amplification and longer persistence in the circulation, and may play an additional pathogenic role.

11. Renal transplantation in patients with biopsy-proven IGAN on native kidneys

In cases which progressed to dialysis, renal transplantation should be a strong option and overall the results are similar to the other recipients matched for age and gender. However, there are two specific situations which have strong pathogenic implication.

First, a silent IgA nephropathy can be present on grafted kidney from apparently normal donors leading to the discovery of mesangial IgA deposits on graft biopsies performed early after transplantation; it was demonstrated in few cases that these deposits can regress and disappear demonstrating a contrario that the disease has a systemic (blood) transmission.

Second, the original disease may reappear (**recurrence**) on the normal grafted kidney after few years and despite immunosuppression [51-59]. The cumulative incidence of clinic-pathological recurrence is high reaching 35 % or more at 10 years post-transplant [56] and may lead to graft losses in up to 17 % at 10 y [57]. The factors associated to recurrence are not well understood: living donors, better HLA matching, short duration of the original disease, etc. There is yet no specific treatment for the recurrent disease; however in a retrospective study [56] we demonstrated that induction treatment with ATG seems able to reduce the incidence of recurrence in comparison to no induction or to induction with Basiliximab. A prospective randomized controlled trial comparing rabbit ATG to Basiliximab has already started, the PIRAT study: Prevention in IgA nephropathy recipients of full Recurrence After renal Transplantation according to induction immunosuppressive therapy: ATG versus Basiliximab. It seems now mandatory to carefully measure the serum levels of the auto-antigen and the auto-antibodies at time of grafting to check for any predicting value of these parameters for recurrence.

12. Conclusions

IgA nephropathy is a frequent disease whose individual prognosis can be totally different: no significant progression for 50 years versus progression to dialysis in few months or years. The clinical challenge is to accurately predict the long term individual prognosis at time of diagnosis (at time of the renal biopsy which is still mandatory for this purpose). We have made significant progress with our new concept: the **Absolute Renal Risk of Dialysis/Death** (ARR); it takes in account the presence or not of three independent, simplified and dichotomous risk factors: - **arterial hypertension**; - **proteinuria ≥1g/d**; and severe histopathological lesions appreciated by the **Global Optical Score ≥ 8** (range from 0 to 20). The cumulative incidence rate of primary event (dialysis or death) at 10 years post-

diagnosis, is 4 % for ARR=0; 8 % for ARR=1; 18 % for ARR=2; and 68 % for ARR=3 in our prospective cohort adequately treated/managed on long term.
The pathogenesis of the disease has also made significant progress: it is an **auto-immune disease** with a known **auto-antigen**, the Galactose-deficient IgA1, which can elicit a specific **auto-antibody** response, IgG and IgA anti-O-GalNac. There is formation of specific **immune complexes** which are **circulating** and then **deposited** in the mesangium with creation of the disease. These recent findings will have significant future applications in the diagnosis and in the treatment.

13. References

[1] Berger J, Hinglais N. Intercapillary deposits of IgA-IgG. J Urol Nephrol 1968;74:694-5.

[2] Berger J. IgA glomerular deposits in renal disease. Transplant Proc 1969; 1: 939-44.

[3] Donadio JV, Grande JP. IgA nephropathy. N Engl J Med 2002; 347: 738-48.

[4] Barratt J, Feehally J. IgA nephropathy. J Am Soc Nephrol 2005; 16: 2088-97.

[5] Berthoux FC, Mohey H, Afiani A. Natural history of primary IgA nephropathy. Semin Nephrol 2008; 28: 4-9.

[6] Alamartine E, Sabatier JC, Guerin C, et al. Prognostic factors in mesangial IgA glomerulonephritis: an extensive study with univariate and multivariate analyses. Am J Kidney Dis 1991; 18:12-9.

[7] Koyama A, Igarashi M, Kobayashi M. Natural history and risk factors for immunoglobulin A nephropathy in Japan. Research Group on Progressive Renal Diseases. Am J Kidney Dis 1997; 29: 526-32.

[8] Radford MG, Donadio JV, Bergstralh EJ, Grande JP. Predicting renal outcome in IgA nephropathy. J Am Soc Nephrol 1997; 8:199-207.

[9] D'Amico G. Natural history of idiopathic IgA nephropathy: role of clinical and histological prognostic factors. Am J Kidney Dis 2000; 36: 227-37.

[10] Bartosik LP, Lajoie G, Sugar L, Cattran DC. Predicting progression in IgA nephropathy. Am J Kidney Dis 2001; 38: 728-35.

[11] Li PK, Ho KK, Szeto CC, et al. Prognostic indicators of IgA nephropathy in the Chinese-clinical and pathological perspectives. Nephrol Dial Transplant 2002; 17: 64-9.

[12] Berthoux F, Mohey H, Laurent B, Mariat C, Afiani A, Thibaudin L. Predicting the risk for Dialysis or Death in IgA nephropathy. J Am Soc Nephrol 2011; 22: 752-61.

[13] Alamartine E, Sabatier JC, Berthoux FC. Comparison of pathological lesions on repeated renal biopsies in 73 patients with primary IgA glomerulonephritis : value of quantitative scoring and approach to final prognosis. Clin Nephrol 1990; 34: 45- 51.

[14] Bonnet F, Deprele C, Sassolas A, et al. Excessive body weight as a new independent risk factor for clinical and pathological progression in primary IgA nephritis. Am J Kidney Dis 2001; 37: 720-

[15] Donadio JV, Bergstralh EJ, Grande JP, Rademcher DM. Proteinuria patterns and their association with subsequent end-stage renal disease in IgA nephropathy. Nephrol Dial Transplant 2002; 17: 1197-203.

[16] Syrjänen J, Mustonen J, Pasternack A. Hypertriglyceridaemia and hyperuricaemia are risk factors for progression of IgA nephropathy. Nephrol Dial Transplant 2000; 15:34-42.

[17] Panzer U, Schneider A, Steinmetz OM, et al. The chemokine receptor 5 Delta32 mutation is associated with increased renal survival in patients with IgA nephropathy. Kidney Int 2005; 67:75-81.

[18] Berthoux FC, Berthoux P, Mariat C, et al. CC-chemokine receptor five gene polymorphism in primary IgA nephropathy: the 32 bp deletion allele is associated with late progression to end-stage renal failure with dialysis. Kidney Int 2006; 69: 565-72.

[19] Kannel WB, McGee D, Gordon T. A general cardiovascular risk profile: the Framingham study. Am J Cardiol 1976; 38: 46-51.

[20] D'Agostino RB Sr, Vasan RS, Pencina MJ, et al. General cardiovascular risk profile for use in primary care: the Framingham heart study. Circulation 2008; 117: 743-53.

[21] Haas M. Histologic subclassification of IgA nephropathy: a clinicopathological study of 244 cases. Am J Kidney Dis 1997; 29: 829-42.

[22] Lee HS, Lee MS, Lee SM, et al. Histological grading of IgA nephropathy predicting renal outcome: revisiting H.S. Lee's glomerular grading system. Nephrol Dial Transplant 2005; 20: 342-8.

[23] A working group of the international IgA nephropathy network and the renal pathology society: Cattran DC, Coppo R, Cook HT, et al. The Oxford classification of IgA nephropathy: rationale, clinicopathological correlations, and classification. Kidney Int 2009; 76: 534-45.

[24] A working group of the international IgA nephropathy network and the renal pathology society: Roberts IS, Cook HT, Troyanov S, et al. The Oxford classification of IgA nephropathy: pathology definitions, correlations, and reproducibility. Kidney Int 2009; 76: 546-56.

[25] Praga M, Gutiérrez E, Gonzalez E, et al. Treatment of IgA nephropathy with ACE inhibitors: a randomized and controlled trial. J Am Soc Nephrol 2003; 14: 1578-83.

[26] Dillon JJ; Angiotensin-converting enzyme inhibitors and angiotensin receptor blockers for IgA nephropathy. Semin Nephrol 2004; 24: 218-24.

[27] Kanno Y, Okada H, Saruta T, Suzuki H. Blood pressure reduction associated with preservation of renal function in hypertensive patients with IgA nephropathy: a 3-year follow-up. Clin Nephrol 2000; 54: 360-5.

[28] Reich HN, Troyanov S, Scholey JW, et al. Remission of proteinuria improves prognosis in IgA nephropathy. J Am Soc Nephrol 2007; 18: 3177-83.

[29] Lv J, Zhang H, Chen Y, et al. Combination therapy of prednisone and ACE inhibitor versus ACE-inhibitor therapy alone in patients with IgA nephropathy: a randomized controlled trial. Am J Kidney Dis 2008; 53: 26-32.

[30] Pozzi C, Andrulli S, Del Vecchio L, et al. Corticosteroid effectiveness in IgA nephropathy: long-term results of a randomized, controlled trial. J Am Soc Nephol 2004; 15: 157-63.

[31] Cheng J, Zhang X, Zhang W, et al. Efficacy and safety of glucocorticoids therapy for IgA nephropathy: a meta analysis of randomized controlled trials. Am J Nephrol 2009; 30: 315-22.

[32] Donadio JV Jr, Bergstralh EJ, Offord KP, Spencer DC, Holley KE. A controlled trial of fish oil in IgA nephropathy. Mayo Nephrology Collaborative Group. N Engl J Med 1994; 331:1194-9.

[33] Donadio JV, Grande JP. The role of fish oil / omega-3 fatty acids in the treatment of IgA nephropathy. Semin Nephrol 2004; 24: 225-43.

[34] Conley ME, Cooper MD, Michael AF. Selective deposition of immunoglobulin A1 in immunoglobulin A nephropathy, anaphylactoid purpura nephritis, and systemic lupus erythematosus. J Clin Invest 1980; 66:1432-6.

[35] Hiki Y, Tanaka A, Kokubo T, Iwase H, Nishikido J, Hotta K, Kobayashi Y. Analyses of IgA1 hinge glycopeptides in IgA nephropathy by matrix-assisted laser desorption/ionization time-of-flight mass spectrometry. J Am Soc Nephrol 1998; 9:577-82

[36] Hiki Y, Kokubo T, Iwase H, Masaki Y, Sano T, Tanaka A, Toma K, Hotta K, Kobayashi Y. Underglycosylation of IgA1 hinge plays a certain role for its glomerular deposition in IgA nephropathy. J Am Soc Nephrol 1999; 10:760-9.

[37] Allen AC, Bailey EM, Barratt J, Buck KS, Feehally J. Analysis of IgA1 O-glycans in IgA nephropathy by fluorophore-assisted carbohydrate electrophoresis. J Am Soc Nephrol 1999; 10:1763-71.

[38] Hiki Y, Odani H, Takahashi M, Yasuda Y, Nishimoto A, Iwase H, Shinzato T, Kobayashi Y, Maeda K. Mass spectrometry proves under-O-glycosylation of glomerular IgA1 in IgA nephropathy. Kidney Int 2001; 59:1077-85

[39] Suzuki H, Moldoveanu Z, Hall S, Brown R, Vu HL, Novak L, Julian BA, Tomana M, Wyatt RJ, Edberg JC, Alarcón GS, Kimberly RP, Tomino Y, Mestecky J, Novak J. IgA1-secreting cell lines from patients with IgA nephropathy produce aberrantly glycosylated IgA1. J Clin Invest 2008; 118:629-39.

[40] Allen AC, Bailey EM, Brenchley PE, Buck KS, Barratt J, Feehally J. Mesangial IgA1 in IgA nephropathy exhibits aberrant O-glycosylation: observations in three patients. Kidney Int 2001; 60:969-73

[41] Inoue T, Sugiyama H, Kikumoto Y, Fukuoka N, Maeshima Y, Hattori H, Fukushima K, Nishizaki K, Hiki Y, Makino H. Downregulation of the beta1,3-galactosyltransferase gene in tonsillar B lymphocytes and aberrant lectin bindings to tonsillar IgA as a pathogenesis of IgA nephropathy. Contrib Nephrol 2007; 157:120-4

[42] Li GS, Zhang H, Lv JC, Shen Y, Wang HY. Variants of C1GALT1 gene are associated with the genetic susceptibility to IgA nephropathy. Kidney Int 2007; 71:448-53

[43] Gharavi AG, Moldoveanu Z, Wyatt RJ, Barker CV, Woodford SY, Lifton RP, Mestecky J, Novak J, Julian BA. Aberrant IgA1 glycosylation is inherited in familial and sporadic IgA nephropathy. J Am Soc Nephrol 2008; 19:1008-14

[44] Tomana M, Novak J, Julian BA, Matousovic K, Konecny K, Mestecky J. Circulating immune complexes in IgA nephropathy consist of IgA1 with galactose-deficient hinge region and antiglycan antibodies. J Clin Invest 1999; 104:73-81

[45] Suzuki H, Fan R, Zhang Z, Brown R, Hall S, Julian BA, Chatham WW, Suzuki Y, Wyatt RJ, Moldoveanu Z, Lee JY, Robinson J, Tomana M, Tomino Y, Mestecky J, Novak J. Aberrantly glycosylated IgA1 in IgA nephropathy patients is recognized by IgG antibodies with restricted heterogeneity. J Clin Invest 2009; 119:1668-77

[46] Moldoveanu Z, Wyatt RJ, Lee JY, Tomana M, Julian BA, Mestecky J, Huang WQ, Anreddy SR, Hall S, Hastings MC, Lau KK, Cook WJ, Novak J. Patients with IgA nephropathy have increased serum galactose-deficient IgA1 levels. Kidney Int 2007; 71:1148-54

[47] Novak J, Julian BA, Tomana M, Mestecky J. IgA glycosylation and IgA immune complexes in the pathogenesis of IgA nephropathy. Semin Nephrol. 2008; 28:78-87

[48] Moura IC, Arcos-Fajardo M, Sadaka C, Leroy V, Benhamou M, Novak J, Vrtovsnik F, Haddad E, Chintalacharuvu KR, Monteiro RC. Glycosylation and size of IgA1 are essential for interaction with mesangial transferrin receptor in IgA nephropathy. J Am Soc Nephrol 2004; 15:622-34

[49] Coppo R, Fonsato V, Balegno S, Ricotti E, Loiacono E, Camilla R, Peruzzi L, Amore A, Bussolati B, Camussi G. Aberrantly glycosylated IgA1 induces mesangial cells to produce platelet-activating factor that mediates nephrin loss in cultured podocytes. Kidney Int 2010; 77:417-27.

[50] Launay P, Grossetête B, Arcos-Fajardo M, Gaudin E, Torres SP, Beaudoin L, Patey-Mariaud de Serre N, Lehuen A, Monteiro RC. Fc alpha receptor (CD89) mediates the development of immunoglobulin A (IgA) nephropathy (Berger's disease). Evidence for pathogenic soluble receptor-Iga complexes in patients and CD89 transgenic mice. J Exp Med 2000 ; 5;191:1999-2009.

[51] Berger J, Yaneva H, Nabarra B, Barbanel C. Recurrence of mesangial deposition of IgA after renal transplantation. Kidney Int 1975; 7: 232.

[52] Hariharan S, Peddi VR, Savin VJ, et al. Recurrent and de novo renal diseases after renal transplantation: a report from the renal allograft disease registry. Am J Kidney Dis 1998; 31: 928.

[53] Chandrakantan A, Ratanapanichkich P, Said M, Barker CV, Julian BA. Recurrent IgA nephropathy after renal transplantation despite immunosuppressive regimens with mycophenolate mofetil. Nephrol Dial Transplant 2005; 20: 1214.

[54] Wang AY, Lai FM, Yu AW, et al. Recurrent IgA nephropathy in renal transplant allografts. Am J Kidney Dis 2001;38: 588.

[55] Ponticelli C, Traversi L, Feliciani A, et al. Kidney transplantation in patients with IgA mesangial glomerulonephritis. Kidney Int 2001; 60 (5): 1948.

[56] Berthoux F, El Deeb S, Mariat C, Diconne E, Laurent B, Thibaudin L. Antithymocyte globulin (ATG) induction therapy and disease recurrence in renal transplant recipients with primary IgA nephropathy. Transplantation 2008; 85: 1505.

[57] Briganti EM, Russ GK, Mc Neil JJ, et al. Risk of renal allograft loss from recurrent glomerulonephritis. New Engl J Med 2002; 347: 103

[58] Ponticelli C, Glassock RJ. Posttransplant recurrence of primary glomerulonephritis. Clin J Am Soc Nephrol 2010; 5: 2363-72.

[59] Han SS, Huh W, Park SK, Ahn C, Han JS, Kim S, Kim YS. Impact of recurrent disease and chronic allograft nephropathy on the long-term allograft outcome in patients with IgA nephropathy. Transpl Int 2010; 23:169-75.

5

IgA Nephropathy: Insights into Genetic Basis and Treatment Options

Dimitrios Kirmizis[1], Aikaterini Papagianni[1] and Francesco Paolo Schena[2]
[1]*Aristotle University, Thessaloniki,*
[2]*Renal Unit, University of Bari, Bari,*
[1]*Greece*
[2]*Italy*

In memoriam of Prof. Efstathios Alexopoulos

1. Introduction

IgA nephropathy (IgAN), is the most common primary glomerulonephritis worldwide. On light microscopy the picture can vary from slight mesangial hypertrophy to extra capillary proliferation of glomeruli, with sclerosis and interstitial fibrosis. On immunofluorescence staining of kidney sections the disease is characterized by mesangial deposits of IgA, predominantly polymeric IgA (pIgA) of the IgA1 subclass, and often co-deposition of complement factor C3, properdin and IgG. It is important however to realize that, although IgA mesangial deposits are necessary for the diagnosis of IgAN, the latter is not obligatory in every individual with mesangial IgA deposits. Thus, IgA deposits may also be seen in subjects with no evidence of renal disease [Suzuki et al, 2003; Waldherr et al, 1989] at an incidence that ranges from 3 to 16 percent. Furthermore, there are also a number of reports documenting IgA deposition in other forms of glomerulonephritis, particularly thin basement membrane disease, lupus nephritis, minimal change disease, and diabetic nephropathy, a finding which is most probably casual rather than causal.

IgAN occurs at any age, but most commonly the age of onset is in the second or third decade of life. Males are more often affected than females, with a male:female ratio of 2:1. Most patients with IgAN present microscopic hematuria with or without mild proteinuria. About 40% of patients have episodes of macroscopic hematuria. This is sometimes preceded by infections, most commonly upper respiratory tract infections, a phenomenon known as "synpharyngitic" hematuria. Other infections like gastrointestinal or urinary tract infections have also been reported to precede macroscopic hematuria. Proteinuria is common and can vary from mild proteinuria to nephrotic syndrome.

IgAN has been considered a benign disease for a long time, but nowadays it is clear that 30-40% of patients may develop renal failure with significant socioeconomical consequenses. In Western Europe and the United States of America 7-10% of the patients on renal replacement therapy suffer from IgAN. The severity of histological lesions, especially diffuse proliferative glomerulonephritis, marked capsular adhesions, fibrocellular crescents, glomerular hyalinosis and severe sclerosis, as well as tubulointerstitial damage correlate with poor renal outcome [Schena, 1998]. Next to the gravity of histological lesions, unfavourable outcome is associated with persistent hematuria and proteinuria of more than 1g/day, decreased glomerular filtration rate (GFR) at the time of the diagnosis, and hypertension. Although several laboratory tests have been reported to correlate with clinical outcome, so far no reliable biomarker has been identified to predict outcome in IgAN. Recurrence of IgAN after renal transplantation is common. This finding, along with the observation that IgA depositions disappear from a kidney of an IgAN patient, after transplantation of this kidney to a non IgAN patient, are suggestive of a rather systemic disease.

2. Genetics of IgAN

The strongest evidence for the existence of genetic factors in the development and/or progression of IgAN comes from descriptions of familial IgAN, largely in white populations [Julian et al, 1985], and recent studies suggest that familial and sporadic IgAN may share a common pathogenic mechanism and similar outcomes [Izzi et al, 2006]. The genetic predisposition may be independent of environmental factors and may reflect an inherited susceptibility to develop mesangial glomerulonephritis.

IgAN does not exhibit classic single-gene Mendelian inheritance pattern [Frimat & Kessler, 2002]. The complex genetic pattern of IgAN is reflected by the multiple pathways involved in its immunopathogenesis, namely multiple discrete immunologic abnormalities related to the abnormal overproduction and release of mucosal pIgA1 in the systemic compartment and possibly other protein functional abnormalities related to a propensity for mesangial deposition of pIgA1. It is therefore probable that the disease-associated genetic variations at identified IGAN loci, instead of occuring in the form of "classic" nonsense/missense/splice site mutations and deletions/insertions that affect protein structure and function, may be rather of the type specific single-nucleotide polymorphism (SNP) alleles in non-coding regions or synonymous SNPs in coding regions. The latter function as cis-acting elements that alter the transcriptional activity of a disease gene and/or messenger RNA stability and, therefore, the expression level of the encoded protein. It is interesting that recent studies indicate that 30% to 50% of human genes with coding SNPs can present allelic variation in gene expression [Hoogendoorn et al, 2003; Lo et al, 2003]. From this point of view, the most comprehensive theory is that several genetic loci contribute significantly to the disease susceptibility that underlie the primary immunologic defects observed in IgAN. Each locus may occur at a different prevalence rate in different racial/ethnic groups. Variations at these major genetic loci may not be sufficient for the development and progression of IgAN and the contribution from a potentially large number of modifying genes with modest genetic effects but high prevalence is probably needed as well. The various allelic combinations of these loci may underlie the different disease phenotypes (disease development and progression, nephritic vs. nephrotic clinical presentation, histopathologic subclass, severity of disease, responsiveness of proteinuria to angiotensin-converting enzyme [ACE] inhibitors and/or angiotensin II receptor blockers [ARBs], etc.) observed in IgAN. For diseases with complex genetic pattern, it has been shown that the optimal analysis approach is the combination of linkage, association and sequence approaches. Until now, two basic approaches have been used in genetic studies of IgAN: a) genome-wide linkage analysis study, a methodology that has been used successfully to identify major disease/susceptibility loci, b) candidate-gene association study, mainly used to identify altered genes with modest genetic effects but high prevalence. Recently, a genome-wide association study was carried out in cohorts of Chinese and European IgAN patients (A.G.Gharawi et al, 2011). Five loci (3 in the major histocompatibility complex at chromosome 6p21, a common deletion of CGHR1 and CFHR3 at chromosome 1q32 and one locus at chromosome 22q12) were identified. They explain 4-7% of the disease variance.

2.1 Genome-wide linkage analysis studies

Genome-wide linkage analysis is used successfully to identify major disease/susceptibility genes but has limited power to detect genes of modest effect. Linkage studies involve recruitment of families with multiple affected individuals. In a typical whole-genome linkage scan, up to 400 microsatellites, or equivalently approximately 10,000 SNP markers, equally spaced across the genome, are typed in families to interrogate marker cosegregation with a disease phenotype. The advantage of genome-wide linkage studies is that they do not require a priori assumption about disease pathogenesis. These studies are very sensitive to phenotype misspecification, however their power is limited to detecting rare genetic variants with a relatively large effect on the risk of disease.

Linkage studies of IgAN are faced with multiple challenges. Familial forms of IgAN are frequently underrecognized because the associated urinary abnormalities in affected family members are often mild or intermittent. Moreover, once familial disease is documented, systematic screening by renal biopsy cannot be justified among asymptomatic at-risk relatives, necessitating reliance on less accurate phenotypes, such as microscopic hematuria, to diagnose affection. Additionally, IgAN has been observed to co-occur in families with thin basement membrane disease (TBMD), an autosomal dominant disease caused by heterozygous mutations in the collagen type IV genes (COL4A3/COL4A4) [Frasca et al, 2004]. Short of kidney biopsy or direct sequencing of the very large collagen genes, TBMD cannot be reliably excluded among relatives of IgAN patients. Finally, because urinary abnormalities may manifest intermittently, one also cannot unequivocally classify at-risk relatives as unaffected, necessitating affected-only linkage analysis. The inability to classify affected and unaffected individuals accurately is commonly encountered in linkage studies of complex traits, leading to decreased study power. Increasing sample size by including additional families is also not necessarily helpful in these situations because the diagnosis of IgAN likely encompasses several disease subsets, such that expansion to larger sample size can paradoxically reduce analytic power due to increased heterogeneity [Durner et al, 1992; Cavalli-Sforza & King, 1986].

To date, four genome-wide linkage studies of familial IgAN have been reported [Gharavi et al, 2000; Bisceglia et al, 2006; Paterson et al, 2007, Feehally et al, 2010]. Families in these studies have all been ascertained via at least two cases with biopsy-documented IgAN, with additional family members diagnosed as affected based on clinical evidence (renal failure or multiple documentation of hematuria/proteinuria). In the first study, 30 families with two or more affected members were examined [Gharavi et al, 2000]; multipoint linkage analysis under the assumption of genetic heterogeneity yielded a peak LOD score of 5.6 on chromosome 6q22-23 (locus named IGAN1), with 60% of families linked. The remainder of families linked to chromosome 3p24-23 with a suggestive LOD of 2.8. This study demonstrated that IgAN is genetically heterogeneous but argued for the existence of a single locus with a major effect in some families. In the second genome-wide linkage study 22 Italian IgAN families were enrolled [Bisceglia et al, 2006] (see section 2.3). The third linkage scan was based on a unique large pedigree with 14 affected relatives (two individuals with biopsy defined diagnosis and 12 with hematuria/proteinuria on urine dipstick) [Paterson et al, 2007]. Linkage to chromosome 2q36 was detected with a maximal multipoint LOD score of 3.47. Most reported linkage intervals did not contain obvious candidate genes, but the 2q36 locus encompasses the COL4A3 and COL4A4 genes, which are mutated in TBMD. Together with the high penetrance of hematuria, this finding suggests that affected individuals in the 2q36-linked family may belong to an IgAN subtype that overlaps with TBMD. Finally, the fourth genome-wide analysis, carried out in a cohort of IgAN patients selected from the UK Glomerulonephritis DNA Bank, the region of the MHC (major histocompatibility complex). The strongest association signal included a combination of DQ loci and HLA-B. This study suggests that HLA region contains some alleles that predispose to the disease in the UK population. In conclusion, four genome-wide linkage studies, carried out in four different IgAN patient populations, demonstrate different chromosomal traits linked to the disease.

None of the genes underlying these linkage loci has been identified until now. The underlying reasons are numerous, including the phenotyping difficulties discussed above; the presence of locus heterogeneity, which limits the ability to precisely map the disease interval and find additional linked families to refine loci; the contribution from non-coding susceptibility alleles (e.g. point mutations or structural genomic variants within intronic or promoter regions), which usually escape detection if mutational screening is confined to exonic regions. It is expected that the availability of inexpensive Next-Gen sequencing will enable comprehensive interrogation of linkage intervals, facilitating identification of disease-risk alleles.

In addition, future studies of this kind that aim at dissection of increasingly genetically homogeneous cohorts must consider the importance of defining distinct clinical subtypes of IgAN that may exist within the single pathologic ascertainment criterion currently used to diagnose IgAN: light microscopic evidence of mesangial deposits of IgA by immunofluorescence. As with all family-based genetic studies, there is a high degree of dependency on access to sufficient numbers of clinically well-phenotyped and genetically informative cohorts. To address the paucity of cohorts with biopsy-proven IgAN available for the conduct of linkage-based, association-based, and sequence-based approaches, the European IgAN consortium has published the details of its IgAN Biobank resource [Schena et al, 2005].

2.2 Candidate-gene association studies

Candidate-gene association studies examine polymorphisms in only specific genes that are selected based on a priori assumption about their involvement in the disease pathogenesis, and they are highly sensitive to population stratification, multiple testing, and reporting bias. As a result, most candidate-gene association studies in the literature have not been replicated [Ioannidis et al, 2001; Hsu SI et al, 2000; Hsu SI, 2001; Frimat & Kessler, 2002], an issue which questions the validity and the methodology used in these studies [Hsu & Feehally, 2008]. Not surprisingly, candidate-gene studies for IgAN have also been largely unrevealing. Many candidate genes have been proposed, but for most of them no solid a priori evidence for their involvement in IgAN existed, whereas most were studied in the context of IgAN progression rather than causality. Over the last 15 years, there were more than 120 candidate-gene association studies for IgAN published in the English literature and indexed on PubMed (e.g., components of the renin-angiotensin-aldosterone pathway, mediators of inflammation and/or vascular tone, components of the mesangial matrix, and various receptors for polymeric IgA1 expressed in mesangial cells) [Kiryluk et al, 2010]. Of these, 39 (31%) studies examined genetic polymorphisms in association with susceptibility to IgAN, 40 (32%) examined an association with disease severity, progression, or complications, and 44 (35%) examined both susceptibility and risk of progression. Many candidate-gene association studies are lacking in functional genetics.

Approximately one third of all studies involved polymorphisms in the renin-angiotensin-aldosterone system (RAAS). A widely studied example of the dilemma of repeated non-replication of results is represented by genetic case-control association studies of the angiotensin I–converting enzyme (ACE) gene insertion/deletion (I/D) polymorphism in the development and/or progression of IgAN, as well as a whole host of common human diseases and conditions, including cardiovascular disease, complications of diabetes such as retinopathy and nephropathy, glomerular, tubulointerstitial, and renal cystic renal diseases, and even renal allograft survival [Hsu SI et al, 2000; Hsu SI, 2001; Schena et al, 2001]. The interest in studying the ACE I/D polymorphism is based on evidence for "biologic plausibility." Rigat and colleagues reported in 1990 that the ACE I/D polymorphism in intron 16 of the human ACE gene accounts for half of the variation in serum ACE levels in a white study cohort [Rigat et al, 1990], and this is due to the presence of a transcriptional repressor element in the I allele [Hunley et al, 1996].

There have been numerous population-based studies that either support or refute an association between the D allele and progression of renal disease in these conditions [Hsu SI et al, 2000; Hsu SI, 2001]. Recent meta-analyses have concluded that the D allele is not associated with renal disease progression in patients with IgAN or diabetic nephropathy [Schena et al, 2001; Kunz et al, 1998]. Despite more than a dozen generally small genetic case-control studies of the ACE I/D polymorphism in both white and Asian IgAN cohorts have been done, no definite conclusions can be drawn from them regarding the association between the D allele or DD genotype and development and/or progression of IgAN. Population-based genetic association studies of other genes encoding proteins in the RAAS such as angiotensinogen (AGT) and the angiotensin II type 1 receptor (ATR1), as well as renin (REN) and aldosterone synthase (CYP11b2), have also generated conflicting results, as have similar studies of the "expanded" RAAS that includes 11b-hydroxysteroid dehydrogenase type 2 (11bHSD2) and the mineralocorticoid receptor (MLR) [Poch E et al, 2001]. In general, the approach has been to genotype a single common polymorphism in each gene with the use of polymerase chain reaction/restriction fragment length polymorphism (PCR-RFLP). It is remarkable that to date, the role of the RAAS, whose components ACE and ATR1 are the targets of ACE inhibitors and angiotensin-II receptor blockers (ARB), respectively, has not been convincingly demonstrated by any genetic association study.

In general, most of these studies were of poor quality and severely underpowered and, therefore, negative findings were almost universally inconclusive. Overall, the average size of case–control cohorts per study was 182 cases and 171 controls. Many studies used ad hoc controls derived from unscreened blood donors who were poorly matched to the cases in terms of ancestry and geography. The potential impact of confounding by population stratification was ignored by the majority of studies, despite the fact that the tools for quantification of this problem have been developed. An additional matter of concern is the lack of adequate correction (permutation testing) for multiple, non-independent tests which would be anticipated as long as several of these studies tested several hypotheses (multiple polymorphisms, multiple phenotypes, or multiple genetic models). Other major problems included inadequate or variable SNP coverage of candidate genomic areas, with several studies examining only a single polymorphism. Thus far, only one group attempted to survey the entire genome, yet the results have not been replicated, are inconclusive and difficult to interpret, as long as an underpowered cohort was studied with inadequate coverage of ~80,000 SNPs [Obara et al, 2003; Ohtsubo et al, 2005]. Moreover, 77% of all published candidate-gene studies reported positive findings, an observation that is likely explained by a combination of high rate of false positives and a strong publication bias, whereas the statistical effect of the study of the same patient cohorts for multiple polymorphisms has never been accounted for in the literature [Kiryluk et al, 2010]. Most findings were not reproduced in other populations. None of the above problems is unique to the field of IgAN and for these reasons, new general guidelines aimed at improving the design and execution of genetic association studies have recently been formulated [von Elm et al, 2007; Little et al, 2009].

In the post-genomic era, there has been a renewed interest in conducting genetic association studies, especially SNP-based, whole-genome association studies, to identify genetic variations associated with the development and/or progression of a number of common human diseases. This renewed interest reflects the important finding that linkage disequilibrium (LD), the phenomenon that particular alleles at nearby sites can co-occur on the same haplotype more often than expected by chance [Goldstein, 2001; Wahl et al, 2003] is highly structured into discrete blocks separated by hotspots for recombination. The haplotype block model for LD has important implications for the way in which genetic association studies should now be conducted, and may explain at least in part the problem of repeated non-replication of results that has plagued such studies in the past. Based on the haplotype block model of LD, the ACE I/D polymorphism is a single marker variant in the ACE gene, whereas in unknown yet whether the D allele defines a simple population of subjects at risk for disease or not. The lumping of subgroups defined by haplotypes that share the D allele may explain at least in part the basis for discrepant reports of genetic association with disease.

Nowadays the common SNP haplotype block model is considered essential for the credibility of a study [Couser, 2003] and genetic association studies, especially family based, that employ one or more methodologically valid approaches and satisfy the minimum rigorous conditions for a reliable genetic association study are viewed as studies with solid documentation. These include mainly studies employing biologic plausibility, haplotype relative risk analysis to identify statistically significant "at-risk haplotype[s]" associated with small P values, use of family-based methodologies, such as the transmission equilibrium test (TDT/sib-TDT) or the family-based association test (FBAT) to directly study trios/sib-trios and extended families or to verify the absence of significant population stratification bias (admixture) inherent in population-based case-control association studies, and the study of moderately large i.e., adequately powered] cohorts. To date, very few studies examining candidate genes have employed the family-based TDT study methodology and/or analysis of "at-risk" haplotypes, reflecting the emergence of the first studies to attempt to satisfy minimum criteria for a valid association study.

A family- and haplotype-based association study employing the TDT methodology has shown that 2093C and 2180T SNP variants in the 3'-untranslated region of the *Megsin* gene were significantly more frequently transmitted from heterozygous parents to patients than expected in the extended TDT analysis (increased co-transmission in 232 Chinese families, $P < 0.001$). In addition, haplotype relative risk (HRR) analyses showed that these same SNP alleles were more often transmitted to patients (HRR = 1.568, $P < 0.014$ for the 2093C allele; HRR = 2.114, $P < 0.001$ for the 2180T allele) [Li YJ et al, 2004]. The same group using a similar approach recently reported that the *Megsin* 23167G SNP variant is associated with both susceptibility and progression of IgAN in 435 Chinese patients and their family members using TDT and HRR analyses [Takei et al, 2006]. The GG genotype was found to be associated with severe histologic lesions and disease progression. Megsin is a member of the serpin (serine proteinase inhibitor) superfamily that is upregulated in the context of mesangial proliferation and extracellular matrix expansion in IgAN, and therefore represents a strong candidate gene for susceptibility to IgAN. Lately, the gene encoding Cosmc, a C1Gal-T1 chaperone protein which also mediates IgA O-galactosylation was studied as a candidate gene involved in the pathogenesis of IgAN but no evidence for a role for Cosmc mutations was reported [Malycha et al, 2009].

2.3 IgAN consortium

The IgAN Biobank, coordinated by F.P. Schena, contains at minimum 72 multiplex extended pedigrees, 159 trios, and 1,068 cases and 1,040 matched controls. All subjects enrolled are white and belong to various geographic areas from Germany, Italy, and Greece [Schena et al, 2005]. Aiming at a genome wide linkage study, which has been considered the most promising approach to identify IgAN susceptibility genes, a group of investigators constituted the European IgAN Consortium which was initially funded by the European Union. DNA samples of IgAN patients and relatives belonging to 74 multiple extended pedigrees were collected. Moreover, 166 trios (affected sons or daughters and their healthy parents), 1,085 patients with biopsy-proven IgAN and 1,125 healthy subjects were included in the Biobank. In combination with linkage analysis, family based candidate gene association studies were also applied in an efford to discover responsible genes and overcome obstacles inherent the genetic analysis of complex traits such as IgAN.

Linkage Analysis Studies – The European IgAN Consortium performed the first genome-wide scan involving 22 Italian multiplex IgAN families [Bisceglia L et al, 2006]. A total of 186 individuals (59 affected and 127 unaffected) were genotyped and included in a two-stage linkage analysis. The regions 4q26–31 and 17q12–22 exhibited the strongest evidence of linkage by non-parametric analysis (best p values of 0.0025 and 0.0045, respectively). These localizations were also supported by multipoint parametric analysis where a peak LOD score of 1.83 (α=0.50) and of 2.56 (α=0.65), respectively, were obtained using the affected only dominant model, and by allowing for the presence of genetic heterogeneity. These regions became the second (IGAN2) and third (IGAN3) genetic locus candidates to contain causative and/or susceptibility genes for familial IgAN. Other regions did not reach the threshold of a suggestive or significant LOD score; however, the enrolment of additional IgAN families means that these chromosomal regions may be explored in the near future. The above results provide further evidence for genetic heterogeneity among IgAN families. Evidence of linkage to multiple chromosomal regions is consistent with both an oligo/polygenic and a multiple susceptibility gene model for familial IgAN with small/moderate effects in determining the pathological phenotype. The analysis of the known genes located in these two novel loci (positional information procedure), carried out consulting the National Center for Biotechnology Information, identified some potential candidate genes such as the transient receptor potential channel 3 (TRPC3) gene, the interleukin-2 (IL-2) gene, and the IL-21 gene located in 4q26–31, which could be largely involved in the unbalanced Th1/Th2 immune response reported in IgAN patients. In addition, the histone deacetylase 5 (HD5) gene and the granulin (GRN) gene located on the 17q12–22 region, which could be involved in the immune-response deregulation, will also considered. Family-based association studies, evaluating the distribution of these candidate gene polymorphisms, are in progress.

Microarray Studies – Different high-throughput gene analysis techniques can be used for obtaining transcriptome profiling of renal diseases. Microarray analysis represents the best and the latest approach to gain information on global gene expression. Genome-wide linkage analyses have identified at least three locus candidates containing IgAN susceptibility genes, although no specific gene(s) have been discovered. Microarrays are now in use to fingerprint the pathological process.

A published study postulated that changes in gene expression patterns in circulating leukocytes of IgAN patients may correlate with renal disease activity [Preston et al, 2004]. The investigators identified 14 upregulated genes. The BTG2, NCUBE1, FLJ2948, SRPK1, LYZ, GIG2 and IL-8 genes correlated with serum creatinine levels and the PMAIP1, SRPK1, SSI-3, LYZ and PTGS2 genes correlated with higher values of creatinine clearance, thus implying that the latter group of genes may provide a protective effect, while the overexpression of other genes such as B3GNT5, AXUD1 and GIG-2 indicated a worse prognosis. This gene signature reflected kidney function and did not correlate with hematuria or proteinuria. The authors concluded that studies carried out on large populations of IgAN patients will be necessary to confirm that the leukocyte gene expression profile can be used as a marker for diagnosis and for predicting outcome. The European IgAN Consortium has recently organized a protocol for studying gene expression in peripheral blood mononuclear cells (PBMC) and their subpopulations from IgAN patients with different clinical and histological patterns. Cox et al [2010] conducted a whole-genome expression study to identify genes and pathways differently modulated in peripheral blood leukocytes of IgAN patients. Gene expression of leukocytes demonstrated the hyperactivity of two important pathways as the canonical WNT-β catenin and the PI3k/Akt pathways. The abnormal WNT signalling was also confirmed in IgAN patient's monocytes and to a less extent in B lymphocytes. Low gene expression of inversion and phosphatase and tensin homolog (PTEN) are responsible for the hyperactivation of these two pathways that enhance cell proliferation through lymphoid enhancer factor-1 (LEF-1) of which the gene is located within our previous described region 4q26-31 linked to IgAN [Bisceglia et al, 2006]. Finally, the hyperactivation of the PJ3k/Akt pathway is in linkage with the upregulation of the immunoproteasome in peripheral blood mononuclear cells of IgAN patients, reported by Coppo et al, [2009].

Expression profiling using serial analysis of gene expression (SAGE) and microarray techniques allows global description of expressed genes present in renal tissue. This is a high throughput genomics technology which enables the simultaneous determination of a large number of genes from tissue samples. Preston et al identified 13 upregulated genes in IgAN renal biopsy samples. The cluster analysis identified 3 clusters with 7, 12 and 1 involved gene, respectively [Preston et al, 2004]. The expression levels of these genes were then examined on expanded RNA samples from other renal biopsies, leukocyte samples and cultured primary cells. Data demonstrated the involvement of the genes GABP and STAT3 in cluster I, and gp330 (megalin), MBP45K, MEF2, Oct1 and GABX in cluster II. The use of laser-capture microdissection applied to renal biopsy samples in combination with differential gene expression analysis is expected to provide novel knowledge in the search for IgAN candidate genes.

Candidate genes association studies – The IgAN Consortium takes care of the collection of biological samples from large homogeneous cohorts of IgAN patients, their parents and their first degree relatives, and family-based association studies are preferred to analyze the role of some candidate genes. A family-based association study, including 53 patients, 45 complete trios, 4 incomplete trios and 36 discordant siblings, evaluated the impact of some Th1/Th2/Th3/TR-type lymphocyte and monocyte/macrophage cytokines on IgAN susceptibility [Schena FP et al, 2006]. Cytokine gene polymorphisms with a potential regulatory role on their production were investigated using the family-based association test (FBAT): IFNγ intron-1 CA-repeat at position 1349–1373; IL-13 –1055C/T; TGFβ 915G/C; IL-10 5'-proximal and distal microsatellites; TNFα –308G/A, –238G/A. The FBAT multi-allelic analysis showed an association between IFNγ polymorphism and susceptibility to IgAN (p=0.03). The bi-allelic analysis showed that the 13-CA repeat allele was preferentially transmitted to the affected individuals (p=0.006; Bonferroni p=0.04). The direct sequencing of IFNγ amplicons showed a strict association between the 13-CA repeat allele and the A variant of the +874T/A SNP (rs2430561) directly adjacent to the 5' end of the microsatellite. The in vitro production of IFNγ evaluated in PBMC from 10 genotyped patients demonstrated a correlation between the +874A allele and a lower production of IFNγ (p=0.028). Notably, the +874A variant was associated with transcriptional downregulation of INFγ gene promoter activity, consistent with the known role of NF-κB in the transcriptional regulation of the INFγ gene.

The occurrence of the +874A variant is responsible for the low production of IFNγ and predisposes to a preferential Th2-mediated immune response. The predominance of this variant in individuals with IgAN may be responsible for the onset of the disease. This unbalanced Th2 cytokine production in response to upper respiratory tract infections may be a significant pathogenic factor in human IgAN. The prevalence of Th2 cytokines may also explain the abnormality in IgA1 glycosylation occurring in IgAN patients and the concomitant formation of circulating IgA1-IgG immune complexes. Hyperfunction of Th2 cells and cytokine polarity are linked to a more nephritogenic pattern of IgA1 glycosylation in the animal model, and the decreased glycosylation of IgA1 elicited by Th2 cytokines is blunted in vitro by the addition of IFNγ [Ebihara et al, 2008]. The core 1 β1,3-galactosyltransferase (C1Gal-T1) is suspected to be involved in the abnormal glycosylation process of IgA1 in IgAN. With the genetic characterization of the enzymes responsible for O-glycosylation of IgA1, it has been possible to study changes in the O-glycosylation of IgA1 at a genetic level. Most recently two groups [Pirulli et al, 2009; Li GS et al, 2007] have independently found that SNPs in the C1Gal-T1 gene are associated with a genetic susceptibility to IgAN in Chinese and Italian populations, albeit it is not clear how these polymorphisms relate to changes in the functional activity of C1Gal-T1. The C1Gal-T1 gene complete sequence analysis was performed in 284 IgAN patients and 234 healthy controls. A statistically significant association of the genotype 1365G/G with susceptibility to IgAN (χ^2=17.58, p<0.0001, odds ratio 2.57 [95% CI: 1.64–4.04]), but not with the progression of the disease, was found [Pirulli et al, 2009]. The latter case-control association study demonstrates that the low expression of C1Gal-T1 seems to confer susceptibility to IgAN.

In conclusion, to date the Consortium has identified two loci (located on chromosomes 4q26–31 and 17q12–22), in addition to a previous study which described the first IgAN locus on chromosome 6q22–23. The functional mapping of genes involved in the disease proceeds from the identification of susceptibility loci identified by linkage analysis (step 1) to the isolation of candidate genes within gene disease-susceptibility loci, after obtaining information by microarray analysis carried out on peripheral leukocytes and renal tissue samples (step 2). Next steps will be the design of RNA interference agents against selected genes (step 3) and the application of systematically tested effect of RNA agents on functional cellular assay (step 4). The above combined high-throughput technologies will give information on the pathogenic mechanisms of IgAN. In addition, these data may indicate potential targets for screening, prevention and early diagnosis of the disease and more appropriate and effective treatment.

3. Treatment of IgAN

Treatment strategy for IgAN remains a controversial issue, even more as published randomized controlled trials (RCTs) on this topic are few and most studies are underpowered to provide definitive information. Furthermore, the disease heterogeneity, its clinical course along with the slow rate of GFR decline (1 to 3 mL/min per year) seen in many patients hinders the ability to perform adequate studies. An additional obstacle is the fact that a significant percentage of the patients have only minimal clinical presentation, such as isolated microhematuria, no or minimal proteinuria and normal GFR, and are often not biopsied or even identified. Still no treatment is known to modify mesangial deposition of IgA, which obviously reflects our incomplete knowledge of immunopathogenesis of IgAN [Barratt et al, 2007], and available treatment options are directed mostly at downstream immune and inflammatory events that may lead on to renal scarring. Therefore, as more pathogenetic details, the genetic substrate and heterogeneity of IgAN become increasingly understood, novel treatment strategies with solid therapeutic targets are anticipated, as long as the traditional therapies used until today seem symptomatic rather than etiologic. The discovery and establishment of novel biomarkers associated with the disease activity and outcome will provide the prognostic and therapeutic tool for more accurate and clear therapeutic targeting.

However, there seems to be a consensus regarding patient selection for the different therapeutic approaches. Patient selection for therapy is based in part upon the perceived risk of progressive kidney disease:

- Patients with isolated hematuria, no or minimal proteinuria (<500mg/day), a normal GFR and no signs of progressive disease, such as increasing proteinuria, blood pressure, and/or serum creatinine, are typically not treated.
- Patients with persistent proteinuria (>500 mg/day), normal or only slightly reduced GFR (>50mL/min) that is not declining rapidly, and only mild to moderate histologic findings on renal biopsy are managed with general interventions to slow progression with ACE-inhibitors or angiotensin receptor blockers (ARB) or with combination therapy of corticosteroid (6 months) and ACE-inhibitors forever.

- Patients with more severe or rapidly progressive disease (eg, proteinuria > 1g or proteinuria persisting despite ACE inhibitor/ARB therapy, rising serum creatinine, and/or renal biopsy with more severe histologic findings, but no significant chronic changes) may benefit from immunosuppressive therapy in addition to non-immunosuppressive interventions to slow disease progression.
- In the future, the Oxford histologic classification system, once validated, is anticipated to become a useful prognostic tool that could lead in the future our therapeutic choices [Working Group of the International IgAN Network and the Renal Pathology Society, 2010].

3.1 Monitoring disease activity

Up to date, there are no specific markers to identify continued immunologic activity. Instead, the clinical parameters typically used as the main therapeutic criterion are the urine sediment, protein excretion and the serum creatinine concentration. Persistent hematuria is generally a marker of persistent immunologic activity, but not necessarily of progressive disease. This finding may be a sign of a "smoldering" segmental necrotizing lesion, suggestive of "capillaritis." Hematuria alone does not require any form of therapy. Proteinuria, rather than hematuria alone, is a marker of more severe disease [Donadio et al, 2002]. Increasing proteinuria may be due to one of two factors: ongoing active disease; and secondary glomerular injury due to non-immunologic progression. It is often not possible to distinguish between these two possibilities, except for a rapid increase in protein excretion which is only seen with active disease. Protein excretion most often falls with ACE inhibitor/ARB therapy and the degree of proteinuria is, as described below, one of the end points of such therapy. Protein excretion also may fall spontaneously, particularly during recovery from an acute episode and perhaps in children, and following effective immunosuppressive therapy. Finally, serum creatinine, unless it is rapidly rising, permits an estimation of the GFR. As noted above, most patients with chronic IgAN have stable or slowly progressive disease. The rate of GFR decline is often as low as 1 to 3 mL/min per year, a change that will not detectably raise the serum creatinine above normal levels for many years [Rekola et al, 1991]. Thus, a stable and even normal serum creatinine does not necessarily indicate stable disease.

The establishment of accurate biomarkers is necessary for the optimal categorization and treatment of patients with IgAN. Over the last few years specific urine biomolecules have been proposed as probable biomarkers to be used in the prognosis and therapeutic strategy in patients with IgAN. Two recent studies identified urine epidermal growth factor and monocyte chemoattractant protein-1 as strong independent predictors of renal outcome in patients with IgAN [Torres et al, 2008; Stangou et al, 2009]. These and other biomolecules are being validated as probable biomarkers of IgAN in studies underway.

3.2 Non-immunosuppressive therapies

Three main non-immunosuppressive therapies are in use in IgAN [Barratt & Feehally, 2006; Appel & Waldman, 2006]:

- ACE inhibitors or ARB, to control blood pressure and to slow down progression of the renal disease.
- Statin therapy, for lipid-lowering in selected patients, to lower cardiovascular risk and possibly reduce disease progression.
- Fish oil (omega-3 fatty acids) may also be beneficial in certain cases.

3.2.1 Angiotensin inhibition

The progression of IgAN may be slowed by anti-hypertensive and anti-proteinuric therapy that can minimize secondary glomerular injury [Kanno et al, 2000]. The treatment goals with angiotensin inhibition are the same as those in other forms of proteinuric chronic kidney disease as described in the K/DOQI guidelines [K/DOQI, 2004]. ACE inhibitors and ARBs act by reducing the intraglomerular pressure and by directly improving the size-selective properties of the glomerular capillary wall, both of which contribute to reducing protein excretion [Remuzzi et al, 1991; Maschio et al, 1994].

Both observational studies [Cattran et al, 1994; Kanno et al, 2005] and small randomized trials [Maschio et al, 1994; Praga et al, 2003; Li PK et al, 2006] have provided suggestive evidence that ACE inhibitors or ARBs are more effective than other antihypertensive drugs in slowing the progressive decline in GFR in IgAN as they are in other forms of chronic proteinuric kidney disease. Praga et al in their randomized trial in 44 IgAN patients with proteinuria (≥0.5 g/day, mean 1.9 g/day) and a serum creatinine concentration ≤1.5 mg/dL at baseline, found a significant decrease in proteinuria in the enalapril group (1.9 g/day at baseline to 0.9 g/day at the last visit) and a significantly higher renal survival, defined as less than a 50 percent increase in the serum creatinine concentration, at 6 years of follow up [Praga et al, 2003]. More recently, Li et al in their double-blind randomized placebo-controlled HKVIN trial in 109 Chinese patients with protein excretion ≥1 g/day (mean ~2.0 g/day), found a better renal survival, defined as doubling of serum creatinine or ESRD, a significant improvement in proteinuria (33 % reduction in proteinuria) and a slower rate of decline in GFR (4.6 versus 6.9 mL/min per year) in the valsartan group compared to placebo [Li PK et al, 2006]. Similarly, the IgACE trial in 65 young patients with moderate proteinuria (between 1 and 3.5 grams/day per 1.73 m²) and creatinine clearance >50 mL/min per 1.73 m² revealed a better renal survival (fewer patients with >30% decline in renal function) and significant improvement in proteinuria at 38 months of follow-up in the benazepril group compared to the placebo group [Coppo, 2007].

Normotensive patients who excrete less than 500 mg of protein per day are not typically treated with angiotensin inhibition. However, because most patients progress slowly over time, monitoring of the serum creatinine and protein excretion at yearly intervals is recommended. Angiotensin inhibition should be started if there is evidence of progressive disease and protein excretion above 500 mg/day.

The addition of an ARB to an ACE inhibitor in patients with IgAN seems to exert a further antiproteinuric effect [Russo et al, 1999, 2001], albeit there are no randomized trials showing that this regimen improves renal outcomes. This finding is consistent with meta-analyses of trials in different glomerular diseases, the largest of which found a significant 18 to 25% greater reduction in proteinuria with combined ACE inhibitors and ARBs compared to monotherapy [Kunz et al, 2008; Catapano et al, 2008]. The rationale for this combination therapy is the assumption that ARBs would counteract theAT1-mediated effect of residual angiotensin II formation by non-ACE enzymes like chymase, whereas ACE inhibitors would additionally increase the level of kinins. Furthermore, ACE inhibitors as well as ARBs would synergistically elevate the levels of angiotensin, which also might promote vasodilation. Finally, combining both drug classes might simply provide a higher degree of blockade of the classic renin-angiotensin system pathways [Alexopoulos, 2004]. However, any anticipated benefits from this combination should be weighted against possible adverse effects in individual patients; this is important especially given the findings from the ONTARGET trial in 25,620 patients with vascular disease or diabetes, where an increase in adverse side effects (including a possible increase in mortality) in patients who received combination therapy with an ACE inhibitor and ARB was shown, compared to those who received monotherapy [ONTARGET Investigators, 2008; Mann et al, 2008].

3.2.2 Lipid-lowering therapy
Chronic kidney disease is associated with a marked increase in cardiovascular risk, and is now considered a coronary artery disease risk equivalent. Furthermore, lipid-lowering with statins has been associated with a slower rate of loss of GFR in patients in some patients with mild to moderate CKD, and there are indications for such a beneficial effect of statins in patients with IgAN as well [Kano et al, 2003]. Therefore, it seems rational that all patients with decreased kidney function and/or hypercholesterolemia should receive lipid-lowering therapy with a statin, with treatment goals similar to that in patients with underlying coronary heart disease.

3.2.3 Fish oil
The rationale for using fish oil (omega-3 fatty acids) in IgAN is based on the premise that they may limit the production or action of cytokines and eicosanoids evoked by the initial or by repeated immunologic renal injury, and the resulting production of mediators involved in renal damage [Donadio, 1991]. Randomized controlled trials evaluating fish oil in patients with IgAN have reported conflicting results [Donadio et al, 1994; Alexopoulos et al, 2004; Donadio et al, 1999, 2001; Bennett et al, 1989; Pettersson et al, 1994; Hogg et al, 2006; Ferraro et al, 2009]. In the largest and most well documented and conducted randomized trial in 106 patients with baseline creatinine clearance 80 mL/min and protein excretion of 2.5 to 3 g/day, Donadio et al found better patient and renal outcomes at 4 years, extended also at >6 years, in patients having received 12g of fish oil for 2 years, compared to patients having received a similar amount of olive oil [Donadio et al, 1994, 1999]. Similarly, in a controlled study of 14 IgAN patients and 14 controls, a low dose of fish oil (0.85 g eicosapentaenoic acid and 0.57 g phytohemaglutinin) was found effective in slowing renal progression in high-risk patients with IgAN and particularly those with advanced renal disease [Alexopoulos et al, 2004]. On the other hand, in the randomized controlled trial by the Southwest Pediatric Nephrology Study Group in 96 patients with IgAN, mean GFR >100 mL/min per 1.73 m^2 and proteinuria 1.4 to 2.2 g/day, no significant benefit in the renal outcome was found in patients assigned to omega-3 fatty acids (4 g/day) for two years compared to the patients assigned to either alternate day prednisone or placebo [Hogg et al, 2006]. On the basis of the existing data, fish oil can be tried in addition to ACE inhibitors or ARBs in patients with protein excretion >500 to 1000 mg/day, a gradual reduction in GFR, and mild to moderate histologic lesions [Alexopoulos E, 2004].

3.3 Immunosuppressive therapy
The optimal role of immunosuppressive therapy in IgAN is uncertain [Barratt & Feehally, 2006; Appel & Waldman, 2006]. A variety of regimens have been used, mostly consisting of corticosteroids alone or with other immunosuppressive drugs. The available studies are not conclusive since most are relatively small and have limited follow-up, and the results are sometimes conflicting [D'Amico, 1992; Alamartine et al, 1991; Alexopoulos, 2004; Strippoli et al, 2003; Laville & Alamartine, 2004; Ballardie, 2004; Julian, 2000; Dillon, 2001]. There is

rather consensus that mild, stable, or very slowly progressive IgAN should not be treated with corticosteroids or other immunosuppressive therapies, given the limited evidence of benefit and their known toxicity from chronic use [Floege & Eitner, 2005; Locatelli et al, 1999]. Corticosteroid or other immunosuppressive therapy should only be attempted in patients with clinical and histologic evidence of active inflammation (eg, hematuria and/or proliferative or necrotizing glomerular changes). Patients with chronic kidney disease with significant tubulointerstitial fibrosis and glomerulosclerosis are not likely to benefit from such therapy and are likely to be harmed from the side effects.

3.3.1 Corticosteroids

Current evidence regarding the potential benefit of corticosteroid therapy in IgAN are rather limited, as long as most of the studies performed are uncontrolled retrospective observations; moreover, the few available randomized controlled trials are rather small and in most of them the standard recommendations for proteinuria and blood pressure goals were not followed, limiting thus the applicability of the findings to current practice. Whatsoever, these studies point towards a beneficial effect of corticosteroid therapy (administered for 6 up to >24 months) in proteinuria and perhaps in renal survival [Floege & Eitner, 2005; Nolin & Courteau, 1999; Kobayashi Y et al, 1989, 1996; Pozzi et al, 1999, 2004; Tamoura et al, 2001; Katafuchi et al, 2003; Hotta et al, 2001; Moriyama et al, 2004; Lv et al, 2009, Manno et al, 2009], probably preferentially in individuals with preserved kidney function (eg, creatinine clearance above 50 mL/min) [Kobayashi et al, 1989, 1996; Pozzi et al, 1999, 2004]. Two randomised clinical trials demonstrated the benefit of the combination therapy with corticosteroids and ACE inhibitors on long-term follow-up in proteinuric IgAN patients. Lv et al (2009) evaluated the efficacy of the combination therapy versus ACE-inhibitors alone in a small number of IgAN patients with mild or moderate histologic lesions and with a follow-up period that was too short to evaluate the renal survival. Data demonstrated that the combination therapy reduced better the urinary protein excretion than the administration of ACE-inhibitors alone.

Even more, Manno et al enrolled 97 IgAN patients with moderate histologic lesion (see IgAN classification of F.P. Schena in Manno et al., 2007) daily proteinuria more than 1.0g and estimated GFR more than 50 ml/min/1.73m². Patients were randomly allocated to receive a 6-month course of oral prednisone plus ramipril or ramipril alone for the total duration of the follow-up (96 months). The combination of corticosteroids and ramipril provided less probability of renal disease progression because induced the decline of GFR and daily proteinuria. In an interesting recent meta-analysis of randomized and quasi-randomized controlled trials of corticosteroid treatment in IgAN against treatment without steroids, Zhou et al found that steroid therapy, especially long-term, is associated with a significant benefit in proteinuria and renal survival [Zhou et al, 2011].

In addition, the IgAN patients seemingly to benefit from prednisone therapy are those with nephrotic syndrome, little or no hematuria, preserved kidney function, minimal glomerular changes on light microscopy, and diffuse fusion of glomerular epithelial cell foot processes on electron microscopy. These histologic findings are characteristic of minimal change disease, and these patients behave accordingly, frequently developing a remission with corticosteroids and occasionally requiring cytotoxics for frequently relapsing proteinuria [Mustonen et al, 1983; Lai KN et al, 1986; Cheng et al, 1989]. Mesangial IgA deposits in these patients often disappear or are greatly reduced following steroid-induced remission [Cheng et al, 1989]. Nephrotic syndrome can also occur with severe chronic IgAN and relatively advanced disease on renal biopsy. These patients do not seem to benefit from corticosteroid therapy alone [Mustonen et al, 1983; Lai KN et al, 1986].

3.3.2 Combined immunosuppressive therapy

Combined immunosuppressive therapy should only be attempted in patients with more severe active disease as defined by a more rapidly progressive clinical course and/or histologic evidence of severe active inflammation (eg, crescent formation). Early therapy is important because improvement is rare when the baseline serum creatinine concentration is greater than 3.0 mg/dL in the absence of crescentic glomerulonephritis [Alexopoulos E, 2004].

Corticosteroids plus azathioprine — Whether the addition of azathioprine provide any benefit to that of corticosteroids is still debatable. In a multicenter randomized trial by Pozzi et al in 207 patients with plasma creatinine ≤ 2.0 mg/dL and protein excretion >1.0 g/day, at a median follow-up of 4.9 years, there was no difference neither in renal survival time, defined as the time to 50% increase in plasma creatinine from baseline, nor in the decrease in proteinuria between patients who received corticosteroids alone or along with azathioprine (1.5 mg/kg /day for six months) [Pozzi et al, 2010]. However, in the above study, only a rather small percentage of patients were receiving either ACE inhibitors or ARBs, and even fewer patients were receiving statins. Most recently, Stangou et al published a randomized, yet underpowered study in 22 patients with IgAN and eGRF≥30mL/min, urine protein ≥1g/day, blood pressure <130/80mmHg, who failed to respond to previous treatment with renin-angiotensin system inhibitors and poly-unsaturated fatty acids administered for at least 6 months. During the 5th year after the diagnosis was made, the patients were randomized to receive either methylprednisolone alone, or methyl-prednisolone in combination with azathioprine, for 12months, while treatment with renin-angiotensin system inhibitors and poly-unsaturated fatty acids continued unchanged in both groups. Both, steroid treatment alone, or steroids in combination with azathioprine were found to be equally effective in reducing the severity of proteinuria and stabilizing renal function [Stangou et al, 2011].

Corticosteroids plus cyclophosphamide — There are evidence suggesting that patients with severe or progressive disease (eg, rising creatinine, nephrotic range proteinuria, and/or marked proliferation without crescents) who do not have significant chronic damage on kidney biopsy may benefit from combined immunosuppressive therapy with prednisone and cyclophosphamide. This regimen was evaluated in a study of Ballardie et al in 38 patients with IgAN and initially impaired renal function (baseline serum creatinine between 1.5 and 2.8 mg/dL, mean baseline protein excretion 4.0 to 4.5 g/day, no crescents on biopsy) that was declining at a relatively moderate rate (by at least 15% per year). Compared with the control group, the patients treated with combination therapy (prednisolone 40mg/day tapered to 10mg/day by two years plus low-dose cyclophosphamide for 3 months followed by low-dose azathioprine for at least 2 years) had a significant reduction in protein excretion during the first six months of therapy that persisted during follow-up (eg, reached 1.8 g/day in treatment group versus unchanged at 4.4 g/day in controls at one year). Renal survival was significantly higher in the treatment group at two (82 versus 68 percent) and five years (72 versus 6 percent). [Ballardie et al, 2002].

Uncontrolled reports in patients with crescentic, rapidly progressive glomerulonephritis suggest possible benefit from regimens similar to those used in idiopathic crescentic glomerulonephritis: intravenous pulse methylprednisolone followed by oral prednisone, intravenous or oral cyclophosphamide, and/or plasmapheresis [Welch et al, 1988; Lai KN et al, 1987a; Rocatello et al, 1995; McIntyre et al, 2001; Tumlin et al, 2003]. Corticosteroids may act in this setting by diminishing acute inflammatory injury rather than by correcting the abnormality in IgA production [Galla, 1995]. In a study by Rocatello et al, although a substantial clinical improvement was found with the administration of aggressive combination therapy (including pulse methylprednisolone, oral cyclophosphamide, and plasmapheresis) for 2 months in six patients with crescentic glomerulonephritis due to IgAN [Rocatello et al, 1995], yet cellular crescents failed to remit in repeat renal biopsy, whereas the disease continued to progress in half of the patients after therapy was discontinued. Limited data for a more prolonged course of aggressive immunosuppressive therapy (pulse methylprednisolone 15mg/kg/day for 3 days, followed by oral prednisolone 1 mg/kg/ day for 60 days gradually tapered, along with monthly iv cyclophosphamide (0.5 g/m²) for 6 months) point towards a significant improvement in the serum creatinine and in protein excretion along with a significant reversion of cellular crescents and endocapillary proliferation [Tumlin et al, 2003].

These limited data suggest that patients with active crescentic glomerulonephritis who do not have significant chronic damage on kidney biopsy may benefit from therapy that initially includes intravenous cyclophosphamide. This is consistent with the benefit noted with a similar regimen in other forms of crescentic glomerulonephritis.

3.3.3 Other immunosuppressive agents

Cyclosporine – Cyclosporine has been investigated in small studies, and resulted in reduced proteinuria. In a recent study, Shin et al reported a significant benefit of cyclosporine therapy in proteinuria reduction and renal pathology regression in 14 children with IgAN and near normal creatinine clearance [Shin et al, 2010]. However, there are important issues of concern regarding its use in IgAN treatment, with most important the associated nephrotoxicity, which can lead to harmful effects on renal function [Lai KN et al, 1987b; Cattran, 1991], as well as the rapid disease relapse after drug discontinuation.

Mycophenolate mofetil – Small, prospective placebo-controlled randomized trials of mycophenolate mofetil (MMF) in which the patients were also treated with ACE inhibitors, have produced conflicting results, ranging from no benefit [Maes et al, 2004; Frisch et al, 2005] to a reduction in proteinuria and decrease in rate of decline of GFR [Tang et al, 2010]. A short course (< 6 months) of MMF in patients with persistent proteinuria (>1.5 g/day) and well-maintained renal function (serum creatinine <1.5 mg/dL) in addition to ACE inhibitor/ARB therapy may be considered in patients with well-preserved renal histology on biopsy. Current evidence does not support the use of MMF in patients with advanced disease (serum creatinine >2.5 to 3 mg/dL) [Cattran & Appel, 2011].

3.4 Other possible interventions

Tonsillectomy – Several retrospective studies have suggested that tonsillectomy, usually in combination with some immunosuppressive therapy, is associated with improved renal survival among patients with relatively mild renal injury [Hotta et al, 2001; Xie et al, 2003; Komatsu et al, 2008]. These non-randomized studies provide some evidence that tonsillectomy may be effective in inducing remission of proteinuria and hematuria in patients with IgAN (ie, proteinuria >500 mg/day). However, there are no randomized trials of tonsillectomy in IgAN, the design of the above studies precludes any definitive conclusions regarding the overall efficacy of tonsillectomy in IgAN, while other studies reported negative results [Rasche et al, 1999].

Low antigen diet — The rationale for using a low antigen diet in IgAN, ie diet free of gluten, dairy products, eggs, and most meats, is that dietary macromolecules may be responsible for activating the mucosal IgA system. When given to 21 consecutive patients with IgAN, protein excretion fell markedly in all 12 patients whose baseline rate was more than 1g/day. In addition, repeat renal biopsy showed significant reductions in mesangial IgA and complement deposition and mesangial cellularity [Ferri et al, 1993]. However, the benefits in the above study have not been confirmed and a report using a gluten-free diet alone for several years was unable to document improvement in either proteinuria or renal function despite a reduction in the level of circulating IgA-containing immune complexes [Coppo et al, 1990].

Intravenous immune globulin — At least part of the rationale for intravenous immune globulin (IVIG) therapy in IgAN comes from the observation that a partial IgG deficiency, which could be corrected with IVIG, may predispose to infections that trigger flare-ups of the renal disease [Rostoker et al, 1989, 1994]. Despite the promising findings from two small studies with the administration of high-dose IVIG in severe IgAN, characterized by heavy proteinuria and a relatively rapid decline in GFR (reduction in protein excretion, prevention of GFR decline, decreased inflammatory activity and IgA deposition on repeat renal biopsy) [Rostoker et al, 1994; Rasche et al, 2006], these findings need to be confirmed by larger studies.

4. Conclusion

Genetic susceptibility for IgAN exhibits a complex genetic pattern. To date various groups and the European IgAN Consortium have identified several loci. The extensive genetic studies under way with the use of delicate, high-throughput technologies will give information on the pathogenic mechanisms of IgAN. In addition, these data may indicate potential targets for screening, prevention and early diagnosis of the disease and more appropriate and effective treatment.

Summarizing the most updated data, following are concise treatment guidelines:

- Patients with isolated hematuria, no or minimal proteinuria (<0.5g/day), and a normal GFR need no treatment. Such patients should be periodically monitored at 6 to 12 month intervals to assess disease progression that might warrant therapy.
- Patients with persistent proteinuria (>0.5 or >1 g/day), should be treated with angiotensin inhibition (ACE inhibitor or ARB), with a target of a minimum reduction in protein excretion of at least 50 to 60% from baseline values and a goal protein excretion of <0.5 or <1 g/day.
- All patients who meet criteria for angiotensin inhibition may also be considered as candidates to receive fish oil.
- Patients with persistent nephrotic syndrome and/or chronic kidney disease who have dyslipidemia should be treated with a statin, primarily for cardiovascular protection.
- Corticosteroid therapy for at least 6 months is indicated in the following cases:

a. In patients with acute onset of nephrotic syndrome and minimal changes beyond mesangial IgA deposits on renal biopsy (as in patients with minimal change disease).

b. In patients with moderate renal lesions (eg, hematuria with persistent proteinuria >1 g/day and/or GFR>50ml/min) in association with ACE inhibitors or ARBs.

• For patients with severe disease at baseline (defined as initial serum creatinine >1.5 mg/dL) or progressive disease (eg, increasing serum creatinine and/or protein excretion) who do not have significant chronic damage on kidney biopsy, therapy with oral prednisone and cyclophosphamide is recommended.

5. References

Alamartine E, Sabatier JC, Guerin C, et al (1991). Prognostic factors in mesangial IgA glomerulonephritis: an extensive study with univariate and multivariate analyses. *Am J Kidney Dis*, 18, 1, 12-19.

Alexopoulos E, Stangou M, Pantzaki A, et al (2004). Treatment of severe IgA nephropathy with omega-3 fatty acids: the effect of a "very low dose" regimen. *Ren Fail*, 26, 4, 453-459.

Alexopoulos E (2004). Treatment of primary IgA nephropathy. *Kidney Int*, 65, 1, 341-355.

Allen AC, Bailey EM, Brenchley PE, et al (2001). Mesangial IgA1 in IgA nephropathy exhibits aberrant O-glycosylation: observations in three patients. *Kidney Int*, 60, 3, 969-973.

Appel GB, Waldman M (2006). The IgA nephropathy treatment dilemma. *Kidney Int*, 69, 11, 1939-1944.

Ballardie FW, Roberts IS (2002). Controlled prospective trial of prednisolone and cytotoxics in progressive IgA nephropathy. *J Am Soc Nephrol*, 13, 1, 142-148.

Ballardie FW (2004). IgA nephropathy treatment 25 years on: can we halt progression? The evidence base. *Nephrol Dial Transplant*, 19, 5, 1041-1046.

Barratt J, Feehally J (2006). Treatment of IgA nephropathy. *Kidney Int*, 69, 11, 1934-1938.

Barratt J, Smith AC, Molyneux K, Feehally J (2007). Immunopathogenesis of IgAN. *Semin Immunopathol*, 29, 4, 427-443.

Bennett WM, Walker RG, Kincaid-Smith P (1989). Treatment of IgA nephropathy with eicosapentanoic acid (EPA): a two-year prospective trial. *Clin Nephrol*, 31, 3, 128-131.

Bisceglia L, Cerullo G, Forabosco P, et al (2006). Genetic heterogeneity in Italian families with IgA nephropathy: suggestive linkage for two novel IgA nephropathy loci. *Am J Hum Genet*, 79, 6, 1130-1134.

Catapano F, Chiodini P, De Nicola L, et al (2008). Antiproteinuric response to dual blockade of the renin-angiotensin system in primary glomerulonephritis: meta-analysis and metaregression. *Am J Kidney Dis*, 52, 3, 475-485.

Cattran DC (1991). Current status of cyclosporin A in the treatment of membranous, IgA and membranoproliferative glomerulonephritis. *Clin Nephrol*, 35 Suppl 1, S43-47.

Cattran DC, Greenwood C, Ritchie S (1994). Long-term benefits of angiotensin-converting enzyme inhibitor therapy in patients with severe immunoglobulin a nephropathy: a comparison to patients receiving treatment with other antihypertensive agents and to patients receiving no therapy. *Am J Kidney Dis*, 23, 2, 247-254.

Cattran DC (2007). Is proteinuria reduction by angiotensin-converting enzyme inhibition enough to prove its role in renal protection in IgA nephropathy? *J Am Soc Nephrol*, 18, 6, 1633-1634.

Cavalli-Sforza LL, King MC (1986). Detecting linkage for genetically heterogeneous diseases and detecting heterogeneity with linkage data. *Am J Hum Genet*, 38, 5, 599–616.

Cheng IK, Chan KW, Chan MK (1989). Mesangial IgA nephropathy with steroid-responsive nephrotic syndrome: disappearance of mesangial IgA deposits following steroid-induced remission. *Am J Kidney Dis*, 14, 5, 361-364.

Coppo R, Roccatello D, Amore A, et al (1990). Effects of a gluten-free diet in primary IgA nephropathy. *Clin Nephrol*, 33, 2, 72-86.

Coppo R, Peruzzi L, Amore A, et al (2007). IgACE: a placebo-controlled, randomized trial of angiotensin-converting enzyme inhibitors in children and young people with IgA nephropathy and moderate proteinuria. *J Am Soc Nephrol*, 18, 6, 1880-1888.

Coppo R, Camilla R, Alfarano A, Balegno S, Mancuso D, Peruzzi L, Amore A, Dal Canton A, Sepe V, Tovo P. (2009) Upregulation of the immunoproteasome in peripheral blood mononuclear cells of patients with IgA nephropathy. Kidney Int. 75: 536-41.

Couser WG (2003). Revisions to instructions to JASN authors regarding articles reporting studies using DNA arrays, DNA polymorphisms and randomized controlled clinical trials. *J Am Soc Nephrol*, 14, 2686–2687.

Cox SN, Sallustio F, Serino G, Pontrelli P, Verrienti R, Pesce F, Torres DD, Ancona N, Stifanelli P, Zaza G, Schena FP. (2010) Altered modulation of WNT-beta-catenin and PI3K/Akt pathways in IgA nephropathy. Kidney Int. 78: 396-407.

D'Amico G (1992). Influence of clinical and histological features on actuarial renal survival in adult patients with idiopathic IgA nephropathy, membranous nephropathy, and membranoproliferative glomerulonephritis: survey of the recent literature. *Am J Kidney Dis*, 20, 4, 315-323.

Dillon JJ (2001). Treating IgA nephropathy. *J Am Soc Nephrol*, 12, 4, 846-847.

Donadio JV Jr (1991). Omega-3 polyunsaturated fatty acids: a potential new treatment of immune renal disease. *Mayo Clin Proc*, 66, 10, 1018–1028.

Donadio JV Jr, Bergstralh EJ, Offord KP, et al (1994). A controlled trial of fish oil in IgA nephropathy. Mayo Nephrology Collaborative Group. *N Engl J Med*, 331, 18, 1194-1199.

Donadio JV Jr, Grande JP, Bergstralh EJ, et al (1999). The long-term outcome of patients with IgA nephropathy treated with fish oil in a controlled trial. Mayo Nephrology Collaborative Group. *J Am Soc Nephrol*, 10, 8, 1772-1777.

Donadio JV Jr, Larson TS, Bergstralh EJ, Grande JP (2001). A randomized trial of high-dose compared with low-dose omega-3 fatty acids in severe IgA nephropathy. *J Am Soc Nephrol*, 12, 4, 791-799.

Donadio JV, Bergstralh EJ, Grande JP, Rademcher DM (2002). Proteinuria patterns and their association with subsequent end-stage renal disease in IgA nephropathy. *Nephrol Dial Transplant*, 17, 7, 1197-1203.

Durner M, Greenberg DA, Hodge SE (1992). Inter- and intrafamilial heterogeneity: effective sampling strategies and comparison of analysis methods. *Am J Hum Genet*, 51, 4, 859–870.

Ebihara I, Hirayama K, Yamamoto S, et al (2001). Th2 predominance at the single-cell level in patients with IgA nephropathy. *Nephrol Dial Transplant*, 16, 9, 1783–1789.

Feehally J, Farrall M, Boland A, Gale DP, Gut I, Heath S, Kumar A, Peden JF, Maxwell PH, Morris DL, Padmanabhan S, Vyse TJ, Zawadzka A, Rees AJ, Lathrop M, Ratcliffe PJ. (2010) HLA has strongest association with IgA nephropathy in genome-wide analysis. J Am Soc Nephrol. 21: 1791-7.

Ferraro PM, Ferraccioli GF, Gambaro G, et al (2009). Combined treatment with renin-angiotensin system blockers and polyunsaturated fatty acids in proteinuric IgA nephropathy: a randomized controlled trial. *Nephrol Dial Transplant*, 24, 1, 156-160.

Ferri C, Puccini R, Longombardo G, et al (1993). Low-antigen-content diet in the treatment of patients with IgA nephropathy. *Nephrol Dial Transplant*, 8, 11, 1193-1198.

Floege J, Eitner F (2005). Present and future therapy options in IgA-nephropathy. *J Nephrol*, 18, 4, 354-361.

Frasca GM, Soverini L, Gharavi AG, et al (2004). Thin basement membrane disease in patients with familial IgA nephropathy. *J Nephrol*, 17, 6, 778–785.

Frimat L, Kessler M (2002). Controversies concerning the importance of genetic polymorphism in IgA nephropathy. *Nephrol Dial Transplant*, 17, 4, 542–545.

Frisch G, Lin J, Rosenstock J, et al (2005). Mycophenolate mofetil (MMF) vs placebo in patients with moderately advanced IgA nephropathy: a double-blind randomized controlled trial. *Nephrol Dial Transplant*, 20, 10, 2139-2145.

Galla JH (1995). IgA nephropathy. *Kidney Int*, 47, 2, 377-387.

Gharavi AG, Yan Y, Scolari F, et al (2000). IgA nephropathy, the most common cause of glomerulonephritis, is linked to 6q22-23. *Nat Genet*, 26, 3, 354–357.

Gharavi AG, Kiryluk K, Choi M, Li Y, Hou P, Xie J, Sanna-Cherchi S, Men CJ, Julian BA, Wyatt RJ, Novak J, He JC, Wang H, Lv J, Zhu L, Wang W, Wang Z, Yasuno K, Gunel M, Mane S, Umlauf S, Tikhonova I, Beerman I, Savoldi S, Magistroni R, Ghiggeri GM, Bodria M, Lugani F, Ravani P, Ponticelli C, Allegri L, Boscutti G, Frasca G, Amore A, Peruzzi L, Coppo R, Izzi C, Viola BF, Prati E, Salvadori M, Mignani R, Gesualdo L, Bertinetto F, Mesiano P, Amoroso A, Scolari F, Chen N, Zhang H, Lifton RP. (2011) Genome-wide association study identifies susceptibility loci for IgA nephropathy. Nat Genet. 43: 321-7.

Goldstein DB (2001). Islands of linkage disequilibrium. *Nat Genet*, 29, 2, 109–111.

Hogg RJ, Lee J, Nardelli N, et al (2006). Clinical trial to evaluate omega-3 fatty acids and alternate day prednisone in patients with IgA nephropathy: report from the Southwest Pediatric Nephrology Study Group. *Clin J Am Soc Nephrol*, 1, 3, 467-474.

Hoogendoorn B, Coleman SL, Guy CA, et al (2003). Functional analysis of human promoter polymorphisms. *Hum Mol Genet*, 12, 18, 2249–2254.

Hotta O, Miyazaki M, Furuta T, et al (2001). Tonsillectomy and steroid pulse therapy significantly impact on clinical remission in patients with IgA nephropathy. *Am J Kidney Dis*, 38,4, 736-743.

Hsu SI, Ramirez SB,Winn MP, et al (2000). Evidence for genetic factors in the developmen, and progression of IgA nephropathy. *Kidney Int*, 57, 5, 1818–1835.

Hsu SI (2001). The molecular pathogenesis and experimental therapy of IgA nephropathy: Recent advances and future directions. *Curr Mol Med*, 1, 2, 183–196.

Hsu S, Feehally J. The Molecular Basis of IgA Nephropathy, Mount DB, Pollak MR (eds): *Molecular and Genetic Basis of Renal Disease, A Companion to Brenner & Rector's The Kidney*, 481-498, Saunders Elsevier, 2008, Philadelphia, U.S.A.

Hunley TE, Julian BA, Phillips JA 3rd, et al (1996). Angiotensin converting enzyme gene polymorphism: potential silencer motif and impact on progression in IgA nephropathy. *Kidney Int*, 49, 2, 571-577.

Ioannidis JP, Ntzani EE, Trikalinos TA, Contopoulos-Ioannidis DG (2001). Replication validity of genetic association studies. *Nat Genet*, 29, 3, 306–309.

Izzi C, Ravani P, Torres D, et al (1985). IgA nephropathy: the presence of familial disease does not confer an increased risk for progression. *Am J Kidney Dis*, 47, 5, 761-769.

Julian BA, Quiggins PA, Thompson JS, et al (1985). Familial IgA nephropathy. Evidence of an inherited mechanism of disease. *N Engl J Med*, 312, 4, 202–208.

Julian BA (2000). Treatment of IgA nephropathy. *Semin Nephrol*, 20, 3, 277-285.

Kano K, Nishikura K, Yamada Y, Arisaka O (2003). Effect of fluvastatin and dipyridamole on proteinuria and renal function in childhood IgA nephropathy with mild histological findings and moderate proteinuria. *Clin Nephrol*, 60, 2, 85-89.

Kanno Y, Okada H, Saruta T, Suzuki H (2000). Blood pressure reduction associated with preservation of renal function in hypertensive patients with IgA nephropathy: a 3-year follow-up. *Clin Nephrol*, 54, 5, 360-365.

Kanno Y, Okada H, Yamaji Y, et al (2005). Angiotensin-converting-enzyme inhibitors slow renal decline in IgA nephropathy, independent of tubulointerstitial fibrosis at presentation. *QJM*, 98, 3, 199-203.

Katafuchi R, Ikeda K, Mizumasa T, et al (2003). Controlled, prospective trial of steroid treatment in IgA nephropathy: a limitation of low-dose prednisolone therapy. *Am J Kidney Dis*, 41, 5, 972-983.

Kidney Disease Outcomes Quality Initiative (K/DOQI) (2004). K/DOQI clinical practice guidelines on hypertension and antihypertensive agents in chronic kidney disease. *Am J Kidney Dis*, 43, 5, Suppl 1, S1-290.

Kiryluk K, Julian BA, Wyatt RJ, et al (2010). Genetic studies of IgA nephropathy: past, present, and future. *Pediatr Nephrol*, 25, 11, 2257–2268

Kobayashi Y, Hiki Y, Fujii K, et al (1989). Moderately proteinuric IgA nephropathy: prognostic prediction of individual clinical courses and steroid therapy in progressive cases. *Nephron*, 53, 3, 250-256.

Kobayashi Y, Hiki Y, Kokubo T, et al (1996). Steroid therapy during the early stage of progressive IgA nephropathy. A 10-year follow-up study. *Nephron*, 72, 2, 237-242.

Komatsu H, Fujimoto S, Hara S, et al (2008). Effect of tonsillectomy plus steroid pulse therapy on clinical remission of IgA nephropathy: a controlled study. *Clin J Am Soc Nephrol*, 3, 5, 1301-1307.

Kunz R, Bork JP, Fritsche L, et al (1998). Association between the angiotensin-converting enzyme-insertion/deletion polymorphism and diabetic nephropathy: A methodologic appraisal and systematic review. *J Am Soc Nephrol*, 9, 9, 1653–1663.

Kunz R, Friedrich C, Wolbers M, Mann JF (2008). Meta-analysis: effect of monotherapy and combination therapy with inhibitors of the renin angiotensin system on proteinuria in renal disease. *Ann Intern Med*, 148, 1, 30-48.

Lai KN, Lai FM, Ho CP, Chan KW (1986). Corticosteroid therapy in IgA nephropathy with nephrotic syndrome: a long-term controlled trial. *Clin Nephrol*, 26, 4, 174-180.

Lai KN, Lai FM, Leung AC, et al (1987). Plasma exchange in patients with rapidly progressive idiopathic IgA nephropathy: a report of two cases and review of literature. *Am J Kidney Dis*, 10, 1, 66-70.

Lai KN, Lai FM, Li PK, Vallance-Owen J (1987). Cyclosporin treatment of IgA nephropathy: a short term controlled trial. *Br Med J (Clin Res Ed)*, 295, 6607, 1165-1168.

Laville M, Alamartine E (2004). Treatment options for IgA nephropathy in adults: a proposal for evidence-based strategy. *Nephrol Dial Transplant*, 19, 8, 1947-1951.

Li, GS, Zhang, H, Lv, JC, et al (2007). Variants of C1GALT1 gene are associated with the genetic susceptibility to IgA nephropathy. *Kidney Int*, 71, 5, 379-381.

Li PK, Leung CB, Chow KM, et al (2006). Hong Kong study using valsartan in IgA nephropathy (HKVIN): a double-blind, randomized, placebo-controlled study. *Am J Kidney Dis*, 47, 5, 751-760.

Li YJ, Du Y, Li CX, et al (2004). Family-based association study showing that immunoglobulin A nephropathy is associated with the polymorphisms 2093C and 2180T in the 3′ untranslated region of the Megsin gene. *J Am Soc Nephrol*, 15, 7, 1739–1743.

Little J, Higgins JP, Ioannidis JP, et al (2009). STrengthening the REporting of Genetic Association Studies (STREGA)-an extension of the STROBE statement. *Genet Epidemiol*, 33, 7, 581–598.

Lo HS, Wang Z, Hu Y, et al (2003). Allelic variation in gene expression is common in the human genome. *Genome Res*, 13, 8, 1855–1862.

Locatelli F, Del Vecchio L, Pozzi C (1999). The patient with IgA glomerulonephritis--what is the role of steroid treatment? *Nephrol Dial Transplant*, 14, 5, 1057-1060.

Lv J, Zhang H, Chen Y, et al (2009). Combination therapy of prednisone and ACE inhibitor versus ACE-inhibitor therapy alone in patients with IgA nephropathy: a randomized controlled trial. *Am J Kidney Dis*, 53, 1, 26-32.

Maes BD, Oyen R, Claes K, et al (2004). Mycophenolate mofetil in IgA nephropathy: results of a 3-year prospective placebo-controlled randomized study. *Kidney Int*, 65, 5, 1842-1849.

Malycha F, Eggermann T, Hristov M, et al (2009). No evidence for a role of cosmc-chaperone mutations in European IgA nephropathy patients. *Nephrol Dial Transplant*, 24, 1, 321-324.

Mann JF, Schmieder RE, McQueen M, et al (2008). Renal outcomes with telmisartan, ramipril, or both, in people at high vascular risk (the ONTARGET study): a multicentre, randomised, double-blind, controlled trial. *Lancet*, 372, 9638, 547-553.

Manno C, Strippoli GF, D'Altri C, Torres D, Rossini M, Schena FP. A novel simpler histological classification for renal survival in IgA nephropathy: a retrospective study. Am J Kidney Dis. 2007; 49: 763-75.

Manno C, Torres DD, Rossini M, Pesce F, Schena FP. Randomized controlled clinical trial of corticosteroids plus ACE-inhibitors with long-term follow-up in proteinuric IgA nephropathy. Nephrol Dial Transplant. 2009; 24: 3694-701.

Maschio G, Cagnoli L, Claroni F, et al (1994). ACE inhibition reduces proteinuria in normotensive patients with IgA nephropathy: a multicentre, randomized, placebo-controlled study. *Nephrol Dial Transplant*, 9, 3, 265-269.

McIntyre CW, Fluck RJ, Lambie SH (2001). Steroid and cyclophosphamide therapy for IgA nephropathy associated with crescenteric change: an effective treatment. *Clin Nephrol* 56, 3, 193-198.

Moriyama T, Honda K, Nitta K, et al (2004). The effectiveness of steroid therapy for patients with advanced IgA nephropathy and impaired renal function. *Clin Exp Nephrol*, 8, 3, 237-243.

Mustonen J, Pasternack A, Rantala I (1983). The nephrotic syndrome in IgA glomerulonephritis: response to corticosteroid therapy. *Clin Nephrol*, 20, 4, 172-176.

Nolin L, Courteau M (1999). Management of IgA nephropathy: evidence-based recommendations. *Kidney Int Suppl*, 70, S56-62.

Obara W, Iida A, Suzuki Y, et al (2003). Association of single-nucleotide polymorphisms in the polymeric immunoglobulin receptor gene with immunoglobulin A nephropathy (IgAN) in Japanese patients. *J Hum Genet*, 48, 6, 293–299.

Ohtsubo S, Iida A, Nitta K, et al (2005). Association of a single-nucleotide polymorphism in the immunoglobulin mu-binding protein 2 gene with immunoglobulin A nephropathy. *J Hum Genet*, 50, 1, 30–35.

ONTARGET Investigators, Yusuf S, Teo KK, et al (2008). Telmisartan, ramipril, or both in patients at high risk for vascular events. *N Engl J Med*, 358, 15,1547-1559.

Paterson AD, Liu XQ, Wang K, et al (2007). Genome-wide linkage scan of a large family with IgA nephropathy localizes a novel susceptibility locus to chromosome 2q36. *J Am Soc Nephrol*, 18, 8, 2408–2415.

Pettersson EE, Rekola S, Berglund L, et al (1994). Treatment of IgA nephropathy with omega-3-polyunsaturated fatty acids: a prospective, double-blind, randomized study. *Clin Nephrol*, 41, 4, 183-190.

Pirulli D, Crovella S, Ulivi S, et al (2009). Genetic variant of C1GalT1 contributes to the susceptibility to IgA nephropathy. *J Nephrol*, 22, 1, 152-159.

Poch E, Gonzalez D, Giner V, et al (2001). Molecular basis of salt sensitivity in human hypertension. Evaluation of reninangiotensin- aldosterone system gene polymorphisms. *Hypertension*, 38, 5, 1204–1209.

Pozzi C, Bolasco PG, Fogazzi GB, et al (1999). Corticosteroids in IgA nephropathy: a randomised controlled trial. *Lancet*, 353, 9156, 883-887.

Pozzi C, Andrulli S, Del Vecchio L, et al (2004). Corticosteroid effectiveness in IgA nephropathy: long-term results of a randomized, controlled trial. *J Am Soc Nephrol*, 15,1,157-163.

Pozzi C, Andrulli S, Pani A, et al (2010). Addition of azathioprine to corticosteroids does not benefit patients with IgA nephropathy. *J Am Soc Nephrol*, 21, 10, 1783-1790.

Praga M, Gutierrez-Millet V, Navas JJ, et al (1985). Acute worsening of renal function during episodes of macroscopic hematuria in IgA nephropathy. *Kidney Int*, 28, 1, 69-74.

Praga M, Gutiérrez E, González E, et al (2003). Treatment of IgA nephropathy with ACE inhibitors: a randomized and controlled trial. *J Am Soc Nephrol*, 14, 6, 1578-1583.

Preston GA, Waga I, Alcorta DA, et al (2004). Gene expression profiles of circulating leukocytes correlate with renal disease activity in IgA nephropathy. *Kidney Int*, 65, 2, 420-430.

Rasche FM, Schwarz A, Keller F (1999). Tonsillectomy does not prevent a progressive course in IgA nephropathy. *Clin Nephrol*, 51, 3, 147-152.

Rasche FM, Keller F, Lepper PM, et al (2006). High-dose intravenous immunoglobulin pulse therapy in patients with progressive immunoglobulin A nephropathy: a long-term follow-up. *Clin Exp Immunol*, 146, 1, 47-53.

Reich HN, Troyanov S, Scholey JW, et al (2007). Remission of proteinuria improves prognosis in IgA nephropathy. J Am Soc Nephrol, 18, 12, 3177-3183.

Rekola S, Bergstrand A, Bucht H (1991). Deterioration of GFR in IgA nephropathy as measured by 51Cr-EDTA clearance. *Kidney Int*, 40, 6, 1050-1054.

Remuzzi A, Perticucci E, Ruggenenti P, et al (1991). Angiotensin converting enzyme inhibition improves glomerular size-selectivity in IgA nephropathy. *Kidney Int*, 39, 6, 1267-1273.

Rigat B, Hubert C, Alhenc-Gelas F, et al (1990). An insertion/deletion polymorphism in the angiotensin I-converting enzyme gene accounting for half the variance of serum enzyme levels. *J Clin Invest*, 86, 4, 1343-1346.

Roccatello D, Ferro M, Coppo R, et al (1995). Report on intensive treatment of extracapillary glomerulonephritis with focus on crescentic IgA nephropathy. *Nephrol Dial Transplant*, 10, 11, 2054-2059.

Rostoker G, Pech MA, Del Prato S, et al (1989). Serum IgG subclasses and IgM imbalances in adult IgA mesangial glomerulonephritis and idiopathic Henoch-Schoenlein purpura. *Clin Exp Immunol*, 75, 1, 30-34.

Rostoker G, Desvaux-Belghiti D, Pilatte Y, et al (1994). High-dose immunoglobulin therapy for severe IgA nephropathy and Henoch-Schönlein purpura. *Ann Intern Med*, 120, 6, 476-484.

Russo D, Pisani A, Balletta MM, et al (1999). Additive antiproteinuric effect of converting enzyme inhibitor and losartan in normotensive patients with IgA nephropathy. *Am J Kidney Dis*, 33, 5, 851-856.

Russo D, Minutolo R, Pisani A, et al (2001). Coadministration of losartan and enalapril exerts additive antiproteinuric effect in IgA nephropathy. *Am J Kidney Dis*, 38, 1, 18-25.

Schena F.P. IgA nephropathies, In: *Oxford Textbook of Clinical Nephrology*, A.M. Davison, J. S. Cameron, J.-R. Gruenfeld, D.N.S. Kerr, E. Ritz, C. G. Winearls (Ed.), 537-570, Oxford University Press, 2nd ed., 1998, New York, U.S.A.

Schena FP, D'Altri C, Cerullo G, et al (2001). ACE gene polymorphism and IgA nephropathy: an ethnically homogeneous study and a meta-analysis. *Kidney Int*, 60, 2, 732-740.

Schena FP, Cerullo G, Torres DD, et al (2005). The IgA nephropathy Biobank. An important starting point for the genetic dissection of a complex trait. *BMC Nephrol*, 6, 14.

Schena FP, Cerullo G, Torres DD, et al, on behalf of the European IgA Nephropathy Consortium (2006). Role of interferon-gamma gene polymorphisms in susceptibility to IgA nephropathy: a familybased association study. *Eur J Hum Genet*, 14, 4, 488–496.

Shin JI, Lim BJ, Kim PK, Lee JS, Jeong HJ, Kim JH. (2010). Effects of cyclosporin A therapy combined with steroids and angiotensin converting enzyme inhibitors on childhood IgA nephropathy. *J Korean Med Sci*, 25, 5, 723-727.

Stangou M, Alexopoulos E, Papagianni A, et al (2009). Urinary levels of epidermal growth factor, interleukin-6 and monocyte chemoattractant protein-1 may act as predictor markers of renal function outcome in immunoglobulin A nephropathy. *Nephrology (Carlton)*, 14, 6, 613-620.

Stangou M, Ekonomidou D, Giamalis P, et al (2011). Steroids and azathioprine in the treatment of IgA nephropathy. *Clin Exp Nephrol*, Epub ahead of print.

Strippoli GF, Manno C, Schena FP (2003). An "evidence-based" survey of therapeutic options for IgA nephropathy: assessment and criticism. *Am J Kidney Dis*, 41, 6, 1129-1139.

Suzuki K, Honda K, Tanabe K, et al (2003). Incidence of latent mesangial IgA deposition in renal allograft donors in Japan. *Kidney Int*, 63, 6, 2286-2294.

Takei T,Hiraoka M, Nitta K, et al (2006). Functional impact of IgA nephropathy-associated selectin gene haplotype on leukocyte-endothelial interaction. *Immunogenetics*, 58, 5-6, 355–361.

Tamura S, Ueki K, Ideura H, et al (2001). Corticosteroid therapy in patients with IgA nephropathy and impaired renal function. *Clin Nephrol* 55, 3, 192-195.

Tang SC, Tang AW, Wong SS, et al (2010). Long-term study of mycophenolate mofetil treatment in IgA nephropathy. *Kidney Int*, 77, 6, 543-549.

Torres DD, Rossini M, Manno C, et al (2008). The ratio of epidermal growth factor to monocyte chemotactic peptide-1 in the urine predicts renal prognosis in IgA nephropathy. *Kidney Int*, 73, 3, 327-333.

Tumlin JA, Lohavichan V, Hennigar R (2003). Crescentic, proliferative IgA nephropathy: clinical and histological response to methylprednisolone and intravenous cyclophosphamide. *Nephrol Dial Transplant*, 18, 7, 1321-1329.

von Elm E, Altman DG, Egger M, et al (2007). The Strengthening the Reporting of Observational Studies in Epidemiology (STROBE) statement: guidelines for reporting observational studies. *Lancet*, 370, 9596, 1453– 1457.

Wahl JD, Pritchard JK (2003). Haplotype blocks and linkage disequilibrium in the human genome. *Nat Rev Genet*, 4, 8, 587–597.

Waldherr R, Rambausek M, Duncker WD, Ritz E (1989). Frequency of mesangial IgA deposits in a non-selected autopsy series. *Nephrol Dial Transplant*, 4, 11, 943-946.

Welch TR, McAdams AJ, Berry A (1988). Rapidly progressive IgA nephropathy. *Am J Dis Child*, 142, 7, 789-793.

Working Group of the International IgA Nephropathy Network and the Renal Pathology Society, Coppo R, Troyanov S, et al (2010). The Oxford IgA nephropathy clinicopathological classification is valid for children as well as adults. *Kidney Int,* 77, 10, 921-927.

Xie Y, Nishi S, Ueno M, et al (2003). The efficacy of tonsillectomy on long-term renal survival in patients with IgA nephropathy. *Kidney Int,* 63, 5, 1861-1867.

Zhou YH, Tang LG, Guo SL, et al (2011). Steroids in the treatment of IgA nephropathy to the improvement of renal survival: a systematic review and meta-analysis. *PLoS One,* 6, 4, e18788.

6

Rapidly Progressive Glomerulonephritis

Maria Pia Rastaldi
Renal Research Laboratory,
Fondazione IRCCS Ca' Granda Ospedale Maggiore
Policlinico & Fondazione D'Amico per la Ricerca sulle Malattie Renali Milano,
Italy

1. Introduction

Rapidly Progressive Glomerulonephritis are a group of renal diseases which are still posing serious threat to human health and survival. They are all characterised by acute and rapid deterioration of renal function. Renal biopsy reveals extracapillary glomerulonephritis, most frequently circumferential and diffuse, and immunofluorescence findings continue to represent the most important clue toward precise diagnosis. In the last years, with the development of new technologies and more targeted animal models, several discoveries have been made, that can help in better understanding the pathogenesis and perspectively defining new molecular targets for novel therapies, which are still required to improve the prognosis of these patients.

2. Definition

Introduced for the first time by Ellis in 1942 (Ellis, 1942), the term Rapidly Progressive Glomerulonephritis (RPGN) clinically describes a heterogeneous group of glomerulonephritis characterised by worsening of kidney function that, if not adequately and timely treated, rapidly progresses to end stage renal disease. From the pathological point of view, these diseases are classified as extracapillary or crescentic glomerulonephritis, generally showing extracapillary proliferation in more than 50% of glomeruli. Besides renal biopsy, which is mandatory to make the diagnosis and guide therapeutic decisions, clinical symptoms, biochemical exams, and the observation of the urinary sediment are relevant to the diagnostic process.

Observation of the urinary sediment in the acute phase of disease allows to detect in the vast majority of cases marked erythrocytic cylindruria, mild to moderate leukocyturia, presence of tubular epithelial cells and tubular epithelial cell casts. Fatty casts and leukocyte casts can be detected in about one third of cases (Fogazzi, 2009). Progressive disappearance of these features follows successful therapeutic intervention, and their reappearance frequently precedes disease relapses, making the urinary sediment an important exam not only at diagnosis but also during the patient's follow-up.

Despite the amelioration of prognosis obtained with introduction of high doses of steroids, immunosuppressive agents, and plasma exchange, these diseases are still life-threatening and a high percentage of subjects have a poor renal outcome.

3. Classification

Along the years, different schemes for classifying RPGN have been proposed. Among them, the classification which is still largely accepted and mostly utilised was proposed by Couser (Couser, 1988), and defines disease groups on the basis of immunofluorescent findings. Clinical features and haematological exams are as well very important in reaching a precise diagnosis (Table 1).

Light microscopy	Necrotising extracapillary or pure extracapillary glomerulonephritis		
Immuno-fluorescence	Linear IgG staining	None or minimal deposits	Granular deposits
Hemato-chemical exams	Circulating anti-GBM antibodies	ANCA	Autoantibodies Complement components
Clinical features	Lung haemorrhage	Systemic symptoms	Systemic symptoms
Diagnosis	Anti-GBM disease Goodpasture's syndrome	Wegener's granulomatosis Microscopic polyangiitis Renal limited vasculitis Churg-Strauss syndrome	Post-streptococcal GN Post-infectious GN SLE nephritis IgA GN/HS syndrome Primary MPGN Other primary GN

Table 1. Classification of RPGN according to immunofluorescence findings

Linear deposition of IgG along the glomerular basement membrane associated to circulating anti-GBM antibodies allow the diagnosis of anti-GBM disease. If pulmonary haemorrhage is present, the diagnosis becomes of Goodpasture's Syndrome.

When immunofluorescence on renal biopsy material demonstrates absence of immune deposits or scanty immune deposition in the glomerulus, in association to the presence of circulating ANCA antibodies, a diagnosis of pauci-immune ANCA-associated renal vasculitis is made. In these cases, necrotising crescentic GN can be associated to clinical symptoms of systemic vasculitis. A prevalent involvement of the upper respiratory tract is highly suggestive for a diagnosis of Wegener's Granulomatosis, whereas the presence of only general systemic symptoms, such as fever, is highly suggestive of Renal Limited Vasculitis. Rarely presenting as RPGN, Churg-Strauss syndrome is diagnosed when asthma and increased circulating eosinophils are present.

Importantly, there is a percentage (10-30%, according to the literature) (Chen, 2009) of renal vasculitis which are negative for ANCA antibodies. A part from subjects with circulating AECA (anti-endothelial cell antibodies), that according to a recent study may be present in about 50% of cases (Cong, 2008), diagnosis is mainly based on clinical and biopsy findings and exclusion of other causes.

Among cases of RPGN with granular immune deposition in glomeruli, the most frequent are Post-Streptococcal/post-infectious nephritis and extracapillary GN observed in cases of Lupus Nephritis. In these diseases, besides clinical symptoms, diagnosis is made thanks to the presence of autoantibodies (ASLO and anti-DNAseB in PSGN, and ANA in SLE).

RPGN can also complicate any primary form of GN, most frequently MPGN and IgA nephropathy. A part from the immunofluorescence findings, diagnosis is also guided by clinical and biochemical exams, such as the evaluation of complement components for the diagnosis of MPGN, and the presence of purpura in cases of Henoch-Schoenlein syndrome. It remains to be said, as a word of caution, that it is not infrequent to find a completely negative immunofluorescence or immunofluorescence findings particularly difficult to interpret in cases with very severe extracapillary proliferation or necrotic lesions, because of the consequent compression or destruction of the glomerular tuft.

4. Morphological findings

Though the common element characterising this group of diseases is the presence of extracapillary proliferation, morphological findings can be very diverse, according to the stage of the disease and also to the underlying disease, likely reflecting the different pathogenesis of glomerular lesions.

4.1 Anti-GBM nephritis and Goodpasture's Syndrome
By light microscopy, variable degrees of necrotising extracapillary lesions can be observed, which range from focal and segmental to global and diffuse (Fig 1).

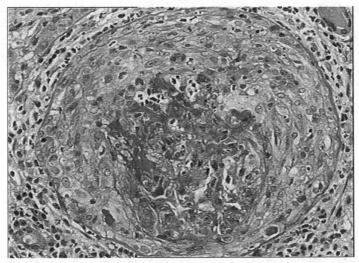

Fig. 1. Anti-GBM nephritis. A large area of necrosis of the glomerular tuft is surrounded by a circumferential crescent. Inflammatory cells surround the glomerulus.

Extracapillary lesions are composed by monocytes, epithelioid macrophages and epithelial cells. Glomeruli not involved by these lesions and the parts of the glomerulus not affected by necrosis can present normal features, but more commonly they show mild to moderate mesangial proliferation, some degree of mesangial matrix expansion, and increased leukocyte infiltration. Intraglomerular inflammatory cells are mostly monocyte-macrophages with variable numbers of T-lymphocytes (Ferrario, 1985; Bolton, 1987).
In about 50% of cases, multinucleated giant cells can be detected either in the crescent or in the periglomerular inflammatory infiltrate, forming the so-called granuloma-like lesions.

Generally well corresponding to the degree of glomerular damage, the tubulointerstitium shows variable extents of tubular atrophy, oedema, and interstitial inflammation. If the biopsy is timely performed, no interstitial fibrosis is observed.

Vascular lesions are not common, though necrotising arteritis and thrombotic microangiopathy have been reported occasionally in the literature (Dean, 1991; Stave, 1984).

Immunofluorescence is diagnostic, with the linear deposition of IgG along the glomerular basement membrane. This aspect can be best appreciated in glomeruli not particularly damaged, whereas it is more difficult to be seen when the glomerular capillary is largely destroyed by necrosis or compressed by extensive cellular crescents.

A combination of IgG and C3 can also be found, as well as a linear deposition of IgA or IgM (Gris, 1991; Peto, 2011) has been reported.

Linear IgG staining can be also detected along the Bowman's capsule, and along the tubular basement membranes. Additionally, the fibrinogen antiserum strongly stains the areas of necrosis in the tuft and within the crescents.

4.2 ANCA-associated renal vasculitis

Irrespective of diagnosis, identical renal microscopy features can be observed in Wegener's granulomatosis, microscopic polyangiitis, and renal limited vasculitis. Necrotising glomerulonephritis and extracapillary proliferation are the renal hallmark of these diseases, and can be found with variable degrees of association. Necrosis can be present alone in cases when renal biopsy is early performed, but more commonly is associated with segmental areas of extracapillary proliferation. Particularly compromised glomeruli show instead large areas of necrosis of the tuft and circumferential crescents, with frequent rupture of the Bowman's capsule and intense periglomerular leukocyte infiltration, so that the limit of the glomerular area is no more distinguishable (Fig 2), and the area has the aspect of a granulomatous reaction.

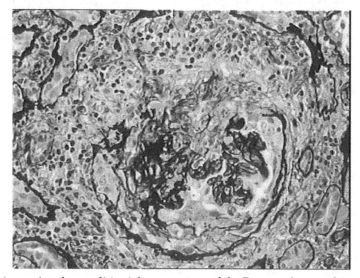

Fig. 2. ANCA-associated vasculitis. A large rupture of the Bowman's capsule can be observed.

Extracapillary and granuloma-like lesions are mainly made by inflammatory cells, mostly acutely activated monocyte-macrophages (Fig. 3, Fig 4) (Rastaldi, 1996; Rastaldi, 2000), whose entrance into the glomerulus seems to be facilitated by the de novo expression of the adhesion molecule VCAM-1 (Fig 5).

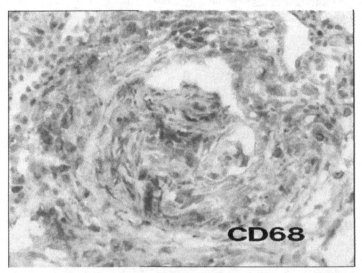

Fig. 3. ANCA-associated vasculitis. Glomerular damage and periglomerular granuloma-like reaction are mainly composed by monocyte-macrophages, as witnessed by the positivity for the marker CD68.

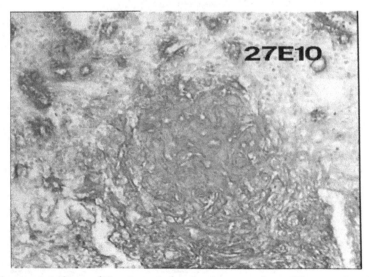

Fig. 4. ANCA-associated vasculitis. A vast glomerular granuloma-like reaction is strongly positive for the marker of acutely activated monocyte-macrophages 27E10.

The acute activation of cells composing the glomerular granuloma-like reaction differentiates this type of alteration from other kind of tissue granulomas, where acute macrophages have not been found (Bhardwaj, 1992).

Differently from those observed in other diseases, monocyte-macrophages present in renal vasculitis are proliferating cells, as we have shown by staining with antibodies against PCNA (Fig 6) and Ki67 (Rastaldi, 2000).

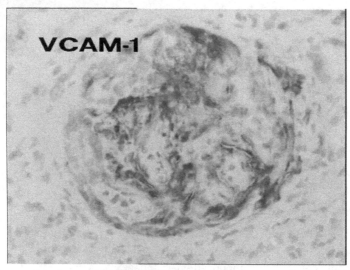

Fig. 5. ANCA-associated vasculitis. VCAM-1 de novo expression in damaged areas of the glomerulus.

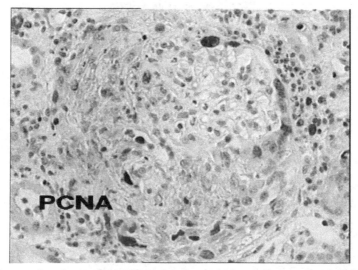

Fig. 6. ANCA-associated vasculitis. PCNA labels numerous cells in and around the glomerulus.

Depending on the timing of renal biopsy, glomeruli can be affected by active lesions or by more sclerotic alterations. It is not infrequent to observe both types of lesions in the same renal biopsy and even in the same glomerulus (Fig 7).

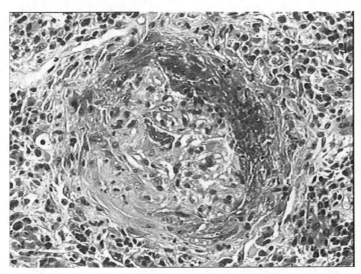

Fig. 7. ANCA-associated vasculitis. The glomerulus shows evident necrotic damage in the upper part of the crescent, whereas the lower part is already fibrous.

Besides periglomerular infiltrates, focal perivascular inflammatory cells are frequently detected in the interstitium, and a diffuse interstitial leukocyte infiltration is also present, whose degree well corresponds to the extent of glomerular damage. Interstitial cells are mainly monocyte-macrophages and T-lymphocytes.

Prevalence of eosinophils, in association to the clinical symptoms of asthma, and increased numbers of circulating eosinophils, stand for a diagnosis of Churg-Strauss syndrome.

By definition, in ANCA-associated renal vasculitis immune deposits are absent or few and scattered, hence the term pauci-immune glomerulonephritis. Instead, the fibrinogen antiserum strongly stains areas of necrosis of the tuft and fibrin deposits into the crescents.

4.3 Post-infectious glomerulonephritis

Either post-streptococcal and other post-infectious glomerulonephritis can present with a rapidly progressive course, which is indicative of a poor prognosis.

Several systemic infections, especially occult, such as infective endocarditis, infected atrio-ventricular shunts, visceral abscesses, and infected vascular prostheses, can be at the origin of RPGN. Blood levels of complement can be reduced.

By light microscopy necrotising lesions, but more frequently extracapillary damage without necrosis of the tuft are observed.

Especially in case of streptococcal infections, the presence of numerous intraglomerular granulocytes (so-called glomerular exudative lesions) (Fig 8) is useful for diagnostic purposes.

In post-streptococcal GN, granular IgG and C3 deposits are the most common finding. IgG, C3, and IgM deposits can be observed in other post-infectious GN, at various locations, but primarily subendothelial and mesangial.

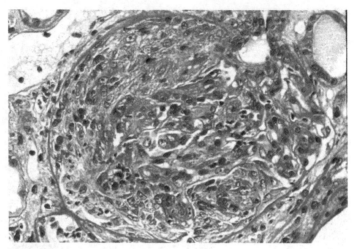

Fig. 8. Post-streptococcal GN. Numerous granulocytes can be observed in the glomerular tuft and in the crescent.

4.4 RPGN complicating primary and secondary glomerular diseases

Though rarely, any primary or secondary glomerular diseases can be complicated by a rapidly progressive course and display necrotising crescentic glomerulonephritis at light microscopy. Very recently, a report has shown for the first time the appearance of RPGN complicating the course of AL amyloidosis (Crosthwaite, 2010). Cases of association of primary or secondary glomerulonephritis and anti-GBM disease or renal vasculitis have also been published, as well as cases of association of anti-GBM disease and ANCA-positive renal vasculitis (Curioni, 2002; O'Connor, 2010). Diagnosis in these patients requires skilful and careful analysis of clinical features, renal biopsy findings, and hematochemical exams.

4.4.1 IgA nephropathy and Henoch-Schonlein purpura

Less than 10% of patients with primary IgA nephropathy or Henoch-Schonlein syndrome have been reported with a truly rapidly progressive course (Ferrario, 1997).

Clinical features of cutaneous purpura or abdominal and joint pain, accompanied by the finding of a small vessel leukocytoclastic vasculitis, most frequently detected in skin biopsies, help in making a diagnosis of systemic disease.

Focal segmental or global and diffuse necrotising and extracapillary lesions of the glomerulus can be found, or extracapillary lesions can be present without necrosis of the glomerular tuft (Fig 9), which always presents variable degrees of mesangial proliferation and expansion of the mesangial matrix.

Immunofluorescence shows prevailing IgA mesangial deposits, possibly in combination with IgG and C3 deposition, especially in the systemic disease.

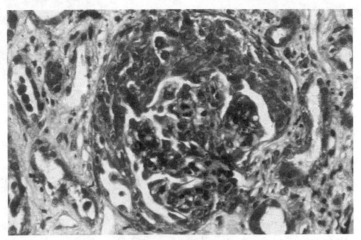

Fig. 9. Primary IgA nephropathy. A circumferential crescent surrounds a glomerulus affected by mesangial proliferation and mesangial expansion.

4.4.2 Systemic lupus erythematosus

Among the histological classes of SLE nephritis (Weening, 2004), RPGN is more frequently observed in classes III and IV. In these cases the occurrence of antineutrophil cytoplasmic antibodies is not uncommon and is thought to contribute to the development of necrotising and crescentic glomerular lesions (Sen, 2003).

Extensive extracapillary proliferation has been rarely reported (Fig 10), whereas segmental necrotising extracapillary alterations are a rather common finding, but not always translate in a RPGN clinical phenotype.

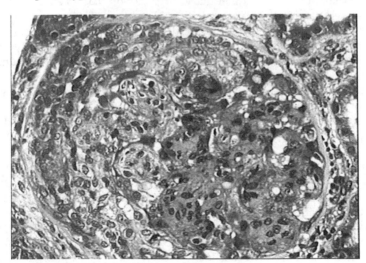

Fig. 10. Rapidly progressive class IV SLE nephritis. A circumferential crescent surrounds a glomerulus affected by intense intracapillary proliferation, mesangial expansion, and leukocyte infiltration.

Immunofluorescence has the typical findings of lupus nephritis, according to the class of disease, with frequent "full house" deposition, and fibrinogen positivity in necrotic areas and crescents.

5. Pathogenesis and experimental models

In recent years, thanks to the possibilities offered by molecular modelling, genetic studies, and the generation of novel animal models better reproducing human disease features, important advances have been made in understanding pathogenetic mechanisms underlying certain forms of RPGN, especially anti-GBM nephritis and ANCA-associated renal vasculitis.

Instead, it continues to be less clear why a rapidly progressive course can complicate virtually any type of primary and secondary glomerulonephritis.

5.1 Anti-GBM nephritis and Goodpasture's disease

The seminal discovery in understanding the pathogenesis of the disease was the identification of the antigen that causes production of pathogenic autoantibodies (Saus, 1988).

Thereafter, injection of the recombinant antigen, i.e. the noncollagenous domain (NC1) of the alpha3chain of collagen type IV, was shown to induce a severe glomerulonephritis in Wistar-Kyoto rats (Sado, 1998), hence proving a direct relationship between the self-antigen sustaining autoantibody production and the disease.

More recently, a second class of autoantibodies has been described, which are specific for the alpha5NC1 domain, occur in 70% of affected patients, and seem to be associated with a worse renal prognosis (Pedchenko, 2010).

In the normal glomerular basement membrane, the NC1 domain is assembled in alpha345NC1 hexamers, whose quaternary organisation has been shown in a three-dimensional model (Vanacore, 2008) as an ellipsoid-shaped structure composed by two NC1 trimers joined at the base by hydrophobic and hydrophilic interactions and reinforced by sulfilimine bonds. This crosslinked alpha345NC1 hexamer is inert to antibody binding. Anti-GBM antibodies in fact can bind only to dissociated monomer and dimer subunits that form after alteration of the hexamer and expose pathogenic neoepitopes. This explains why passive transfer of antibodies to the mouse, where hexamers in the GBM are completely crosslinked, does not result in glomerulonephritis (Luo, 2010).

The major epitopes within the alpha3 and alpha5 subunits have been identified as well, and named EA-alpha3, EA-alpha5, and EB-alpha3 (Netzer, 1999; Hellmark, 1999; Pedchenko, 2010).

Several questions, primarily regarding the causes of hexamer alteration that induce epitope exposure and antibody production, need to be answered. At present, the most accredited hypothesis is that environmental factors act in genetically predisposed subjects, leading to epitope alteration and antibody formation.

As for genetic predisposition, positive and negative associations with HLA molecules have been found, especially with the MHC class II HLA-DRB1*1501 allele (Yang, 2009), which is strongly associated to anti-GBM disease.

A number of experimental data are in favour of a role played by FcγR gene and the complement system, though their precise role in humans is still unclear.

Instead, several experimental models implicate T-cell mediated immunity in the pathogenesis of anti-GBM disease, which is based on the following findings. In rats, anti-GBM disease can be induced by injecting alpha3(IV)NC1-specific CD4+Tcells (Wu, 2002). Anti-CD8 monoclonal antibodies reduce disease severity and antigen-specific CD8+Tcell clones have been found in diseased patients (Reynolds, 2002). Invariant natural killer cells (iNKT) could have a role as well, because the disease has a worse course in iNKT cell-deficient mice (Mesnard, 2009). Finally, mice deficient in IL-23, which is important for the maintenance of Th17 cells, the CD4+Tcell subset producing IL17, are protected from anti-GBM disease (Ooi, 2009).

5.2 ANCA-associated renal vasculitis

The discovery of ANCAs (Falk, 1988) radically changed not only the diagnosis of small vessel vasculitis, but also introduced an important element for the study of the etiology and pathogenesis of this group of diseases. Major ANCA autoantigens are two proteins contained in azurophil granules of neutrophil granulocytes, MPO and PR3, which are mainly expressed during neutrophil development at the myeloblast and promyelocytic stage (Cowland, 1999). They are aberrantly expressed in mature neutrophils of ANCA patients, whereas are silenced in mature neutrophils of healthy subjects (Yang, 2004).

In vivo first evidence for a pathogenetic role of ANCA was demonstrated by injection of anti-MPO antibodies or anti-MPO lymphocytes, causing a pauci-immune focal necrotising extracapillary glomerulonephritis (Xiao, 2002). Subsequent research then showed that in this model neutrophil granulocytes are required, because mice depleted of neutrophils do not develop the disease, and disease worsening is obtained by priming neutrophils using a pro-inflammatory stimulus (Xiao, 2005). The model has been also useful in investigating the role of the alternative complement pathway, because the disease does not occur in C5 or Factor B null mice, but it fully develops in C4-KO animals (Xiao, 2007).

In an additional model, MPO-KO mice were first immunised with mouse MPO, determining production of anti-MPO antibodies. These mice having circulating anti-MPO antibodies were then irradiated and subsequently transplanted with MPO-wild type or MPO-KO bone marrow cells. A pauci-immune necrotising-crescentic glomerulonephritis developed only in mice engrafted with MPO-wild type cells, indicating the requirement for bone marrow derived cells in disease development (Schreiber, 2006).

5.3 Cells involved in crescent formation

Along the years, composition of glomerular extracapillary proliferation has been, and still remains, the object of intense investigation and discussion.

Though the exact mechanism/s of crescent formation remain elusive, novel animal models have recently added important information, that will lead to further clarification of the molecular pathways involved and the potential identification of possible novel therapeutic targets.

A word has first to be spent in stating that, morphologically speaking, extracapillary proliferation is a heterogeneous phenomenon. It has been shown by several investigators that presence or absence of necrosis of the glomerular capillary is relevant to the type of crescent. When necrosis is present, the crescent is more inflammatory, and mainly formed by monocyte-macrophages. In absence of tuft necrosis, the crescent has more epithelial and less inflammatory features.

If the presence of inflammatory cells and epithelioid macrophages has never been questioned either in animal models and in human disease, opposite data have been obtained when attempting to define the epithelial cell composition.

Until some years ago, both experimental and human studies aiming to study the cells contained in the crescents were mostly based on morphological findings and immunostaining. The conflicting results produced by these studies were due not only to the specific type of experimental model or of human disease under analysis, but especially to a dysregulated phenotype with loss of specific markers. In fact, both podocytes and parietal epithelial cells are likely to change their original resting phenotype once they start proliferating and filling the Bowman's space.

The advent of novel experimental models, though not generating unifying and conclusive data, is providing more convincing proofs of the participation of either podocytes or parietal epithelial cells, based on tagged expression of specific molecules.

Convincing evidence of podocyte contribution to crescent formation has been shown in a podocyte specific mouse model of Vhlh gene knockout (Ding, 2006). These mice showed rapidly progressive glomerulonephritis by 4 weeks of age and died by terminal renal failure after 3-4 weeks. Histology displayed a crescentic glomerulonephritis, and podocytes expressing tagged-ZO1 were found into the crescents. A part from showing podocyte participation in crescent formation, the model also identified a novel pathway potentially operating in extracapillary glomerulonephritis; deletion of Vhlh in fact resulted in stabilisation of hypoxia inducible factor-aplha (HIF1alpha) and consequent upregulation of target genes, among them the chemokine receptor CXCR4. Further, podocyte-specific expression of CXCR4 was sufficient to induce podocyte proliferation and crescent formation, and CXCR4 positivity was observed in glomeruli of human biopsies with necrotising extracapillary lesions, suggesting that the VHLH-HIF-CXCR4 pathway may have functional relevance also in humans.

The contribution of parietal epithelial cells to crescent formation has been recently shown in a mouse model where a construct containing 3 kb of the human podocalyxin (hPODXL1) 5' flanking region and 0.3 kb of the rabbit Podxl1 5' untranslated region were used to drive expression of rabbit podocalyxin, and transgene expression was detected exclusively within PECs but not in podocytes. In this model, injection of nephrotoxic serum caused extracapillary glomerulonephritis and cells within crescents could be clearly identified as of parietal origin (Smeets, 2009, a).

As a final consideration, recent work has demonstrated that the Bowman's capsule contains renal progenitors mainly located at the urinary pole of the glomerulus (Ronconi, 2009). If it is true that these cells are able to regenerate either tubular cells and podocytes, then their participation to crescent formation can be viewed as the pathological consequence of a tentative to repair glomerular damage in the course of inflammatory conditions (Smeets, 2009, b).

6. Conclusion

RPGN still constitute a threat for human health and survival. Despite numerous improvements in understanding the pathogenesis of these diseases, numerous questions still remain unanswered and will need clarification before providing targeted, pathway-based, novel therapeutics.

7. Acknowledgment

All images in this chapter are taken from "Ferrario F, Rastaldi MP. Histopathological Atlas of Renal Diseases", which is publicly available at www.fondazionedamico.org. Fondazione D'Amico per la Ricerca sulle Malattie Renali is gratefully acknowledged.

8. References

Bhardwaj, R.S., Zotz, C., Zwadlo-Klarwasser, G., Roth, J., Goebeler, M., Mahnke, K., Falk, M., Meinardus-Hager, G., & Sorg, C. (1992). The calcium-binding proteins MRP8 and MRP14 form a membrane-associated heterodimer in a subset of monocytes/macrophages present in acute but absent in chronic inflammatory lesions. *Eur J Immunol*, Vol. 22, No. 7, pp. 1891-1897.

Bolton, W.K., Innes, D.J. Jr, Sturgill, B.C., & Kaiser, D.L. (1987). T-cells and macrophages in rapidly progressive glomerulonephritis: clinicopathologic correlations. *Kidney Int*, Vol. 32, No. 6, pp. 869-876.

Chen, M., Kallenberg, C.G., & Zhao, M.H. (2009). ANCA-negative pauci-immune crescentic glomerulonephritis. *Nat Rev Nephrol*, Vol. 5, No. 6, pp. 313-318.

Cong, M., Chen, M., Zhang, J. J., Hu, Z. & Zhao, M. H. (2008). Anti-endothelial cell antibodies in antineutrophil cytoplasmic antibodies negative pauci-immune crescentic glomerulonephritis. *Nephrology (Carlton)* Vol. 13, No. 3, pp. 228–234.

Couser, W.G. (1988). Rapidly progressive glomerulonephritis: classification, pathogenetic mechanisms, and therapy. *Am J Kidney Dis,* Vol. 11, No. 6, pp. 449-464.

Cowland. J,B, & Borregaard, N. (1999). The individual regulation of granule protein mRNA levels during neutrophil maturation explains the heterogeneity of neutrophil granules. *J Leukoc Biol*, Vol. 66, No. 6, pp. 989–995.

Crosthwaite, A., Skene, A., & Mount, P. (2010). Rapidly progressive glomerulonephritis complicating primary AL amyloidosis and multiple myeloma. *Nephrol Dial Transplant*, Vol. 25, No. 8, pp. 2786-2789.

Curioni, S., Ferrario, F., Rastaldi, M.P., Colleoni, N., Colasanti, G., & D'Amico, G. (2002). Anti-GBM nephritis complicating diabetic nephropathy. *J Nephrol*, Vol. 15, No. 1, pp. 83-87.

Dean, S.E., Saba, S.R., & Ramírez, G. (1991). Systemic vasculitis in Goodpasture's syndrome. *South Med J*, Vol. 84, No. 11, pp. 1387-1390.

Ding, M., Cui, S., Li, C., Jothy, S., Haase, V., Steer, B.M., Marsden, P.A., Pippin, J., Shankland, S., Rastaldi, M.P., Cohen, C.D., Kretzler, M., & Quaggin, S.E. (2006). Loss of the tumor suppressor Vhlh leads to upregulation of Cxcr4 and rapidly progressive glomerulonephritis in mice. *Nat Med*, Vol. 12, No. 9, pp. 1081-1087.

Ellis, A. (1942). Natural history of Bright's disease. Clinical, histological and experimental observations. *Lancet*, Vol. 239, No. 6176, pp. 34-36

Falk, R.J., & Jennette, J.C. (1988). Anti-neutrophil cytoplasmic autoantibodies with specificity for myeloperoxidase in patients with systemic vasculitis and idiopathic necrotizing and crescentic glomerulonephritis. *N Engl J Med*, Vol. 318, No. 25, pp. 1651-1657.

Ferrario, F., Castiglione, A., Colasanti, G., Barbiano di Belgioioso, G., Bertoli, S., & D'Amico, G. (1985). The detection of monocytes in human glomerulonephritis. *Kidney Int*, Vol. 28, No. 3, pp. 513-519.

Ferrario, F., & Rastaldi, M.P. (1997). Pathology of rapidly progressive glomerulonephritis, In: *Rapidly Progressive Glomerulonephritis*, Pusey C, Rees A., pp. 59-107, Oxford University Press, UK.

Fogazzi, G.B. (2009). The Urinary sediment in the main diseases of the kidney and of urinary tract, In: *The Urinary Sediment. An Integrated view*, Fogazzi GB, pp. 177-210, Elsevier Srl, Italy.

Gris, P., Pirson, Y., Hamels, J., Vaerman, J.P., Quoidbach, A., & Demol, H. (1991). Antiglomerular basement membrane nephritis induced by IgA1 antibodies. *Nephron*, Vol. 58, No. 4, pp. 418-424.

Hellmark, T., Burkhardt, H., & Wieslander, J. (1999). Goodpasture disease. Characterization of a single conformational epitope as the target of pathogenic autoantibodies. *J Biol Chem*, Vol. 274, No. 36, pp. 25862-25868.

Luo, W., Wang, X.P., Kashtan, C.E., & Borza, D.B. (2010). Alport alloantibodies but not Goodpasture autoantibodies induce murine glomerulonephritis: protection by quinary crosslinks locking cryptic α3(IV) collagen autoepitopes in vivo. *J Immunol*, Vol. 185, No. 6, pp. 3520-3528.

Mesnard, L., Keller, A.C., Michel, M.L., Vandermeersch, S., Rafat, C., Letavernier, E., Tillet, Y., Rondeau, E., & Leite-de-Moraes, M.C. (2009). Invariant natural killer T cells and TGF-beta attenuate anti-GBM glomerulonephritis. *J Am Soc Nephrol*, Vol. 20, No. 6, pp. 1282–1292.

Netzer, K.O., Leinonen, A., Boutaud, A., Borza, D.B., Todd, P., Gunwar, S., Langeveld, J.P., & Hudson, B.G. (1999). The goodpasture autoantigen. Mapping the major conformational epitope(s) of alpha3(IV) collagen to residues 17-31 and 127-141 of the NC1 domain. *J Biol Chem*, Vol. 274, No. 16, pp. 11267-11274.

O'Connor, K., Fulcher, D., & Phoon, R.K. (2010). Development of anti-glomerular basement membrane disease after remission from perinuclear ANCA-associated glomerulonephritis in a patient with HLA susceptibility. *Am J Kidney Dis*, Vol. 55, No. 3, pp. 566-569.

Ooi, J.D., Phoon, R.K., Holdsworth, S.R., & Kitching, A.R. (2009). IL-23, not IL -12, directs autoimmunity to the Goodpasture antigen. *J Am Soc Nephrol*, Vol. 20, No. 5, pp. 980–989.

Pedchenko, V., Bondar, O., Fogo, A.B., Vanacore, R., Voziyan, P., Kitching, A.R., Wieslander, J., Kashtan, C., Borza, D.B., Neilson, E.G., Wilson, C.B., & Hudson, B.G. (2010). Molecular architecture of the Goodpasture autoantigen in anti-GBM nephritis. *N Engl J Med*, Vol. 363, No. 4, pp. 343-354.

Peto, P., & Salama, A.D. (2011). Update on antiglomerular basement membrane disease. *Curr Opin Rheumatol*, Vol. 23, No. 1, pp. 32-37.

Rastaldi, M.P., Ferrario, F., Tunesi, S., Yang, L., & D'Amico, G. (1996). Intraglomerular and interstitial leukocyte infiltration, adhesion molecules, and interleukin-1 alpha expression in 15 cases of antineutrophil cytoplasmic autoantibody-associated renal vasculitis. *Am J Kidney Dis*, Vol. 27, No. 1, pp. 48-57.

Rastaldi, M.P., Ferrario, F., Crippa, A., Dell'Antonio, G., Casartelli, D., Grillo, C., & D'Amico, G. (2000). Glomerular monocyte-macrophage features in ANCA-positive renal vasculitis and cryoglobulinemic nephritis. *J Am Soc Nephrol*, Vol. 11, No. 11, pp. 2036-2043.

Reynolds, J., Norgan, V.A., Bhambra, U., Smith, J., Cook, H.T., & Pusey, C.D. (2002). Anti-CD8 monoclonal antibody therapy is effective in the prevention and treatment of experimental autoimmune glomerulonephritis. *J Am Soc Nephrol*, Vol. 13, No. 2, pp. 359–369.

Ronconi, E., Sagrinati, C., Angelotti, M.L., Lazzeri, E., Mazzinghi, B., Ballerini, L., Parente, E., Becherucci, F., Gacci, M., Carini, M., Maggi, E., Serio, M., Vannelli, G.B., Lasagni, L., Romagnani, S., & Romagnani, P. (2009). Regeneration of glomerular podocytes by human renal progenitors. *J Am Soc Nephrol*, Vol. 20, No. 2, pp. 322-332.

Sado, Y., Boutaud, A., Kagawa, M., Naito, I., Ninomiya, Y., & Hudson, B.G. (1998). Induction of anti-GBM nephritis in rats by recombinant alpha 3(IV)NC1 and alpha 4(IV)NC1 of type IV collagen. *Kidney Int*, Vol. 53, No. 3, pp. 664-671.

Saus, J., Wieslander, J., Langeveld, J.P., Quinones, S., & Hudson, B.G. (1988). Identification of the Goodpasture antigen as the alpha 3(IV) chain of collagen IV. *J Biol Chem*, Vol. 263, No. 26, pp. 13374-13380.

Schreiber, A., Xiao, H., Falk, R.J., & Jennette, J.C. (2006). Bone marrow-derived cells are sufficient and necessary targets to mediate glomerulonephritis and vasculitis induced by anti-myeloperoxidase antibodies. *J Am Soc Nephrol*, Vol. 17, No. 12, pp. 3355–3364.

Sen, D., & Isenberg, D.A. (2003). Antineutrophil cytoplasmic autoantibodies in systemic lupus erythematosus. *Lupus*. Vol. 12, No. 9, pp. 651–658.

Smeets, B., Uhlig, S., Fuss, A., Mooren, F., Wetzels, J.F., Floege, J., & Moeller, M.J. (2009, a). Tracing the origin of glomerular extracapillary lesions from parietal epithelial cells. *J Am Soc Nephrol*, Vol. 20, No. 12, pp. 2604-2615.

Smeets, B., Angelotti, M.L., Rizzo, P., Dijkman, H., Lazzeri, E., Mooren, F., Ballerini, L., Parente, E., Sagrinati, C., Mazzinghi, B., Ronconi, E., Becherucci, F., Benigni, A., Steenbergen, E., Lasagni, L., Remuzzi, G., Wetzels, J., & Romagnani, P. (2009, b). Renal progenitor cells contribute to hyperplastic lesions of podocytopathies and crescentic glomerulonephritis. *J Am Soc Nephrol*, Vol. 20, No. 12, pp. 2593-2603.

Stave, G.M., & Croker, B.P. (1984). Thrombotic microangiopathy in anti-glomerular basement membrane glomerulonephritis. *Arch Pathol Lab Med*, Vol. 108, No. 9, pp. 747-751.

Vanacore, R.M., Ham, A.J., Cartailler, J.P., Sundaramoorthy, M., Todd, P., Pedchenko, V., Sado, Y., Borza, D.B., & Hudson, B.G. (2008). A role for collagen IV cross-links in conferring immune privilege to the Goodpasture autoantigen: structural basis for the crypticity of B cell epitopes. *J Biol Chem*, Vol. 283, No. 33, pp. 22737-22748.

Weening, J.J., D'Agati, V.D., Schwartz, M.M., Seshan, S.V., Alpers, C.E., Appel, G.B., Balow, J.E., Bruijn, J.A., Cook, T., Ferrario, F., Fogo, A.B., Ginzler, E.M., Hebert, L., Hill, G., Hill, P., Jennette, J.C., Kong, N.C., Lesavre, P., Lockshin, M., Looi, L.M., Makino, H., Moura, L.A., & Nagata, M. (2004). The classification of glomerulonephritis in systemic lupus erythematosus revisited. *J Am Soc Nephrol*, Vol. 15, No. 2, pp. 241-250.

Wu, J., Hicks, J., Borillo, J., Glass, W.N., & Lou, Y.H. (2002). CD4(+) T cells specific to a glomerular basement membrane antigen mediate glomerulonephritis. *J Clin Invest*, Vol. 109, No. 4, pp. 517-524.

Xiao, H., Heeringa, P., Hu, P., Liu, Z., Zhao, M., Aratani, Y., Maeda, N., Falk, R.J., & Jennette, J.C. (2002). Antineutrophil cytoplasmic autoantibodies specific for myeloperoxidase cause glomerulonephritis and vasculitis in mice. *J Clin Invest*, Vol. 110, No. 7, pp. 955-963.

Xiao, H., Heeringa, P., Liu, Z., Huugen, D., Hu, P., Maeda, N., Falk, R.J., & Jennette, J.C. (2005). The role of neutrophils in the induction of glomerulonephritis by anti-myeloperoxidase antibodies. *Am J Pathol*, Vol. 167, No. 1, pp. 39-45.

Xiao, H., Schreiber, A., Heeringa, P., Falk, R.J., & Jennette, J.C. (2007). Alternative complement pathway in the pathogenesis of disease mediated by anti-neutrophil cytoplasmic autoantibodies. *Am J Pathol*, Vol. 170, No. 1, pp. 52-64.

Yang, J.J., Pendergraft, W.F., Alcorta, D.A., Nachman, P.H., Hogan, S.L., Thomas, R.P., Sullivan, P., Jennette, J.C., Falk, R.J., & Preston, G.A. (2004). Circumvention of normal constraints on granule protein gene expression in peripheral blood neutrophils and monocytes of patients with antineutrophil cytoplasmic autoantibody associated glomerulonephritis. *J Am Soc Nephrol*, Vol. 15, No. 8, pp. 2103-2114.

Yang, R., Cui, Z., Zhao, J., & Zhao, M.H. (2009). The role of HLA-DRB1 alleles on susceptibility of Chinese patients with anti-GBM disease. *Clin Immunol*, Vol. 133, No. 2, pp. 245–250.

Part 2

Infectious Glomerulopathies and Related Disorders

7

S. pyogenes Infections and Its Sequelae

L. Guilherme[1,3], S. Freschi de Barros[1,3]
A.C. Tanaka[1], M.C. Ribeiro Castro[4] and J. Kalil[1,2,3]
*[1]Heart Institute (InCor), School of Medicine,
University of São Paulo, São Paulo,
[2]Clinical Immunology and Allergy Division, School of Medicine,
University of São Paulo, São Paulo,
[3]Immunology Investigation Institute, National Institute for Science and Technology,
University of São Paulo, São Paulo,
[4]Nephrology Division, School of Medicine,
University of São Paulo, São Paulo,
Brazil*

1. Introduction

Suppurative streptococcal infections of the throat and the skin generate stimuli that lead Rheumatic fever (RF) in 1 to 5% of susceptible children. The disease manifests initially as polyarthritis, carditis/valvulitis, Sydenham`s chorea, erythema marginatum and/or subcutaneous nodules. Chronic renal disease can also occur.

RF occurs at an early phase of life (3 to 19 years of age); thus, heart damage (carditis) can appear in very young children. Rheumatic carditis usually presents as pancarditis, affecting the endocardium, myocardium and pericardium. Recurrent acute cardiac lesions frequently evolve into chronic rheumatic heart disease (RHD), of which valvular deformities are the most important sequelae; these deformities lead to mitral and aortic regurgitation and/or stenosis. Valve replacement surgery is usually the only treatment for chronic RHD patients and incurs high costs for both public and private health systems.

Here, we will present three cases of young RHD patients who underwent valve replacement and the autoimmune reactivity that triggered the heart-tissue rheumatic lesions.

Post-streptococcal glomerulonephritis (PSGN) is another immune sequelae that presents a latency period of one to three weeks after scarlet fever, streptococcal pharyngitis and purulent skin infections.

PSGN has become a rare disease, especially in adults in developed countries, due to an improved standard of living, earlier treatment of pharyngeal infections and widespread use of antibiotics (Rodriguez-Iturbe & Musser, 2008). Despite decades of research, the pathogenesis of PSGN remains obscure. It is still unclear whether or to what extent autoimmune reactions are involved, but several studies have shown that different streptococcal antigens are detectable by immunohistology in the diseased kidneys (Rodriguez-Iturbe & Batsford, 2007). These data are in favor of direct contributions of streptococcal nephritogenic factors to PSGN pathogenesis, although intact bacteria have never been found in affected kidneys. Two PSGN cases will also be presented.

2. Epidemiology

2.1 Acute rheumatic fever

The incidence of ARF in some developing countries exceeds 50 cases per 100,000 children (Carapetis et al., 2005). The worldwide incidence of RHD is at least 15.6 million cases and is responsible for around 233,000 deaths / year. However, these estimates are based on conservative assumptions, so the true disease burden is probably substantially higher (Carapetis et al., 2005). The incidence of ARF can vary from 0.7 to 508 per 100,000 children per year in different populations from several countries (Carapetis et al., 2005). In Brazil, according to the WHO epidemiological model and data from IBGE (Brazilian Institute of Geography and Statistics), the number of Streptococcal pharyngitis infections is around 10 million cases, which could lead to 30,000 new cases of RF, of which around 15,000 could develop cardiac lesions (Barbosa et al.,2009).

2.2 Post-streptococcal glomerulonephritis (PSGN)

PSGN has become a rare disease, especially in adults in developed countries, due to an improved standard of living, earlier treatment of pharyngeal infections and widespread use of antibiotics (Rodriguez-Iturbe & Musser, 2008). However, the occurrence of acute post-infection glomerulonephritis (APIGN) has emerged as a major risk in diabetic patients all over the world (Nars et al., 2008).

The global incidence of acute PSGN was estimated at 472,000 cases per year, of which 456,000 occurred in less-developed countries (Carapetis, 2005). In agreement with these data, the incidence of PSGN ranges from 9.5 to 28.5 new cases per 100,000 individuals per year in developing countries (Rodríguez-Iturbe, 2008).

3. Autoimmunity is the major mechanism leading to both diseases

3.1 Rheumatic fever and rheumatic heart disease

The autoimmune reactions in RF and RHD are controlled by several genes related to both the innate and adaptive immune responses (Guilherme et al., 2011). Briefly, in the last 50 years, several genetic markers from different populations have been studied, and the susceptibility of developing RF/RHD was first associated with some alleles of HLA (human leukocytes antigens) class II genes (DRB1, DQB and DQA), which are located on human chromosome 6. HLA alleles are involved in antigen recognition by T lymphocytes through the T cell receptor (TCR). Later, some studies showed that the TNF-α gene, located in the same region of this chromosome was also associated with the disease. The TNF-α gene encodes the inflammatory TNF alpha protein, which is involved in the inflammatory process mediating heart-tissue lesions in RHD. Several other associations have been established based on gene variability by studying single nucleotide polymorphisms (SNPs). These genes code for other proteins also involved with the immune response (innate and adaptive pathways) (see Diagram 1) (Guilherme et al., 2011).

3.1.1 Molecular mimicry

Molecular mimicry mediates cross-reactivity between streptococcal antigens and human proteins. Several autoantigens have been identified, including cardiac myosin epitopes, vimentin and other intracellular proteins.

Several streptococcal and human cross-reactive antibodies have been found in the sera of RF patients and immunized rabbits and mice over the last 50 years and have been recently reviewed. Briefly, antibodies against N-acetyl β-D-glucosamine, a polysaccharide present in both the streptococcal cell wall and heart valvular tissue displayed cross reactivity against laminin, an extracellular matrix alpha-helical coiled-coil protein that surrounds heart cells and is also present in the valves (Cunningham, 2000; Guilherme et al., 2005).

Among human proteins, cardiac myosin and vimentin seem to be the major target antigens. By using affinity-purified anti-myosin antibodies, Cunningham´s group identified a five amino acid residue (Gln-Lys-Ser-Lys-Gln) epitope of the N-terminal M5 and M6 proteins as cross-reactive with cardiac myosin (Cunningham et al., 1989).

Cunningham´s group found that streptococcal and human cross-reactive antibodies upregulate the adhesion molecule VCAM-1 after binding to the endothelial surface, leading to inflammation, cellular infiltration and valve scarring (Gavin et al., 2000, Roberts et al, 2001). These data established the role of the heart–tissue cross-reactive antibodies (anti-cardiac myosin and laminin) in the early stages of inflammation and T cell infiltration in RHD lesions.

Studies performed in the last 25 years showed that CD4+ cells are the major effectors of autoimmune reactions in the heart tissue in RHD patients (Raizada et al., 1984; Kemeny et al.,1989; Guilherme et al., 1995). However, the role of T cells in the pathogenesis of RF and RHD was demonstrated through the analysis of heart-tissue infiltrating T cell clones (Guilherme et al., 1995). Immunodominant peptides of the M5 protein (residues 81-96 and 83-103) displayed cross-reactivity with valvular proteins and cardiac myosin peptides by molecular mimicry (Faé et al., 2006; Yoshinaga et al., 1995; Guilherme et al, 1995). These M5 epitopes were also preferentially recognized by peripheral T lymphocytes from RHD patients when compared with normal individuals, mainly in the context of HLA-DR7 (Guilherme et al., 2001). Analysis of the T cell receptors (TCR) of peripheral and intralesional T cells from RHD patients showed several antigen-driven oligoclonal T cell expansions at the site of heart-tissue lesions (Guilherme et al, 2000). These autoreactive cells are CD4+ and produce inflammatory cytokines (TNFα and IFNγ). IL-4+ cells are found in the myocardium; however, these cells are very scarce in the valve lesions of RHD patients. IL-4 is a Th2-type cytokine and plays a regulatory role in the inflammatory response mediated by Th1 cytokines. These findings indicate that the Th1/Th2 cytokine balance has a role in healing myocarditis, while the low numbers of IL-4-producing cells in the valves probably induced progressive and permanent valve damage (Guilherme et al, 2004).

Three cases of RHD patients (clinical, surgical data) will be presented. Histological and immunological data obtained from peripheral blood and T-cell lines and T cell clones derived from heart-tissue infiltrating T cells of these patients are summarized in Tables 1 and 2.

Patients	Mitral Valve					Myocardium (LA)	
	Inflammation	Rheumatic Activity	Neovasc	Fibrosis	Calcification	Inflammation	Rheumatic Activity
Case 1	(++)	AB-PR(+) VER(+)	(+)	(+)	(−)	AB-PR (+)	(+)
Case 2-	(+)	(−)	(−)	(++)	(−)	(−)	(−)
Case 3- 1st surgery						(+)	AB(−)
2nd surgery	(+)					(+)	(−)

LA-left atrium; AB-PR- Achoff Bodies in proliferative phase; Ver- verrucae, (-) negative;(+) mild; (++) moderate

Table 1. Histological data of Rheumatic Heart Disease patients

| | Heart-tissue Infiltrating Cells/field | | | Antigens recognized by T cell clones from myocardium and/or mitral valve | |
HLA Class II	CD4+	CD8+	M5 protein peptides	Myocardium derived- proteins	Valve derived proteins
Case # 1	15,7, 52, 53	9.4	3.3	M5 (81-96) M5 (83-103) M5 (163-177)	30-44 kDa; 24-30 kDa LMM25(1607-1624)	>150 kDa, 90-150 kDa; 65-90 kDa;43-65 kDa 30-43 KDa 90-150 kDa; 30-43 KDa
Case # 2	9, 11, 52,53	6.1	1.2	M5(11-25) M5 (81-96) M5 (83-103)		43-65 kDa 90-150 kDa, 43-65 kDa 90-150 kDa; 43-65 kDa
Case # 3	17, 13, 52,	4.5	0.9	M5 (83-103)	>150 kDa LMM10(1413-1430) LMM12(1439-1456)	90-150 kDa; 43-65 kDa; 30-43 KDa

Amino acid sequences of M5 protein were based on sequence published by Philips et al, 1981 and Manjula et al, 1985. M5 (81-96)-DKLKQQRDTLSTQKET; M5 (83-103)-LKQQRDTLSTQKETLEREVQN; M5-(163-177) ETIGTLKKILDETVK; cardiac myosin beta chain sequences published by Diederich et al, 1989: LMM 10 (1413-1430) CSSLEKTKHRLQNEIEDL; LMM12 (1439-1456) AAAAALDKKRNFDKILA; LMM25 (1607-1624) RSRNEALRVKKKMEGDLN, (Guilherme et al, 1995, Faé et al, 2006).

Table 2. T cells from heart-tissue of Rheumatic Heart Disease patients recognize streptococcal peptides and cardiac proteins.

Case # 1

Male 4 years old, presented mitral, aortic and tricuspid regurgitation, left ventricular diastolic diameter of 51 mm and systolic diameter of 34 mm, ejection fraction (LVEF) of 78%, left atrium (LA) of 40 mm, thickened pericardium.

At surgery, mitral valve prolapse was observed with very long strings and small tears of rope. Mitral annulus was dilated. A mitral valve replacement was done. Heart biopsy showed chronic valvulitis with areas of mucoid collagen degeneration and papillary muscles with Aschoff nodules in the granulomatous stage (Table 1).

Case # 2

Male 6 years old, presented clinical features of fever, polyarthritis and carditis with mitral valve involvement. On this occasion, patient showed evidence of inflammatory activity; Gallium 67 positive scintigraphy; endomyocardial biopsy suggestive of rheumatic carditis. A left ventricular diastolic diameter of 59 mm, left ventricular systolic diameter of 39 mm, ejection fraction (LVEF) of 71% and left atrium (LA) of 52 mm were observed. Two valve correction surgeries were performed. Pathological examination of the mitral valve showed sequelae of chronic valvulitis with intense fibrosis and mucoid degeneration.

Case #3

Male 10 years old, presented clinical features of fever, polyarthritis and carditis with progressive cardiac heart failure and mitral and aortic shortcomings as well as relapses of acute outbreak by irregular use of secondary prophylaxis with benzathine penicillin and progression to chronic atrial fibrillation, culminating in death at 18 years of life. Increased left ventricular diastolic diameter (67/43 mm) and left atrial diameter of 62 mm, significant mitral regurgitation, aortic insufficiency and moderate impact tricuspid regurgitation with mild rebound were found. Subjected to two surgeries, first for mitral valve repair and prosthetic aortic and tricuspid valves, then for exchange of the mitral and aortic bioprostheses, and tricuspid valve repair.

3.2 Post Streptococcal Glomerulonephritis (PSGN)

Acute glomerulonephritis can occur sporadically or endemically as a result of infections of both the upper airways and skin by group A streptococcus strains.

Genetic susceptibility factors are likely involved with the development of the disease. HLA class II alleles (DR4 and DRB1* 03011) have been found to be associated with PSGN compared to healthy controls. Genetic association with endothelial nitric oxide synthase intron 4 a/b (eNOSa/b) defined by variable numbers of tandem repeats (VNTR) polymorphism was also described (Ahn & Ingulli, 2008).

The disease is mediated by immune complexes and complement pathway activation. Several theories seek to explain the formation of immune complexes in glomeruli. The most accepted one is that a streptococcal antigen, with affinity for the glomerular structures, can be deposited in the glomerulus, activating the host immune response and initiating development of immune complexes *in situ* (Rodriguez-Iturbe & Bastford, 2007).

Apparently, molecular mimicry between streptococcal antigens and glomerular proteins leads to tissue damage. Two antigens have been investigated as potential causes of PSGN: the plasmin receptor linked to nephritis (NAPlr), identified as glyceraldehyde 3-phosphate dehydrogenase, and a protein known as streptococcal pyrogenic exotoxin B (SpeB). Both are present in renal biopsies of patients with PSGN and are capable of activating the alternative pathway of the complement system. In addition, they are capable of promoting enhanced expression of adhesion molecules, facilitating inflammatory reactions mediated by cytokines (IL-6, TNF α, IL-8 and TGF ß). It seems that the nephritogenic properties of NAPlr and SpeB are related to the binding ability of plasmin, which facilitates the deposition of immune complexes (IgG and C3, properdin and C5) in the glomeruli and subsequent inflammation (Rodriguez-Iturbe & Bastford, 2007; Rodriguez-Iturbe & Musser, 2008).

Molecular mimicry, as mentioned above, leads to the recognition of streptococcal antigens and laminin, collagen and glomerular basement membrane (GBM). Sub-epithelial localization of immune complexes and complement factors in the injured glomeruli points towards a crucial role of the host immune system in tissue destruction.

As mentioned before, renal inflammation may result from a myriad of insults and is often characterized by the presence of infiltrating inflammatory leukocytes within the glomerulus or tubular interstitium. Accumulating evidence indicates that infiltrating leukocytes are the key to the induction of renal injury.

Two cases of PSGN are presented in which anti-streptolysin O (ASO) was positive, indicating a previous infection by *S. pyogenes.*

Case #1

Male 6 years old, presented swollen eyes followed by bilateral periorbital edema followed by progression of lower limb edema and increased abdominal size, decreased urine volume and urine darkness. Lab tests detected hematuria, increased serum levels of urea (63.0 mg/dl) and creatinine (1.2 mg/dl). Decreased levels of complement (16.1 mg/dl) and fractions C3 and C4 (both 11.7 mg/dl) were found. The patient also presented increased levels of ASO (1055 IU).

Case # 2

Male 15 years old, presented edema, hypertension, and gross hematuria and reported a skin abscess in the left leg 20 days before hospital admission. No previous signs of disease or significant co-morbidities were identified. Physical examination showed a 2+ lower edema, with no signs of current skin infections. Laboratory tests revealed 24 hr urine protein 2.4 g/day, serum creatinine 2.9 mg/dl, hematuria, and positive ASO (> 200 IU). Renal ultrasound showed normal kidneys. After introducing antibiotic and controlling edema and hypertension with diuretics and anti-hypertensive drugs, the patient was subjected to a renal biopsy that showed a diffuse proliferative pattern, with focal endocapillary and mesangial proliferation with no cellular crescents.

4. Frequencies of *S. pyogenes* strains collected at Clinical Hospital of the School of Medicine of the University of Sao Paulo

Diverse *S. pyogenes* strains are related with the development of RF/RHD or PSGN and are considered as rheumatogenic and nephritogenic, respectively.

We analyzed 177 samples obtained from diverse biological sources. Most samples were recovered from blood, throat and wound (Table 3).

Source	n° of cases	Strains identified									
		emm1	emm87	emm22	emm12	emm77	emm6	emm75	emm89	st2904	others
Throat	30	6	-	5	1	-	2	1	-	2	13
Blood	58	10	6	3	7	5	3	2	1	-	21
Wound	15	3	2	-	-	-	-	-	1	2	7
Sputum	8	2	-	1	-	2	1	-	-	-	2
Surgical wound	5	-	-	1	1	1	-	-	-	-	2
Ascitis	3	-	-	-	-	-	-	1	-	-	2
Catheter	3	-	-	1	-	-	-	-	-	-	2
Lymph node	3	1	2	-	-	-	-	-	-	-	-
Ocular discharge	3	2	-	-	-	-	-	-	-	-	1
Synovial fluid	2	2	-	-	-	-	-	-	-	-	-
Liquor	2	1	-	-	-	-	-	-	1	-	-
Others	11	3	2	-	-	1	-	1	1	-	3

Table 3. Distribution of *emm* types according to biological source.

The M1 type was more frequently observed. Figure 1 shows the frequencies of all strains analyzed. Our results are similar to those previously published (Table 4). It is interesting to note that studies done by Schulman et al., 2004 and Ma et al., 2009 showed variability of frequencies for some streptococcus strains over different periods, probably due to seasonal influence.

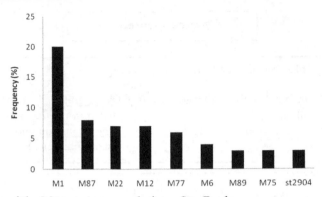

Fig. 1. Prevalence of the M types in a sample from São Paulo
Beta-hemolytic samples (177) obtained from diverse biological sites at the Clinical Hospital,
University of Sao Paulo during the period of 2001-2008.

Country	Year	N° isolates	N° of *emm* types identified	Source	More frequent *emm* types	References
Germany	2003-2007	586	49	invasive	1, 28, 3, 12, 89, 4, 77, 6, 75, 11, 118, 2, 83	Imöhl et al., 2010
United States	1995-1999	1586	17	invasive	1, 28, 12, 3, 11, 4, 114, 89, 17, 77, 33	O'Brien et al., 2002
North America	1nd-2000-2001 2 nd-2001-2002	1nd -975 2nd- 1076	1 nd -29 2 nd - 31	Non invasive	1nd-12, 1, 28, 4, 3, 2 2nd- 1, 12, 4, 28, 3, 2	Schulman et al., 2004
Barcelona	1999-2003	126	29	invasive and non invasive	1, 3, 4, 12, 28, 11, 77	Rivera et al., 2006
Sweden	1986-2001	92	28	invasive and non invasive	1, 2, 4, 8, 12, 28, 66, 75	Maripuu *et al.*, 2008
Australia	2001-2002	107	22	invasive and non invasive	1, 4, 12, 28, 75	Commons et al., 2008
Hungary	2004-2005	26	8	invasive	1, 80, 4, 28, 66, 81.1, 82, 84	Krucsó et al, 2007
China	1nd-1993-1994 2 nd-2005-2006	1 nd -137 2 nd -222	1 nd -24 2 nd - 9	invasive and non invasive	1 nd -3, 1, 4, 12, st1815, 6 2 nd 12, 1	Ma et al., 2009
Denmark	2003-2004	278	29	invasive	28, 1, 3, 89, 12	Luca-Harari et al., 2008
Norway	2006-2007	262	29	invasive	28, 1, 82, 12, 4, 3, 87, 89, 6	Meisal et al., 2010

Two studies were reported for North America and China.

Table 4. Distribution of *emm* types around the world

```
┌─────────────────────────────────────┐
│       S. pyogenes - Infections       │
└─────────────────────────────────────┘
```

Genetic Susceptible Untreated Children and Teenagers	
Genetic markers	**Role**
• MBL, TLR2, FCN2, Fcγ RIIA alleles	Innate immunity
• HLA class II alleles	Adaptive immune response
• Cytokines genes: TNF-α, TGF ß1, IL-1Ra, IL-10	Mediators of inflammatory reactions (agonist or antagonist)

Peripheral Blood
- Streptococcal and human proteins: cross-reactions mediated by both antibodies and CD4+T cells
- Inflammatory cytokines: IL-1, IL-6, IL-10, TNF- α, IFN- γ
- Circulating immune complexes

Heart Tissue (RHD)
- Anti-laminin and/or cardiac myosin antibodies upregulate the VCAM-1 molecule in the endothelium surface leading to inflammation, cellular infiltration and valve scarring
- Infiltrating T cells are predominantly CD4+ (~80%)
- Antigen-driven oligoclonal T cells are expanded in the myocardium and valves
- Intralesional T cell clones recognize streptococcal M peptides and heart-tissue proteins and cardiac myosin peptides (LMM)
- High numbers of TNF-α and IFN-γ secreting mononuclear cells are mediators of myocardium and valvular inflammation
- Low numbers of mononuclear cells IL-4+ in the valves probably lead to permanent and progressive valvular damage

Kidney (Glomerulonephritis)
- Streptococcal anti – SpeB crossreactive antibodies recognize NAPlr, laminin, collagen and the glomerular basement membrane (GBM) antigens
- Sub-epithelial deposition of immune complex and complement factors

Diagram 1. Major events leading autoimmune reactions on both RHD and Glomerulonephritis

5. Prospective vaccines against *S. pyogenes*

Many studies have focused on developing a vaccine against *S. pyogenes* in order to prevent infection and its complications. There are four anti-group A streptococci (GAS) vaccine candidates based on the M protein and eight more candidates based on other streptococcal antigens, including group A CHO, C5a peptidase (SCPA), cysteine protease (Spe B), binding proteins similar to fibronectin, opacity factor, lipoproteins, Spes (super antigens) and streptococcal pili (Steer et al, 2009).

We developed a vaccine epitope (StreptInCor) composed of 55 amino acid residues of the C-terminal portion of the M protein that encompasses both T and B cell protective epitopes

(Guilherme et al, 2006). The structural, chemical and biological properties of this peptide were evaluated, and we have shown that StreptInCor is a very stable molecule, an important property for a vaccine candidate (Guilherme et al, 2011). Furthermore, experiments with mice showed that this construct is immunogenic and safe (Guilherme et al, 2011).

6. Conclusions

The knowledge acquired in the last 25 years pointed out the molecular mimicry mechanism as one of the most important leading autoimmune reactions in RHD and PSGN. Although both diseases are triggered by *S. pyogenes,* RHD is mediated by both antibodies and T cells while PSGN is mainly due to immune complex deposition in the glomeruli.
Several streptococcal cross reactive autoantigens were identified in both diseases.
Many proteins and cardiac myosin epitopes were identified as putative cross-reactive autoantigens in RHD and collagen, glomerular basement membrane in PSGN. Laminin, another autoantigen is also involved in the cross reactivity in both diseases.
Diagram 1 illustrates the major events leading to RHDand PSGN.

7. Acknowledgements

We acknowledge all of the people at the Heart Institute (InCor) School of Medicine from the University of Sao Paulo that contributed to the scientific data published elsewhere and described in this review. This work was supported by grants from "Fundação de Amparo à Pesquisa do Estado de São Paulo (FAPESP)" and "Conselho Nacional de Desenvolvimento Científico e Tecnológico (CNPq)".

8. References

Ahn, S.Y.& Ingulli, E. Acute poststreptococcal glomerulonephritis: an update (2008). *Curr Opin Pediatr.* Vol. 20, No2 (April 2008), pp.157-62, Review.
Barbosa, P.J.B.;Muller, R.E.; Latado, A.l., et al. (2009) Brazilian Guidelines for diagnostic, treatment and prevention of Rheumatic Fever. *Arq Bras Cardiol.*Vol.93 (2009), pp.1-18.
Carapetis, J.R.; Steer, A.C.; Mulholland, E.K. & Weber., M. (2005). The global burden of group A streptococcal disease. *Lancet Infect Dis* Vol.5 (November 2005), pp.685-694.
Commons, R.; Rogers, S.; Gooding, T. Danchin, M.; Carapetis, J.; Robins-Browne, R. & Curtis, N. (2008) Superantigen genes in group A streptococcal isolates and their relationship with *emm* types. *J Med Microbiol.* Vol. 57 (October 2008) pp. 1238-1246.
Cunningham, M.W.(2000) Pathogenesis of group A streptococcal infections. *Clin Microbiol Rev.* Vol.13, No 3 (July 2000) pp. 470-511.
Cunningham, M.W.; McCormack, J.M.; Fenderson, P.G.; Ho M.K.; Beachey, E.H. & Dale, J.B.(1989). Human and murine antibodies cross-reactive with streptococcal M protein and myosin recognize the sequence GLN-LYS-SER-LYS-GLN in M protein. *J Immunol.* Vol. 143, No 8 (october 1989), pp.2677-2683.
Fae, K.C.; Silva, D.D.; Oshiro, S.E.; Tanaka, A.C.; Pomerantzeff, P.M.; Douay, C.; Charron, D.; Toubert, A.; Cunningham, M.W.; Kalil, J. & Guilherme, L. (2006) Mimicry in Recognition of Cardiac Myosin Peptides by Heart-Intralesional T Cell Clones from Rheumatic Heart Disease. *J. Immunol,* Vol.176, No9 (May 2006), pp. 5662-70 (2006).

Galvin J.E.; Hemric, M.E.; Ward. K. & Cunningham, M.W. (2000) Cytotoxic mAb from rheumatic carditis recognizes heart valves and laminin. *J Clin Invest*, Vol. 106, No2 (July 2000), pp. 217-224.

Guilherme, L.; Cunha-Neto, E.; Coelho, V.; Snitcowsky, R.; Pomerantzeff, P.M.; Assis, R.V.; Pedra, F.; Neumann, J.; Goldberg, A.; Patarroyo, M.E.; Pileggi, F.& Kalil, J. (1995). Human heart-infiltrating T-cell clones from rheumatic heart disease patients recognized both streptococcal and cardiac proteins. *Circulation*, Vol.92, No3 (August, 1995), pp. 415-420.

Guilherme, L.; Dulphy, N.; Douay, C.; Coelho, V.; Cunha-Neto, E.; Oshiro, S.E.; Assis, R.V.; Tanaka, A.C.; Pomerantzeff, P.M.; Charron, D.; Toubert, A. & Kalil, J. (2000) Molecular evidence for antigen-driven immune responses in cardiac lesions of rheumatic heart disease patients. *Int Immunol.* Vol.12, No.7 (July 2000) pp.1063-1074.

Guilherme, L.; Oshiro, S.E.; Fae, K.C.; Cunha-Neto, E.; Renesto, G.; Goldberg, A.C.; Tanaka, A.C.; Pomerantzeff, P.M.; Kiss, M.H.; Silva, C.; Guzman, F.; Patarroyo, M.E.; Southwood, S.; Sette, A. & Kalil. J. (2001) T cell reactivty against streptococcal antigens in the periphery mirrors reactivity of heart infiltrating T lymphocytes in rheumatic heart disease patients. *Infect Immunity.*, Vol 69, No 9 (September 2001), pp. 5345-5351.

Guilherme, L.; Cury, P.; Demarchi, L.M.; Coelho, V.; Abel, L.; Lopez, A.P.; Oshiro, S.E.; Aliotti, S.; Cunha-Neto, E.; Pomerantzeff, P.M.; Tanaka, A.C. & Kalil, J. (2004) Rheumatic heart disease: proinflammatory cytokines play a role in the progression and maintenance of valvular lesions. *Am J Pathol.* Vol.165, No.5 (November 2004), pp. 1583-1591.

Guilherme, L.; Faé, K.; Oshiro, S.E. & Kalil, J. (2005). Molecular pathogenesis of rheumatic fever and rheumatic heart disease. *Exp Rev Mol Immunol.* Vol. 7 (December 2005), pp.1- 15.

Guilherme, L., Faé, K. C., Higa, F., Chaves, L., Oshiro, S. E., Freschi de Barros, S., Puschel, C., Juliano, M. A., Tanaka, A. C., Spina, G., and Kalil, J.(2006) Towards a vaccine against rheumatic fever. *Clin Dev Immunol.*, Vol.13 (June-December 2006), pp.125-132.

Guilherme. L.; Postol, E.; Freschi de Barros, S.; Higa, F.; Alencar, R.; Lastre, M.; Zayas, C.; Puschel, C.R.; Silva, W.R.; Sa-Rocha, L.C.; Sa-Rocha, V.M.; Perez, O. & Kalil, J.(2009). A vaccine against *S. pyogenes*: design and experimental immune response. *Methods*, Vol. 49, No.4 (December2009), pp.316-321.

Guilherme, L.; Alba, M.P.; Ferreira, F.M.; Oshiro, S.E.; Higa, F.; Patarroyo, M.E.& Kalil, J.(2010). Anti-group A streptococcal vaccine epitope: structure,stability and its ability to interact with HLA class II molecules. *Biol Chem.*, Vol.286, No.9 (March 2010), pp. 6989-6998.

Guilherme, L.; Köhler, K.F.& Kalil, J.(2011). Rheumatic Heart Disease: mediation by complex immune events. *Advances in Clinical Chemistry.* Vol.53 (January 2011) pp. 31-50. Review.

Imöhl, M.; Reinert, R.R.; Ocklenburg, C. & Van der Linden, M.(2010) Epidemiology of invasive *Streptococcus pyogenes* disease in Germany during 2003-2007. *FEMS Immunol Med Microbiol.* Vol.58, No. 3 (April 2010), pp.389-396.

Kemeny, E. ; Grieve, T. ; Marcus, R. ; Sareli, P. & Zabriskie, J.B. (1989) Identification of mononuclear cells and T cell subsets in rheumatic valvulitis. *Clin Immunol Immunopathol*, Vol.52, No2 (August 1989), pp. 225-237.

Krucsó, B.; Gacs, M.; Libisch, B.; Hunyadi, Z.V.; Molnár, K.; Füzi, M. & Pászti, J. (2007) Molecular characterisation of invasive *Streptococcus pyogenes* isolates from Hungary obtained in 2004 and 2005. *Eur J Clin Microbiol Infect Dis*. Vol.26, No.11 (November 2007) pp. 807-811.

Luca-Harari, B.; Ekelund, K.; van der Linden, M.; Staum-Kaltoft, M.; Hammerum, A.M.& Jasir, A. (2008) Clinical and epidemiological aspects of invasive *Streptococcus pyogenes* infections in Denmark during 2003 and 2004. *J Clin Microbiol*. Vol.46, No1 (January 2008), pp. 79-86

Ma, Y.; Yang, Y.; Huang, M.; Wang, Y.; Chen, Y.; Deng, L.; Yu, S.; Deng, Q.; Zhang, H.; Wang, C.; Liu, L.& Shen, X.(2009) Characterization of emm types and superantigens of *Streptococcus pyogenes* isolates from children during two sampling periods. *Epidemiol Infect*. Vol. 137, No. 10 (October 2009), pp. 1414-1419.

Manjula, B.N.; Acharya, A.S.; Mische, M.S.; Fairwell, T. & Fischetti, V.A. (1984) The complete amino acid sequence of a biologically active 197 -residue fragment of M protein isolated from type 5 group A streptococci. *J Biol Chem.*, Vol. 259, pp.3686-3693.

Maripuu, L.; Eriksson, A. & Norgren, M.(2008) Superantigen gene profile diversity among clinical group A streptococcal isolates. *FEMS Immunol Med Microbiol*. Vol.54, No.2 (November 2008), pp. 236-244.

Meisal, R.; Andreasson, I.K.; Høiby, E.A.; Aaberge, I.S.; Michaelsen, T.E.& Caugant, D.A.(2010) *Streptococcus pyogenes* isolates causing severe infections in Norway in 2006 to 2007: *emm* types, multilocus sequence types, and superantigen profiles. *J Clin Microbiol*. Vol. 48, No.3 (March 2010), pp.842-851.

Nasr, S.H.; Markowitz, G.S.; Stokes, M.B.; Said, S.M.; Valeri, A.M. & D'Agati, V.D. (2008) Acute postinfectious glomerulonephritis in the modern era: experience with 86 adults and review of the literature. *Medicine* (Baltimore), Vol. 8, No 1(January, 2008), pp.21-32.

O'Brien, K.L.; Beall, B.; Barrett, N.L.; Cieslak, P.R.; Reingold, A.; Farley, M.M.; Danila, R.; Zell, E.R.; Facklam, R.; Schwartz, B. & Schuchat, A.(2002) Epidemiology of invasive group a streptococcus disease in the United States, 1995-1999. *Clin Infect Dis*. Vol. 35, No.3 (August 2002), pp. 268-276.

Phillips, J.G.N.; Flicker, P.F.; Cohen, C.; Manjula, B.N. & Fischetti, V.A. (1981) Streptococcal M protein: alpha-helical coiled-coil structure and arrangement on the cell surface. Proc. Natl. Acad. Sci. USA., Vol.78, pp.4689-4693.

Raizada, V.; Williams, R.C. Jr.; Chopra, P.; Gopinath, N.; Prakash, K.; Sharma, K.B.; Cherian, K.M.; Panday, S.; Arora, R.; Nigam, M.; Zabriskie, J.B.& Husby, G. (1983). Tissue distribution of lymphocytes in rheumatic heart valves as defined by monoclonal anti-T cells antibodies. Am J Med.Vol.74, No1 (January 1983), pp. 90-96.

Rivera, A.; Rebollo, M.; Miró, E.; Mateo, M.; Navarro, F.; Gurguí, M.; Mirelis, B. & Coll, P.(2006) Superantigen gene profile, *emm* type and antibiotic resistance genes among group A streptococcal isolates from Barcelona, Spain. *J Med Microbiol*. Vol.5 (August 2006), pp. 1115-1123.

Roberts, S.; Kosanke, S.; Dunn, T.S. et al. (2001) Pathogenic Mechanism in Rheumatic Carditis: Focus on Valvular Endothelium. *J Infect Dis*. Vol. 183, pp. 507-511.

Rodríguez-Iturbe, B. & Batsford, S.(2007) Pathogenesis of poststreptococcal glomerulonephritis: a century after Clemens von Pirquet. Kidney Int. Vol. 71, (June 2007), pp.1094-104, Review.

Rodriguez-Iturbe, B. & Musser, J.M. (2008) The current state of poststreptococcal glomerulonephritis. *J Am Soc Nephrol*, Vol.19, No10 (October 2008), pp.1855-1864.

Steer, A.C.; Batzloff, M.R.; Mulholland, K; Carapetis, J.R.(2009) Group A streptococcal vaccines: facts versus fantasy. Curr Opin Infect Dis Vol 22(6) (October 2009):544-52.

Shulman, S.T.; Tanz, R.R.; Kabat, W.; Kabat, K.; Cederlund, E.; Patel, D.; Li, Z.; Sakota, V.; Dale, J.B.& Beall, B. (2004) US Streptococcal Pharyngitis Surveillance Group. Group A streptococcal pharyngitis serotype surveillance in North America, 2000-2002. *Clin Infect Dis*. Vol.39, No.3 (August 2004) pp. 325-32.

Yoshinaga, M.; Figueiroa, F.; Wahid, M.R.; Marcus, R.H.; Suh, E.&. Zabriskie, J.B. (1995). Antigenic specificity of lymphocytes isolated from valvular specimens of rheumatic fever patients. *J. Autoimmun*, Vol.8, No 4 (August 1995) pp. 601-613.

8

Post-Infectious Glomerulonephritis

Gurmeet Singh

Menzies School of Health Research, Cahrles Darwin University, Darwin, NT,
Northern Territory Medical Program, Flinders University, SA,
Australia

1. Introduction

This chapter will provide a comprehensive review of post-infectious glomerulonephritis focusing in particular on the changing epidemiology and long term outcome.

The immunological response of the kidney to an insult results in glomerulonephritis. The insult can result from a large number of conditions, both infectious and non-infectious. Regardless of the initial insult, the outcome is similar in terms of pathology and clinical symptoms. The most common and most-studied cause is post streptococcal Glomerulonephritis (PSGN). A list of causes is presented in Table 1.

INFECTIOUS

Bacterial: Streptococcal (PSGN), methicillin-resistant *Staphylococcus aureus* (MRSA), pneumococcal pneumonia, typhoid, secondary syphilis, meningococcemia, infective endocarditis, shunt nephritis, sepsis

Viral: Hepatitis B, infectious mononucleosis, mumps, measles, varicella, vaccinia, echovirus, parvovirus, and coxsackievirus

Parasitic: Malaria, toxoplasmosis

Fungal: cryptococccus imitis

NON INFECTIOUS

Primary glomerular diseases: Membranoproliferative GN (MPGN), IgA nephropathy, mesangial proliferative GN

Multisystem systemic diseases: Systemic lupus erythematosus, vasculitis, Henoch-Schönlein purpura, Goodpasture syndrome, Wegener granulomatosis

Miscellaneous: Gullian-barre syndrome, pertussis-tetanus vaccine, serum sickness

---

Table 1. Causes of post-Infectious Glomerulonephritis

2. Burden of disease and changing epidemiology

Of all the bacterial pathogens, group A streptococcus (GAS) causes the widest range of illness in humans. These illnesses range from local infections of the skin and throat (impetigo and pharyngitis respectively) to invasive infections as well as the significant post-infectious immunological sequelae such as the well documented acute rheumatic fever and acute post-streptococcal glomerulonephritis and the lesser known PANDAS (Paediatric Autoimmune Neuropsychiatric Disorder Associated with Streptococcus) [1].

While global estimates of the burden of disease due to GAS infections are difficult to get, some estimates have been reported which are based on published population studies. The estimate of 500 000 deaths per year due to GAS makes it a major human Pathogen [2]. This minimal estimate places GAS infections as less common than HIV, *Mycobacterium tuberculosis, Plasmodium falciparum* and *Streptococcus pneumonia* but as common as rotavirus, measles, *Haemophilus influenzae* type b and hepatitis B as a cause of global mortality [2]. In addition there is the long-term morbidity associated with GAS infections.

The global burden of severe group A streptococcal disease is concentrated largely in developing countries and within disadvantaged populations living in developed countries such as Aboriginal Australians. The review of population based studies estimated the prevalence of severe GAS disease at a minimum of 18·1 million cases, with 1·78 million new cases each year [2]. The greatest burden was due to rheumatic heart disease, with a prevalence of at least 15·6 million cases, with 282 000 new cases and 233 000 deaths each year. The burden of invasive GAS diseases was found to be unexpectedly high, with at least 663 000 new cases and 163 000 deaths each year. In addition, there were more than 111 million prevalent cases of GAS pyoderma, and over 616 million incident cases per year of GAS pharyngitis [2]. The review estimated that over 470 000 cases of acute post-streptococcal glomerulonephritis occur annually, with approximately 5000 deaths (1% of total cases), 97% of which were in less developed countries [2].

The global incidence of acute PSGN was estimated at 472,000 cases per year, of which 456,000 (96.6%) occurred in less developed countries [3, 4]. A similar distribution of higher incident cases in less developed countries is also reported in a review of population based studies [2]. A review of 11 population-based studies documenting the incidence of acute PSGN in children from less developed countries or those that included substantial minority populations in more developed countries, estimated 24·3 cases per 100,000 person as the median PSGN incident rate [2]. The same review estimated an incidence in adults of 2 cases per 100,000 person-years for developing countries and 0.3 per 100,000 person-years in developed countries [2]. Due to the paucity of data in adults with PSGN, the estimate for developing countries was based on data from Kuwait and for developed countries on data from Italian Biopsy Registry and the most conservative estimates were reported [2]. Another recent study described a slightly higher incidence of 9.5-28.5 cases per 100,000 person-years in developing countries [5]. These rates represent only the clinical cases. When asymptomatic cases are screened for in household contacts and family members, asymptomatic disease is reported to be 4-19 times greater [5-7].

PSGN can occur sporadically or epidemically. The changing pattern of PSGN over the last few decades has been described in studies from Florida [8] and Singapore [9]. The overall incidence of PSGN has decreased over the last few decades [10]. The reasons for this decline have not been clearly delineated but possible reasons are the widespread use of antibiotics, changes in etiological pathogens, altered susceptibility of the host, better health care delivery and improved socioeconomic and nutritional conditions [8-10]. Nevertheless, epidemics and clusters of cases continue to appear in several regions of the world and sporadic cases of PSGN account for 21% (4.6–51.6%) of children admitted to the hospital with acute renal failure in developing countries [5]. Although epidemic PSGN has decreased dramatically and is almost unknown in the developed world, epidemics of PSGN continue to occur in the developing world, mainly in Africa, West Indies and the Middle East, as well as in Indigenous people living in the developed world [11]. Epidemics are described mainly in "closed" communities, clusters of densely populated dwellings or areas with poor hygienic conditions, both urban and rural. These conditions are especially prevalent in Aboriginal peoples of Australia living in remote communities, in settings with a high burden of infectious disease and overcrowding [11, 12]. Sporadic cases of PSGN occur in the Northern Territory of Australia each year with outbreaks every 5-7 years [13]. PSGN in New Zealand occurs mostly in children of Pacific Island and Maori heritage (>85% of cases) [14]. Sporadic cases of PSGN also continue to be reported from all over the world.

The rates are higher in children than in adults, and PANDAS is described solely in the paediatric age group. PSGN primarily affects children, aged 2-12 years, with clinically detectable cases estimated to be 10% of children with pharyngitis and up to 25% of children with impetigo during epidemics [15, 16]. Children account for 50-90% of epidemic cases, with 5-10% occurring in people > 40 years and 10% in those below 2 years of age [5]. PSGN is uncommon below 3 years of age and rarely seen below 2 years [17]. This low incidence of PSGN is likely to be due to the decreased immunogenicity of children below 2 years of age, for although GAS pharyngitis is uncommon in children of this age, GAS skin infections are common. Decreased immunogenicity likely results in less robust immune complex formation thus leading to less PSGN [18].

Males have more symptomatic disease, but this difference is no longer present when symptomatic and asymptomatic cases are considered together [19]. Spontaneous recovery occurs in almost all patients, including those who develop renal insufficiency during the acute phase [16], with 1% of all paediatric patients developing renal insufficiency.

There are no large scale published studies of bacterial infections associated with GN other than streptococcal infection. These are limited to small cases series and individual cases reports. The most common of these are related to staphylococcal infections, both methicillin sensitive [20] and methicillin resistant [21, 22]. A case series of 10 cases, age range 21-65 years, of MRSA-associated glomerulonephritis reported polyclonal increases of IgA and IgG and massive T cell activation and suggested the role of the enterotoxin as a bacterial super-antigen initiating the immunological response leading to the glomerulonephritis [22]. The histopathologic findings on immunofluorescence in the patients with MRSA infection with nephritis resemble those seen in IgA nephropathy [22]. Nephritis associated with endocarditis and ventricular shunts is associated with staphylococcal infection [22]. A number of infections can cause nephritis as listed in table 1. Most have been reported as case reports, such as a report of nephritis following malaria due to *falciparum vivax* infection in a 7 year old girl [23], and a report of nephritis following pneumococcal pneumonia in an adult male [24].

Hepatitis-B-associated glomerulonephritis (HBGN) is a distinct entity occurring frequently in hepatitis-B-prevalent areas of the world. The disease affects both adults and children who are chronic hepatitis-B-virus (HBV) carriers with or without a history of overt liver disease. The diagnosis is established by serologic evidence of HBV antigens/antibodies, presence of an immune complex glomerulonephritis, immunohistochemical localization of 1 or more HBV antigens and pertinent clinical history [25]. With the high incidence of hepatitis B in Asia, this entity assumes a greater public health importance. A study from China reported 205 cases from a single hospital from September 1995 to November 2008 [26]. In this series, the peak incidence of HBV-GN was between 20 -40 years of age, with a 3:1 predominance of males. The most common clinic manifestation was nephrotic syndrome and the most common pathology was membranous nephropathy. Decreased renal function was present in 10% of cases. The degree of albuminuria correlated with the viral load [26].

Renal disease is not uncommon in those infected with HIV. The most common manifestation of HIV in the kidney is HIV-associated nephropathy (HIVAN). Immunotactoid glomerulonephritis is a rare disorder found in 0.06% of renal biopsies characterized by organized tubular immune complex deposits. This is seen more commonly Caucasians and tends to occur in an older age group. There are 6 reported cases of HIV associated immunotactoid glomerulonephritis [27].

3. Pathogenesis

The kidney has a limited number of ways of responding to injury. Similar pathological signs may be the end result of different processes, produced by different initiating mechanisms and different molecular pathways may perpetuate the injury process. The initiation and development of the inflammatory response of the kidney to infection are still poorly understood.

The pathognomonic feature of PSGN is the deposition of immune complexes in the glomerular basement membrane. A proposed sequence of events is that a nephritogenic antigen(s) leads to the activation of the complement pathway and/or activates plasmin or production of the circulating immune-complexes. These then lead to increased permeability of the glomerular basement membrane, which allows deposition of the immune complexes, and leakage of the protein and red blood cells. The nephritogenic antigen is responsible for the C3 deposition, the recruitment of immune cells, tissue destruction and IgG deposition which further aggravates tissue injury. Complement activation leads to the release of cytokines, such as C5a, which attracts phagocytes, and proliferation of intrinsic cells and formation of a membrane attack complex which also aggravate the process. The definitive nephritogenic antigen has not yet been defined, although a large number of streptococcal factors (M proteins) have been proposed as the triggering factor. M proteins are present on the pili of the organism and more than 100 have been identified so far. Nephritogenic M proteins are types 1, 2, 4, 3, 25, 49, and 12 following skin infections and types 47, 49, 55, 2, 60, and 57 following throat infections [28]. Infections with nephritogenic streptococci have considerable variability in their ability to cause nephritis. The reason for this variability is not known.

Pathology shows typical glomerular changes which include proliferation of mesangial, endothelial and epithelial cells, inflammatory exudate and deposition of C3 early in the disease process followed by deposition of IgG. This immune deposition has been classified into 3 patterns [29]. The "starry sky" pattern represents an irregular and finely granular deposit of C3 and IgG along the glomerular capillary walls and in the mesangium. This occurs early in the course of the disease and is also seen in subclinical cases [28, 29]. The "mesangial pattern" has mainly C3 and some IgG in the mesangium. The "garland pattern" shows dense deposits along the capillary walls, is commonly associated with severe proteinuria and a poor prognosis [28, 29].

The immunological response of the kidney to an insult results in glomerulonephritis. The causal factors that underlie acute GN can be broadly divided into infectious and noninfectious groups. The most common infectious cause of acute GN is infection by *Streptococcus* species (ie, group A, beta-hemolytic). Nonstreptococcal postinfectious GN may also result from infection by other bacteria, viruses, parasites, or fungi. Bacteria besides group A streptococci that can cause acute GN include diplococci, other streptococci, staphylococci, and mycobacteria. *Salmonella typhosa, Brucella suis, Treponema pallidum, Corynebacterium bovis,* and actinobacilli have also been identified.

In the absence of evidence of a recent group A beta-hemolytic streptococcal infection, infections with Cytomegalovirus (CMV), coxsackievirus, Epstein-Barr virus (EBV), hepatitis B virus (HBV) [30], rubella, rickettsiae (as in scrub typhus), and mumps virus may be accepted as causal organisms. Similarly, attributing glomerulonephritis to a parasitic or fungal etiology requires the exclusion of a streptococcal infection. Possible organisms are *Coccidioides immiti*, *Plasmodium malariae*, *Plasmodium falciparum*, *Schistosoma mansoni*, *Toxoplasma gondii*, filariasis, trichinosis, and trypanosomes. While hepatitis B infection has been well documented as a cause of renal involvement and glomerulonephritis [25, 26], acute GN is as a rare complication of hepatitis A [31].

Noninfectious causes of acute GN may be divided into primary renal diseases, systemic diseases, and miscellaneous conditions or agents. The primary renal diseases are membranoproliferative glomerulonephritis (MPGN), IgA nephropathy and mesangial proliferative glomerulonephritis. Multisystem systemic diseases that can cause acute GN are vasculitis such as Wegener granulomatosis, polyarteritis nodosa and hypersensitivity vasculitis, collagen-vascular diseases like systemic lupus erythematosus (SLE) which causes glomerulonephritis through renal deposition of immune complexes, Henoch-Schönlein purpura and Goodpasture syndrome. Miscellaneous noninfectious causes are Guillain-Barré syndrome, Diphtheria-pertussis-tetanus (DPT) vaccine and serum sickness. These are summarised in table 1.

It is important to identify the exact aetiology of the glomerulonephritis as the prognosis differs widely depending on the underlying cause. There are a number of clinical and laboratory features that may help to differentiate between or even point to a particular cause of glomerulonephritis. The latent period between infection and nephritis is helpful in differentiating PSGN from IgA nephropathy. In contrast to the latent period of 2-3 weeks seen in PSGN, the nephritis of IGA nephropathy may occur either at the same time or just 1-2 days after an upper respiratory infection. Similarly, patients with nephritis of chronic infection have an active infection at the time nephritis becomes evident. Despite the chronic nature of the underlying infection, the associated nephritis can present acutely. Circulating immune complexes play an important role in the pathogenesis of acute GN in these diseases.

The failure of the C3 levels to return to normal should prompt consideration of the possibility of MPGN or SLE as the underlying cause. MPGN is a chronic disease which can manifest with an acute nephritic picture. Gross haematuria is unusual in lupus nephritis. Other associated systemic findings may identify the underlying systemic disease, for example, vasculitic lesions of the lower extremities point to an underlying vasculitis as the cause of glomerulonephritis.

4. Clinical presentation

The typical presentation is the abrupt onset of acute nephritis occurring 1-3 weeks after a streptococcal throat infection and 3-6 weeks after skin infection [28]. The nephritis is characterised by the triad of oedema, gross haematuria, and hypertension. The classical presenting feature is the presence of "coca-cola" coloured urine which is characteristic of homogenous gross haematuria [32]. Other common features are facial puffiness and hypertension secondary to fluid overload and urinary abnormalities such as albuminuria and the presence of red cell casts. General features like malaise, weakness, and anorexia may occur in about half the patients and a minority complain of nausea and vomiting. Within a week or so from onset of symptoms, most patients with PSGN begin to experience spontaneous resolution of fluid retention and hypertension and the urine abnormalities begin to subside. The low C3 levels begin to rise and normalise by 8 weeks. Normal urine findings are found by 12 weeks.

Microscopic haematuria is universally present. Of the triad of features, oedema is seen in 85% of cases and is often the presenting symptom, gross haematuria in 40% of cases (range 30-50%) and hypertension in 50-95% of hospitalised cases. Approximately 95% of clinical cases have at least 2 manifestations, and 40% have the full-blown acute nephritic syndrome. The puffiness of the face or eyelids is sudden, usually prominent upon awakening and tends to subside at the end of the day if the patient is active. The oedema is a result of a defect in renal excretion of salt and water leading to fluid overload. The severity of edema does not correlate well with the degree of renal impairment.

In most cases, urinary abnormalities clear by 12 weeks, although proteinuria may persist for 6 months to 3 years and microscopic haematuria from 1 year to 4 years after the onset of nephritis [33]. In some cases, generalized edema and other features of circulatory congestion, such as dyspnea, may be present.

Accompanying this clinical picture is laboratory evidence of streptococcal infection, typically increasing antistreptolysin-O titers (ASOT) or streptozyme titres following throat infections and anti-DNase B titers following skin infections. Complement levels are decreased; low C3 levels are found in almost all patients with acute PSGN and C4 levels may be slightly low. These low levels of C3 usually normalize within 8 weeks after the first sign of PSGN [34], although up to 12 weeks has been reported [33]. The typical accompanying histopathology is one of diffuse cellular proliferation in the glomerulus, an exudate containing neutrophils and monocytes and variable degrees of complement and immunoglobulin deposition. In most cases, hypertension subsides, renal function returns to normal and all urinary abnormalities eventually disappear [33].

There is, however, a wide variation in the clinical presentation as well in the histopathology associated with PSGN. At the severe end of the spectrum is a rapidly rising azotemia with a rapidly progressive nephritic picture associated with severe cell proliferation, massive exudates and crescent formation in biopsy specimens. This is seen in <5% of PSGN cases [19]. The severity of renal failure tends to be directly related to the degree of proliferation and crescent formation, and about 50% of these patients recover renal function [35]. This type of presentation is more common in the elderly. The mild end of the spectrum, represented by subclinical or asymptomatic glomerulonephritis, is more common. Diligent examination of people with acute, trivial or self-limited infections caused by a range of organisms including various bacteria, parasites or viruses reveal subclinical infection in the form of microscopic hematuria, proteinuria and pyuria. Histopathology reveals mesangial proliferation with mesangial deposits of C3 and IgG deposits [19]. Asymptomatic household contacts of PSGN cases show sub-clinical disease 4-5 times more commonly than the acute classical presentation [6, 36]. An older study puts the ratio of asymptomatic cases as high as 19:1 [7].

5. Typical findings on investigations

Urinalysis reveals haematuria in all patients and proteinuria (from trace to 2+ on dipstick testing) is usually present. Proteinuria may be in the nephrotic range and is usually associated with more severe disease. Red blood cell casts are pathognomonic of acute glomerulonephritis. Occasionally other cellular casts and pyuria are present.

Serological evidence of an antecedent streptococcal infection is present in the form of raised ASOT (> 200 IU/ml) and increased anti-DNAse B (which is a better serological marker of preceding streptococcal skin infection). Bacteriological evidence of streptococcal disease may be present in throat or skin swabs.

Complement levels especially C3 are low at the onset of symptoms. C4 is usually within normal limits in post-streptococcal GN. Causes of nephritis with low complement besides PSGN are MPGN, SLE, cryoglobulinemia, Diabetes Mellitus and Hepatitis C Virus. These diseases should be screened for in case of either an atypical presentation or atypical clinical course of the glomerulonephritis.

Renal function tests, blood urea, sodium, potassium and serum creatinine may be elevated in the acute phase and reflect the decrease in the glomerular filtration rate that occurs at this time. These elevations are usually transient. Failure of renal function tests to normalize within several weeks or months suggests that the patient may not have PSGN and indicates the need to seek an alternative diagnosis by further investigation. The full blood count may show anaemia which is usually dilutional and will return to normal once the fluid overload resolves.

Renal ultrasound is not required to make a diagnosis of glomerulonephririts. Renal ultrasound images usually reveal normal-sized kidneys bilaterally. Renal imaging is often done to confirm that there are two kidneys and that they are structurally normal. It may be done as a prelude to a renal biopsy. PSGN is a clinical diagnosis and requires the detection of glomerulonephritis and evidence of preceding streptococcal infection. A renal biopsy is indicated in cases with an atypical presentation, an atypical course, persistence of clinical features, or a persisting low level of complement (C3) or abnormal renal function tests. Features that suggest a diagnosis other than PSGN in the early stages may also indicate a need for a biopsy. These include the absence of the latent period between streptococcal infection and acute glomerulonephritis, anuria, rapidly deteriorating renal function, normal serum complement levels, lack of rise in antistreptococcal antibodies, general symptoms of systemic disease and either persistent hypertension or lack of improvement in glomerular filtration rate for more than 2 weeks. In the recovery phase, persistent low C3 beyond 8 and definitely beyond 12 weeks from the onset of illness would indicate a need to look for alternate causes and for a renal biospsy.

6. Treatment

Treatment of PSGN remains largely supportive. Complete recovery occurs in over 90% of children, but only 60% of adults fully recover. The rest develop hypertension or renal impairment.

Treatment is directed towards monitoring the signs and symptoms, in particular facial puffiness and hypertension, the main cause of which is fluid overload. Treatment when it is required, is mainly directed towards managing the fluid overload, which is responsive to diuresis and sodium restriction. Effective diuresis reduces cardiac congestion and controls hypertension and in most cases no further treatment is required. Strict input-output monitoring is recommended during the acute phase.

As the hypertension is caused by fluid overload, loop diuretics are the first line treatment and may be adequate for control of hypertension. Furosemide in a dose of 40 mg either orally or intravenously is given 12 hourly. Usually treatment is required for less than 48 hours. Sometimes other anti-hypertensive agents may be needed, especially when the blood pressure is very high and it is unsafe to wait for the effect of diuretic therapy. Nifedipine is then given every 4-6 hours in doses of 5-10 mg. Rarely parenteral hydralazine may be required. Captopril has shown to be effective [37, 38] but should be used in caution in the presence of renal failure and hyperkalemia. Occasionally acute renal failure requires dialysis. Pulmonary oedema may be complication of severe fluid overload and needs urgent treatment.

It is important to check serum complement levels 6-8 weeks after initial testing to make sure they have returned to normal. Blood pressure should be monitored every month for 6 months and then 6 monthly. Renal function tests and serum creatinine levels repeated every 3 months after the acute phase for 1 year and then yearly after that. Urine should be checked for hematuria and proteinuria every 3-6 months.

Aggressive therapy using pulse methyprednisolone has been used in adults with poor prognostic factors such as nephritic range proteinuria, cellular crescents on biopsy and renal insufficiency [39]. Plasmapharesis and pulse methyprednisolone was successfully used in a 6 year old girl with garland pattern PSGN [40]. Whether this would benefit all patients with poor prognosis has not been studied.

Penicillin treatment is given to treat any persisting streptococcal infection [41]. Methicillin resistant staphylococcus should be treated with appropriate antibiotics. Specific infections require treatment with specific antibiotics or antiviral agents. Treatment of the underlying infection may resolve the glomerulonephritis as well. A review of six trials (a total of 159 patients) of which five were specified as hepatitis B virus-associated membranous glomerulonephritis (HBV-MN) showed that antiviral therapy for hepatitis B infections including IFN and lamivudine is effective in leading to remission of proteinuria, HBeAg clearance, and HBV-DNA reduction in both children and adults [42].

7. Preventing spread

A case of PSGN has 2 or more of the following clinical manifestations: oedema, macroscopic hematuria or dipstick hematuria of ≥ 2, or diastolic blood pressure of >80mmHg if ≤ 13 years of age and >90 mmHg if >13 years of age, in the presence of a reduced complement level (C3) and evidence of streptococcal infection by either elevated ASO or anti-DNAse B titres or positive cultures of GAS from skin, if sores are present, or from the throat in the absence of skin sores.

There is evidence that outbreaks can be halted by treating all children with any evidence of skin sores with intra-muscular (IM) benzathine penicillin to stop the transmission of the bacteria in the community [43]. In experimental PSGN, the nephritic process is prevented if penicillin is given within 3 days of the streptococcal infection [41]. Prevention of epidemics requires the control of spread of skin sores and infected scabies [44]. Following the identification of a case(s), family and household members are screened for the presence of skin sores and scabies and tested for urinary abnormalities. Those with skin manifestations are treated with penicillin. Those with urinary abnormalities undergo complete investigation for PSGN including urea, electrolytes, C3, ASO, anti-DNAse B and cultures for streptococcal infection.

Prevention of epidemics of PSGN requires a community level control of skin sores and infected scabies. Promotion of regular washing, especially of children, will prevent spread.

Improvement in housing, especially reduction in overcrowding, will hinder spread of infectious disease. The significant decline in PSGN in Singapore children is attributed to an improvement in the socioeconomic status, the health care system and urbanization of the country [9].

Although research into the development of a vaccine is advanced and 3 GAS vaccines have been approved for phase 1 human trials [45], it is unlikely to be available in the near future.

8. Prognosis

In keeping with the clinico-pathological picture, the prognosis of PSGN is also extremely variable, and largely influenced by clinical presentation and histopathology. An episode of PSGN may result in complete recovery, progression of symptoms or progression to renal failure. Persistence of symptoms may represent either a slow recovery, limited injury without further progression or progression to renal failure.

The immediate prognosis is generally good. In general, children are believed to have an excellent prognosis with the majority showing complete recovery [5]. Fewer than 1% of children have elevated serum creatinine values after 10-15 years of follow-up. Adults have a poorer prognosis overall. Early mortality can be as high as 25% in the elderly who have congestive cardiac failure or azotemia in the early phase. In adults approximately 25% will progress to chronic renal failure. These are usually those with massive proteinuria which suggests a worse prognosis and often signifies the garland pattern of immune deposits on pathology.

It is difficult to predict the prognosis in an individual case particularly early in the disease. While a typical presentation and clinical course indicates a good prognosis and an atypical presentation, severe persistent hypertension and abnormal renal function tests, massive proteinuria and older age group suggest a poor prognosis, there is a lack of a clinical or biochemical marker that might differentiate those with a good prognosis from those with a poorer outcome. Neutrophil gelatinase-associated lipocalin (NGAL), is emerging as a promising biomarker of acute kidney injury [46, 47], but has not yet been evaluated in PSGN.

However, some studies have reported persistent urinary abnormalities [8, 11, 19, 48, 49] and subtle abnormalities in renal function, as defined by reduction in renal functional reserve, in patients who had recovered from PSGN without apparent sequelae [50]

Epidemic cases have a better prognosis than sporadic cases [14, 51, 52], but not always. An outbreak of PSGN in Brazil following an epidemic of *Streptococcus equi zooepidemicus* resulted in a high prevalence of renal abnormalities at a mean follow-up of 5.4 years [53, 54]. These were, however, mainly adult patients. A study of Iranian children has shown that even mild PSGN may result in impaired renal function and that a rising diastolic blood pressure may be an early sign of worsening renal function [55].

Elderly people have poorer outcomes as do those with co-morbidities, including diabetes, cardiovascular and liver diseases [5, 28]. In an Aboriginal population with high rates of ESRD, follow-up of children 6-18 years (mean 14.6 years) after epidemic PSGN showed that risk of overt proteinuria was 6 times (95% CI 2.2-16.9) greater than in healthy controls after adjustment of age, sex and birth weight [11, 56]. The Australian Aboriginal population is at considerably higher risk than the general Australian population of developing chronic diseases such as diabetes mellitus, cardiovascular and renal diseases. There is also a greater burden of infectious disease and adverse early life factors such as low birth and infant weights. It is proposed that in this high risk population with multiple adverse renal influences, childhood PSGN might be a more important risk factor for ESRD than it would be in lower risk populations [11, 44, 57].

9. References

[1] Kurlan, R., D. Johnson, and E.L. Kaplan, *Streptococcal infection and exacerbations of childhood tics and obsessive-compulsive symptoms: a prospective blinded cohort study.* Pediatrics, 2008. 121(6): p. 1188-97.

[2] Carapetis, J.R., et al., *The global burden of group A streptococcal diseases.* Lancet Infect Dis, 2005. 5(11): p. 685-94.

[3] Steer, A.C., M.H. Danchin, and J.R. Carapetis, *Group A streptococcal infections in children.* J Paediatr Child Health, 2007. 43(4): p. 203-13.

[4] Jackson, S.J., A.C. Steer, and H. Campbell, *Systematic Review: Estimation of global burden of non-suppurative sequelae of upper respiratory tract infection: rheumatic fever and post-streptococcal glomerulonephritis.* Trop Med Int Health, 2011. 16(1): p. 2-11.

[5] Rodriguez-Iturbe, B. and J.M. Musser, *The current state of poststreptococcal glomerulonephritis.* J Am Soc Nephrol, 2008. 19(10): p. 1855-64.

[6] Rodriguez-Iturbe, B., L. Rubio, and R. Garcia, *Attack rate of poststreptococcal nephritis in families. A prospective study.* Lancet, 1981. 1(8217): p. 401-3.

[7] Sagel, I., et al., *Occurrence and nature of glomerular lesions after group A streptococci infections in children.* Ann Intern Med, 1973. 79(4): p. 492-9.

[8] Ilyas, M. and A. Tolaymat, *Changing epidemiology of acute post-streptococcal glomerulonephritis in Northeast Florida: a comparative study.* Pediatr Nephrol, 2008. 23(7): p. 1101-6.

[9] Yap, H.K., et al., *Acute glomerulonephritis--changing patterns in Singapore children.* Pediatr Nephrol, 1990. 4(5): p. 482-4.

[10] Markowitz, M., *Changing epidemiology of group A streptococcal infections.* Pediatr Infect Dis J, 1994. 13(6): p. 557-60.

[11] White, A.V., W.E. Hoy, and D.A. McCredie, *Childhood post-streptococcal glomerulonephritis as a risk factor for chronic renal disease in later life.* Med J Aust, 2001. 174(10): p. 492-6.

[12] Streeton, C.L., et al., *An epidemic of acute post-streptococcal glomerulonephritis among aboriginal children.* J Paediatr Child Health, 1995. 31(3): p. 245-8.

[13] *Communicable Diseases Surveillance System.* 2002, Centre for Communicable Diseases: Darwin, NT.

[14] Wong, W., M.C. Morris, and J. Zwi, *Outcome of severe acute post-streptococcal glomerulonephritis in New Zealand children.* Pediatr Nephrol, 2009. 24(5): p. 1021-6.

[15] Stetson, C.A., et al., *Epidemic acute nephritis: studies on etiology, natural history and prevention.* Medicine (Baltimore), 1955. 34(4): p. 431-50.

[16] Tejani, A. and E. Ingulli, *Poststreptococcal glomerulonephritis. Current clinical and pathologic concepts.* Nephron, 1990. 55(1): p. 1-5.

[17] Bingler, M.A., D. Ellis, and M.L. Moritz, *Acute post-streptococcal glomerulonephritis in a 14-month-old boy: why is this uncommon?* Pediatr Nephrol, 2007. 22(3): p. 448-50.

[18] Shet, A., et al., *Immune response to group A streptococcal C5a peptidase in children: implications for vaccine development.* J Infect Dis, 2003. 188(6): p. 809-17.

[19] Kanjanabuch, T., W. Kittikowit, and S. Eiam-Ong, *An update on acute postinfectious glomerulonephritis worldwide.* Nat Rev Nephrol, 2009. 5(5): p. 259-69.

[20] Handa, T., et al., *Glomerulonephritis induced by methicillin-sensitive Staphylococcus aureus infection.* Clin Exp Nephrol, 2003. 7(3): p. 247-9.

[21] Kobayashi, M. and A. Koyama, *Methicillin-resistant Staphylococcus aureus (MRSA) infection in glomerulonephritis--a novel hazard emerging on the horizon.* Nephrol Dial Transplant, 1998. 13(12): p. 2999-3001.

[22] Koyama, A., et al., *Glomerulonephritis associated with MRSA infection: a possible role of bacterial superantigen.* Kidney Int, 1995. 47(1): p. 207-16.

[23] Zaki, S.A. and P. Shanbag, *Acute glomerulonephritis: an unusual manifestation of Plasmodium vivax malaria.* Ann Trop Paediatr, 2011. 31(2): p. 181-4.

[24] Kaehny, W.D., et al., *Acute nephritis and pulmonary alveolitis following pneumococcal pneumonia.* Arch Intern Med, 1978. 138(5): p. 806-8.

[25] Venkataseshan, V.S., et al., *Hepatitis-B-associated glomerulonephritis: pathology, pathogenesis, and clinical course.* Medicine (Baltimore), 1990. 69(4): p. 200-16.

[26] Wei, R.B., et al., *[Clinicopathological analysis on hepatitis B virus-associated glomerulonephritis in 205 patients].* Zhonghua Shi Yan He Lin Chuang Bing Du Xue Za Zhi, 2010. 24(6): p. 464-7.

[27] Chen, Y.M., et al., *An unusual cause of membranous glomerulonephritis in a patient with HIV.* Int Urol Nephrol, 2011.

[28] Nordstrand, A., M. Norgren, and S.E. Holm, *Pathogenic Mechanism of Acute Post-Streptococcal Glomerulonephritis.* Scandinavian Journal of Infectious Diseases, 1999. 31(6): p. 523-537.

[29] Sorger, K., et al., *Subtypes of acute postinfectious glomerulonephritis. Synopsis of clinical and pathological features.* Clin Nephrol, 1982. 17(3): p. 114-28.

[30] Safadi, R., et al., *Glomerulonephritis associated with acute hepatitis B.* Am J Gastroenterol, 1996. 91(1): p. 138-9.

[31] Aggarwal, A., D. Kumar, and R. Kumar, *Acute glomerulonephritis in hepatitis A virus infection: a rare presentation.* Trop Doct, 2009. 39(3): p. 186-7.

[32] Pan, C.G., *Evaluation of gross hematuria.* Pediatr Clin North Am, 2006. 53(3): p. 401-12, vi.

[33] Yoshizawa, N., *Acute glomerulonephritis.* Intern Med, 2000. 39(9): p. 687-94.

[34] Pan, C.G., *Glomerulonephritis in childhood.* Curr Opin Pediatr, 1997. 9(2): p. 154-9.

[35] El-Husseini, A.A., et al., *Acute postinfectious crescentic glomerulonephritis: clinicopathologic presentation and risk factors.* Int Urol Nephrol, 2005. 37(3): p. 603-9.

[36] Tasic, V. and M. Polenakovic, *Occurrence of subclinical post-streptococcal glomerulonephritis in family contacts.* J Paediatr Child Health, 2003. 39(3): p. 177-9.

[37] Morsi, M.R., et al., *Evaluation of captopril versus reserpine and frusemide in treating hypertensive children with acute post-streptococcal glomerulonephritis.* Acta Paediatr, 1992. 81(2): p. 145-9.

[38] Parra, G., et al., *Short-term treatment with captopril in hypertension due to acute glomerulonephritis.* Clin Nephrol, 1988. 29(2): p. 58-62.

[39] Raff, A., et al., *Crescentic post-streptococcal glomerulonephritis with nephrotic syndrome in the adult: is aggressive therapy warranted?* Clin Nephrol, 2005. 63(5): p. 375-80.

[40] Suyama, K., Y. Kawasaki, and H. Suzuki, *Girl with garland-pattern poststreptococcal acute glomerulonephritis presenting with renal failure and nephrotic syndrome.* Pediatr Int, 2007. 49(1): p. 115-7.

[41] Bergholm, A.M. and S.E. Holm, *Effect of early penicillin treatment on the development of experimental poststreptococcal glomerulonephritis.* Acta Pathol Microbiol Immunol Scand C, 1983. 91(4): p. 271-81.

[42] Yi, Z., Y.W. Jie, and Z. Nan, *The efficacy of anti-viral therapy on hepatitis B virus-associated glomerulonephritis: A systematic review and meta-analysis.* Ann Hepatol, 2011. 10(2): p. 165-73.

[43] Johnston, F., et al., *Evaluating the use of penicillin to control outbreaks of acute poststreptococcal glomerulonephritis.* Pediatr Infect Dis J, 1999. 18(4): p. 327-32.

[44] Van Buynder, P.G., et al., *Streptococcal infection and renal disease markers in Australian aboriginal children.* Med J Aust, 1992. 156(8): p. 537-40.

[45] Georgousakis, M.M., et al., *Moving forward: a mucosal vaccine against group A streptococcus.* Expert Rev Vaccines, 2009. 8(6): p. 747-60.

[46] Haase, M., et al., *Accuracy of neutrophil gelatinase-associated lipocalin (NGAL) in diagnosis and prognosis in acute kidney injury: a systematic review and meta-analysis.* Am J Kidney Dis, 2009. 54(6): p. 1012-24.

[47] Devarajan, P., *Neutrophil gelatinase-associated lipocalin (NGAL): a new marker of kidney disease.* Scand J Clin Lab Invest Suppl, 2008. 241: p. 89-94.

[48] Wong, W., M. Morris, and J. Zwi, *Outcome of severe acute post-streptococcal glomerulonephritis in New Zealand children.* Pediatric Nephrology, 2009. 24(5): p. 1021-1026.

[49] Buzio, C., et al., *Significance of albuminuria in the follow-up of acute poststreptococcal glomerulonephritis.* Clin Nephrol, 1994. 41(5): p. 259-64.

[50] Cleper, R., et al., *Renal functional reserve after acute poststreptococcal glomerulonephritis.* Pediatr Nephrol, 1997. 11(4): p. 473-6.

[51] Blyth, C.C., P.W. Robertson, and A.R. Rosenberg, *Post-streptococcal glomerulonephritis in Sydney: a 16-year retrospective review.* J Paediatr Child Health, 2007. 43(6): p. 446-50.

[52] Eison, T.M., et al., *Post-streptococcal acute glomerulonephritis in children: clinical features and pathogenesis.* Pediatr Nephrol, 2011. 26(2): p. 165-80.

[53] Sesso, R. and S.W. Pinto, *Five-year follow-up of patients with epidemic glomerulonephritis due to Streptococcus zooepidemicus.* Nephrol Dial Transplant, 2005. 20(9): p. 1808-12.

[54] Sesso, R., S. Wyton, and L. Pinto, *Epidemic glomerulonephritis due to Streptococcus zooepidemicus in Nova Serrana, Brazil.* Kidney Int Suppl, 2005(97): p. S132-6.

[55] Gheissari, A., et al., *Outcome of Iranian children with mild post streptococcal glomerulonephritis.* Saudi J Kidney Dis Transpl, 2010. 21(3): p. 571-4.

[56] Yamagata, K., et al., *Chronic kidney disease perspectives in Japan and the importance of urinalysis screening.* Clin Exp Nephrol, 2008. 12(1): p. 1-8.

[57] Hoy, W., et al., *Stemming the tide: reducing cardiovascular disease and renal failure in Australian Aborigines.* Aust N Z J Med, 1999. 29(3): p. 480-3.

9

Atypical Clinical Manifestations of Acute Poststreptococcal Glomerulonephritis

Toru Watanabe

Department of Pediatrics, Niigata City General Hospital
Japan

1. Introduction

Acute poststreptococcal glomerulonephritis (APSGN) is one of the most common and important renal diseases resulting from a prior infection with group A β-hemolytic streptococcus (GAS) (Ash and Ingulli, 2008). Typical clinical features of the disease include an acute onset with gross hematuria, edema, hypertension and moderate proteinuria (acute nephritic syndrome) 1 to 2 weeks after an antecedent streptococcal pharyngitis or 3 to 6 weeks after a streptococcal pyoderma (Ahn & Ingulli 2008; Rodriguez-Iturbe & Mezzano, 2009). Gross hematuria usually disappears after a few days, while edema and hypertension subside in 5 to 10 days (Rodriguez-Iturbe & Mezzano, 2009). Although the incidence of APSGN appears to be decreasing in industrialized countries, more than 472,000 cases with APSGN are estimated to occur each year worldwide, with 97% of them occurring in developing countries (Carapetis et al., 2005; Eison et al., 2010).

APSGN occurs most commonly in children, 5 to 12 years old (Ahn & Ingulli, 2008), although 5 to 10 percent of the patients are more than 40 years old (Yoshizawa, 2000). The immediate and long-term prognoses of APSGN are excellent for children, assuming it is diagnosed in a timely fashion (Kasahara et al., 2001, Rodriguez-Iturbe & Musser, 2008). In contrast, adult patients with APSGN show markedly worse prognoses both in the acute phase and in the long-term (Rodriguez-Iturbe & Musser, 2008).

The most popular theory of the pathogenic mechanism of APSGN has been the immune-complex theory, which involves the glomerular deposition of nephritogenic streptococcal antigen and subsequent formation of immune complexes *in situ* and/or the deposition of circulating antigen-antibody complexes (Oda et al., 2010). Two antigens have been actively investigated as the potential causes of APSGN (Rodriguez-Iturbe & Musser, 2008): the nephritis-associated plasmin receptor (NAPlr) also known as streptococcal glyceraldehyde-3-phosphate dehydrogenase (Yamakami et al., 2000; Yoshizawa et al., 2004), and a cationic cysteine proteinase known as streptococcal pyogenic exotoxin B (SPEB) (Batsford et al., 2005).

Patients with APSGN sometimes exhibit atypical or unusual clinical manifestations, which may lead to diagnostic delay or misdiagnosis of the disorder (Eison et al. 2011; Pais et al. 2008). Recognition of these unusual manifestations in cases of APSGN is important in order to assure that the patient receives adequate treatment. In this chapter, I review the atypical clinical manifestations of APSGN.

2. Atypical manifestations of APSGN

Atypical manifestations of APSGN can be classified as the following: co-occurrence of immune-mediated diseases; non immune-mediated complications; and unusual clinical presentations or courses (Table 1).

Immune-mediated diseases
    Acute rheumatic fever (ARF)
    Poststreptococcal reactive arthritis (PSRA)
    Vasculitis
    Immune thrombocytopenic purpura (ITP)
    Autoimmune hemolytic anemia (AIHA)
    Diffuse alveolar hemorrhage (DAH)
    Uveitis

Non immune-mediated complications
    Posterior reversible encephalopathy syndrome (PRES)
    Thrombotic microangiopathy (TMA)
    Gallbladder wall thickening

Unusual clinical presentations or courses
    Minimal urinary abnormalities
    Recurrence

Table 1. Atypical manifestations of acute poststreptococcal glomerulonephritis

2.1 Immune-mediated diseases

Immune-mediated diseases most likely result from immune-complex formation between streptococcal antigens and their associated antibodies, and include acute rheumatic fever, poststreptococcal reactive arthritis, vasculitis, immune thrombocytopenic purpura, autoimmune hemolytic anemia, diffuse alveolar hemorrhage and uveitis.

2.1.1 Acute rheumatic fever

Acute rheumatic fever (ARF) is an autoimmune disease that follows infection by GAS and is characterized by inflammation of several tissues that gives rise to typical clinical characteristics (the so-called Jones criteria) including carditis/valvulitis, arthritis, chorea, erythema marginatum, and subcutaneous nodules (Steer & Carapetis, 2009). ARF is rare in developed countries, but it remains common in developing countries and some poor, mainly indigenous populations of wealthy countries (Steer & Carapetis, 2009; Carapetis et al., 2005).

Although both ARF and APSGN develop following GAS infection, the two diseases have different epidemiology, immunology and bacteriology, and simultaneous occurrence of them in the same patient is rare (Lin et al., 2007). Since Gibney et al. first reported a patient with co-occurrence of ARF and histologically proven APSGN (Gibney et al., 1981), seventeen patients with concurrent ARF and APSGN have been reported (Akasheh et al., 1995; Ben-Dov et al., 1985; Castillejos et al., 1985; Imanaka et al., 1995; Kakkera et al., 1998; Kujala et al., 1989; Kula et al., 2003; Kwong et al., 1987; Lin et al., 2003; Mastell et al., 1990; Öner, et al., 1993; Said et al., 1986; Sieck et al., 1992; Sinha et al., 2007).

Fourteen patients were children and ten were male. Eight patients initially presented with ARF preceding APSGN, 3 patients suffered from ARF following the development of APSGN and both ARF and APSGN simultaneously occurred in 6 patients. Although many patients showed carditis (16 out of 17 patients) and polyarthritis (13 out of 17 patients), the remaining characteristics (erythema marginatum, chorea and subcutaneous nodules) developed in only 4 patients, 1 patient and 1 patient, respectively.

Although it remains unclear why simultaneous occurrence of APSGN and ARF is so rare, one explanation may be that only few streptococcal strains have both nephritogenic and rheumatogenic antigenic features (Lin et al., 2003).

2.1.2 Poststreptococcal reactive arthritis

Poststreptococcal reactive arthritis (PSRA) is defined as acute arthritis of more than 1 joint following an episode of GAS infection in a patient whose illness does not fulfill the Jones criteria for the diagnosis of ARF (Barash et al., 2008; Gerber M, 2007). It remains controversial whether or not PRSA and ARF are distinct entities or not (Gerber M, 2007). Mackie and Keat reviewed 188 published cases of PSRA and concluded that PSRA was a heterogenous group of clinical entities (Mackie & Keat, 2004). However, two recent studies suggested that PSRA and ARF were separate disease entities on the basis of the differences in clinical presentation and disease course (Barash et al., 2008; van der Helm-van Mil, 2010). Compared to patients with ARF, patients with PSRA are older, respond poorer to salicylates and have non-migratory and persistent arthritis (Tokura et al., 2008; van der Helm-van Mil, 2010). The precise pathogenic mechanism underlying the development of PSRA is unclear, production of antistreptococcal antibodies that cross-react with human epitopes causing inflammation and tissue damage is a likely pathogenic mechanism for PSRA, as has been proposed for ARF (Niewold & Ghosh, 2003).

Simultaneous occurrence of PSRA and APSGN is rare, with only 3 cases having been reported (Niewold & Ghosh, 2003; Sugimoto et al., 2008; Tokura et al., 2008). Niewold & Ghosh described a 44-year-old man who developed severe PSRA and APSGN after a subclinical streptococcal infection (Niewold & Ghosh, 2003). Tokura et al. reported a 16-year-old man who presented with simultaneous occurrence of APSGN and PSRA with symmetric persistent tenosynovitis in hands and feet (Tokura et al., 2008). Sugimoto et al. described a 61-year-old man who exhibited PSRA and APSGN with marked renal interstitial inflammation after bacterial endophthalmitis due to *Streptococcus pyogenes* (Sugimoto et al., 2008). Arthritis of all the patients improved with corticosteroid therapies without any sequellae.

2.1.3 Vasculitis

Vasculitis is not a well-recognized condition associated with GAS infection, but there have been several reports of Henoch-Schönlein purpura (HSP) (al-Sheyyab et al., 1999) or Henoch-Schönlein purpura with nephritis (HSPN) (Masuda et al., 2003), cutaneous leukocytoclastic vasculitis (Chalkias et al, 2010), vasculitic neuropathy (Traverso et al., 1997), polyarteritis nodosa (PN) (David et al., 1993) and unclassified systemic vasculitis (Lucas & Moxham, 1978). Although the precise pathogenic role of GAS infection contributing to the development of vasculitis remains unclear, an immune complex-mediated mechanism triggered by GAS infection has been postulated (Ritt M. et al., 2006).

Vasculitides including cutaneous vasculitis mimicking HSP, cerebral vasculitis, PN, necrotizing vasculitis and Wegener's granulomatosis have been described to occur in patients with APSGN.

HSP is an IgA immune complex-mediated systemic leukocytoclastic vasculitis of small vessels that primarily affects the skin, gastrointestinal tract, joints and kidney (Dedeoglu & Sundel, 2007; Robson & Leung , 1994). Respiratory infections with GAS preceding the onset of HSP have been reported in up to one-third of cases (Dedeoglu & Sundel, 2007). APSGN patients simultaneously presenting with HSP or vasculitis mimicking HSP are rare and only five patients have been reported. Goodyer et al. described two boys with histologically proven APSGN, in whom cutaneous vasculitis and abdominal symptoms mimicked HSP (Goody et al., 1978). Onisawa et al. reported a patient with concurrent APSGN and cutaneous leukocytoclastic vasculitis without IgA deposition (Onisawa et al., 1989). Maruyama et al. presented a patient with congenital complement 9 deficiency exhibiting biopsy-proven APSGN and clinical symptoms mimicking HSP (Maruyama et al., 1995). Matsukura et al. also described a 20-month-old girl with biopsy-proven APSGN, who presented with cutaneous vasculitis mimicking HSP (Matsukura et al., 2003). All patients recovered completely without any sequellae.

Central nervous system abnormalities of APSGN are usually secondary to acute severe hypertension, electrolyte disturbances or uremia, but can also be attributed to cerebral vasculitis (Dursun et al., 2008; Ritt et al., 2006). To date, five cases of cerebral vasculitis associated with APSGN have been reported (Dursun et al., 2008; Kaplan et al., 1993; Ritt et al., 2006; Rovang et al., 1997; Wong & Morris, 2001), in which 4 patients were children. Clinical features of cerebral vasculitis in APSGN include severe headache with nausea and vomiting, transient focal neurological signs, visual disturbances, and seizures. Although the computed tomography of the brain may not detect abnormalities, the magnetic resonance imaging of the brain often demonstrated multiple supratentorial areas of abnormal signal intensity in the white and adjacent grey matter (Dursun et al., 2008). All patients underwent corticosteroid therapy (three of them commenced on methylprednisolone pulse therapy) and recovered without any neurological sequellae.

PN is a necrotizing vasculitis affecting the medium-sized muscular arteries (Dillon et al., 2010). Five patients with co-occurrence with PN and APSGN have been described. Fordham et al. reported three young adult patients with both PN and APSGN, two of whom died secondary to multi-system organ failure (Fordham et al., 1964). Blau et al. described two children with PN who also had serological and clinical evidence of APSGN (Blau et al., 1977).

Although extremely rare, necrotizing vasculitis other than PN (Bodaghi et al., 1987; Ingelfinger et al., 1977) and Wegener's granulomatosis (Garrett et al., 1993) has also been reported in patients with APSGN.

2.1.4 Immune thrombocytopenic purpura

Immune thrombocytopenic purpura (ITP) is an immune-mediated acquired disorder in which antiplatelet antibodies cause accelerated destruction of platelets, resulting in thrombocytopenia and an increase risk of bleeding (Psaila & Bussel, 2007). Childhood ITP often occurs following an infection with viruses such as varicella zoster, rubella, Epstein-Barr, influenza, or human immunodeficiency virus (Tasic & Polenakovic, 2003), but may also be preceded by a bacterial infection (Muguruma et al., 2000). Recently, a number of studies have suggested an association between *Helicobacter pylori* and ITP (Cooper & Bussel, 2006).

Since Kaplan and Esseltine first reported ITP in two patients with APSGN (Kaplan & Esseltine, 1978), five cases of ITP in patients with APSGN have been reported (Muguruma et al., 2000; Rizkallah et al., 1984; Tasic & Polenakov, 2003). All patients were children (4 to 7 years of age) who underwent corticosteroid therapy and fully recovered from APSGN and

ITP. One patient exhibited a marked increase in platelet-associated immunoglobulin G level (Muguruma et al., 2000). Although the precise pathogenic mechanism for the development of ITP in patients with APSGN is unclear, Muguruma et al. speculated about the pathogenesis of associated diseases through production of autoantibodies cross-reactive against GAS and against platelets (Muguruma et al., 2000).

2.1.5 Autoimmune hemolytic anemia
Anemia is common in APSGN and traditionally it has been attributed solely to volume overload (Eison et al., 2011). However, autoimmune hemolytic anemia (AIHA) has recently been reported in patients with APSGN. AIHA is a clinical condition in which IgG and/or IgM antibodies bind to red blood cells (RBC) surface antigens and initiate RBC destruction via the complement system and the reticuloendothelial system (Gehrs & Friedberg, 2002). Subtypes include warm AIHA, cold AIHA, mixed-type AIHA and drug-induced immune hemolytic anemia. Furthermore, cold AIHA has been categorized into cold agglutinin syndrome (CAS) and paroxysmal cold hemoglobinuria (PCH). Infectious agents associated with CAS or PCH include *Mycoplasma pneumonia*, Epstein-Barr virus, adenovirus, cytomegalovirus, influenza viruses, human immunodeficiency virus, measles, mumps, *Escherichia coli, Listeria monocytogenes, Haemophilus influenza* and *Treponema pallidum* (Gehrs & Friedberg, 2002).
Greenbaum et al. described three children with both APSGN and cold AIHA, two of whom had an anti-I autoantibody and thereby were diagnosed with CAS (Greenbaum et al., 2003). Two patients were transfused and all patients recovered from AIHA and APSGN. Cachat et al. presented a 10-year-old child with concurrent cold AIHA and APSGN, who developed anuric acute renal failure and profound anemia (Cachat et al., 2003). The patient responded well to corticosteroid therapy and had a full renal and hematological recovery.

2.1.6 Diffuse alveolar hemorrhage
Diffuse alveolar hemorrhage (DAH) is sometimes accompanied by glomerulonephritis, and is often referred to as pulmonary-renal syndrome (Papiris et al., 2007). Pulmonary-renal syndromes include Goodpasture's syndrome, antineutrophil cytoplasmic antibody-associated vasculitis, immune complex-associated glomerulopathy and thrombotic microangiopathy (Papiris et al., 2007).
DAH associated with APSGN is extremely rare and only three patients have been reported. Chugh et al. described a 38-year-old-male with concurrent DAH and crescentic APSGN who progressed to end-stage renal failure (Chugh et al., 1981). Gilboa et al. reported a 12-year-old girl who exhibited a noncrescentic APSGN and DAH (Gilboa et al., 1993). Sung et al. recently described a 59-year-old-woman with APSGN and DAH (Sung et al., 2007). DAH in all three patients subsided after intravenous corticosteroid therapies. The pathogenic mechanism of DAH in APSGN remains unclear.

2.1.7 Uveitis
Uveitis is believed to be an immunological response to exogenous and endogenous antigens (Leiba et al., 1998) and can occur following GAS infection, so-called "poststreptococcal uveitis". Since Cokingtin & Han reported the first case of poststreptococcal uveitis in 1991 (Cokingtin & Han, 1991), several patient reports and case series with poststreptococcal uveitis have been presented (Leiba et al., 1998, Ur Rehman et al., 2006).

Feldon et al. recently reported the first case of a child with concomitant APSGN and uveitis, whose uveitis subsided within a few days with topical corticosteroid and mydriatic treatment (Feldon et al., 2010).

2.2 Non immune-mediated complications

Non immune-mediated complications of APSGN include posterior reversible encephalopathy syndrome, thrombotic microangiopathy and gallbladder wall thickening.

2.2.1 Posterior reversible encephalopathy syndrome

Posterior reversible encephalopathy syndrome (PRES), also known as reversible posterior leukoencephalopathy syndrome (RPLS), is a recently described brain disorder associated with findings on neuroimaging that suggest white-matter edema, mostly in the posterior parietal-temporal-occipital regions of the brain (Hinchey et al., 1996). However, radiological lesions in PRES are rarely isolated to these areas, and often involve the cortex, frontal lobes, basal ganglia and brainstem (Fugate et al., 2010) (Fig. 1).

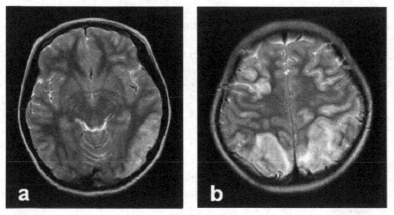

Fig. 1. Magnetic resonance images (MRI) of the brain (T2-weighted image) showing increased intensity in the cortex and subcortical white matter of left occipital (a), bilateral parietal and right frontal lobes (b), consistent with PRES.

The clinical characteristics of the disease include headache, decreased alertness, altered mental functioning, seizures, and visual loss including cortical blindness (Hinchey et al., 1996). The syndrome has been associated with acute hypertension, preeclampsia or eclampsia, glomerulonephritis, sepsis, autoimmune disorders and immunosuppressive or chemotherapeutic treatments (Bartynski, 2008a; Hinchey et al., 1996). Although the underlying pathophysiology of PRES remains elusive, three theories have been proposed: 1) hypertension-induced breakdown in cerebral auto-regulation; 2) cerebrovascular endothelial dysfunction and; 3) vasoconstriction and hypoperfusion with subsequent ischemia and vasogenic edema (Bartynski, 2008b; Fugate et al., 2010). The preferential involvement of the posterior brain in PRES may be caused by its relative paucity of sympathetic innervation in comparison to the anterior circulation (Froehlich et al., 1999). The outcome of PRES is generally favorable, but delay in initiating the appropriate treatment may result in permanent damage to the brain (Fux et al., 2006; Garg, 2001).

While it is estimated that PRES occurs in 5% to 10% of children hospitalized with acute glomerulonephritis of all etiologies, the prevalence of PRES associated with APSGN is unknown (Froehlich et al., 1999). PRES caused by hypertension has been reported in 7 children (from 7 to 15 years of age) with APSGN (Froehlich et al., 1999; Fux et al., 2006; Guputa et al., 2010; Nordby, 1997; Özcakar et al., 2004; Soylu et al., 2001). Six patients complained of headache, 5 exhibited decreased alertness and seizures, and 3 had altered mental functioning and visual loss. All patients exhibited abnormal findings of the brain MRI or CT in the white matter of the parietal and occipital lobes, and recovered without any neurological sequellae following adequate treatment of the associated hypertension.

One patient with APSGN suffered from PRES without severe hypertension (Nordby, 1997). The most important factor in development of pediatric hypertensive PRES is the rapidity of blood pressure elevation and the degree of elevation relative to the patient's baseline pressure (Froehlich et al., 1999). It has been suggested that blood pressures more than 30% above normal for age should alert clinicians to the possibility of hypertensive PRES (Nordby, 1997).

2.2.2 Thrombotic microangiopathy

Thrombotic microangiopathy (TMA) is a pathological term used to describe occlusive microvascular thrombus formation and is most commonly associated with hemolytic uremic syndrome (HUS) and thrombotic thrombocytopenic purpura (TTP) (Keir & Coward, 2010). Pathological features of TMA include vessel wall thickening, swelling and detachment of the endothelial cell from the basement membrane, accumulation of material in the subendothelial space, intraluminal platelet thrombosis, partial or complete vessel luminal obstruction and fragmentation of red blood cells (Keir & Coward, 2010). HUS is defined as the triad of microangiopathic hemolytic anemia, thrombocytopenia, and acute renal injury (Copelovitch & Kaplan, 2008). TTP is characterized by the pentad of microangiopathic hemolytic anemia, thrombocytopenia, fever, acute renal injury, and neurological abnormalities (Copelovitch & Kaplan, 2008).

TMA has been reported in 8 patients with APSGN, consisting of 5 children and 3 adults (Duvic et al., 2000; Izumi, et al., 2005; Laube, et al., 2001; Medani et al., 1987; Proesmans, 1996; Siebels et al., 1995; Tan et al., 1998). All patients exhibited severe hypertension. Hemodialysis or peritoneal dialysis was required in 2 patients. Renal biopsy showed histological features of both APSGN and TMA in 3 patients, and revealed characteristics of APSGN without features of TMA in 5 patients. The outcome in all patients was excellent.

The precise pathogenesis of TMA in patients with APSGN is unclear, although two causes have been postulated: severe hypertension and streptococcal neuraminidase (Duvic et al., 2000; Laube et al., 2001; Izumi et al., 2005). HUS has been reported as a complication of severe hypertension, regardless of the cause (Broyer, 1995). If severe hypertension is transient, histological lesions of TMA are absent. When hypertension becomes malignant, renal histological lesions show features of TMA (Duvic et al., 2000). Another possible cause of TMA in APSGN is alteration of vascular endothelial cells by streptococcal neuraminidase. Circulating neuraminidase causes exposure of the cryptic T-antigen on cell surfaces, to which most people possess a naturally occurring antibody. Therefore antigen-antibody interaction may damage the vascular endothelial cells leading to the clinical manifestations of HUS (Izumi et al., 2005).

2.2.3 Gallbladder wall thickening

Thickening of the gallbladder wall is the most common findings in acute cholecystitis, but it has also been reported in patients with kidney diseases including pyelonephritis (Talarico & Rubens, 1990) and chronic kidney failure (van Breda Vriesman et al., 2007). Only one child with APSGN and gallbladder wall thickening has been reported (Watanabe & Baba, 2009). Although the pathogenesis of this complication is unclear, elevated systemic venous pressure or subclinical vasculitis may have caused edema of the gallbladder wall (Watanabe & Baba, 2009).

2.3 Unusual clinical presentations or courses

Unusual clinical presentations or courses of APSGN include acute nephritic syndrome with minimal urinary abnormalities, and recurrence of the disease.

2.3.1 Minimal urinary abnormalities

Patients with APSGN usually exhibit hematuria and proteinuria. However, Blumberg and Feldman first reported two children with biopsy-proven APSGN without any urinary abnormalities (Blumberg & Feldman, 1962). Thereafter, several authors described biopsy-proven APSGN patients with minimal or no urinary abnormalities including 13 children and 4 adult patients (Albert et al., 1966; Cohen & Levitt, 1963; Dunn, 1967; Fujinaga et al., 2007; Goorno et al., 1967; Grossman et al., 1973; Hoyer et al., 1967; Kandall et al., 1969; Kobayashi et al., 1971). All patients exhibited edema and hypertension, and seven showed pulmonary edema or congestion. Hypertensive encephalopathy occurred in one patient (Hoyer et al., 1967) and acute rheumatic fever developed in another patient (Cohen & Levitt, 1963). All patients recovered completely without any sequellae. The mechanism for the elaboration on normal or minimal urinary abnormalities during the course of APSGN is unclear (Fujinaga et al., 2007; Kandall et al., 1969).

2.3.2 Recurrence

Recurrence of APSGN is a well-recognized, but relatively rare phenomenon, probably due to the relatively limited number of nephritogenic strains of streptococci and the acquisition of protective immunity against a nephritogenic streptococcal antigen after an initial episode of APSGN (Watanabe & Yoshizawa, 2001). Ramberg first mentioned this condition and reported eleven patients with the recurrent attacks out of 152 patients with APSGN (Ramberg, 1947). Thereafter, several clinical studies of APSGN have suggested an incidence of recurrent APSGN that ranges from 0.7% to 7.0% (Baldwin D et al., 1974; Bernstein et al., 1960; Dodge W. et al., 1968; Sanjad et al., 1977; Roy et al., 1969). In addition, a few case reports of recurrent APSGN have been described (Casquero et al., 2006; Derakhshan 2002; Kim et al., 1979; Rosenberg et al., 1984; Velhote et al., 1986; Watanabe & Yoshizawa, 2001). Clinical features and outcomes were well-described in 35 patients including 22 children. Most patients suffered from one recurrent episode, but one patient exhibited 2 recurrent attacks of APSGN (Velhote et al., 1986). Twenty-nine patients recovered completely, whilst 4 patients continued to have some urinary abnormalities and two patients progressed to end-stage renal failure.

Although the exact mechanism leading to recurrence of APSGN has not yet been determined, three possible explanations have been postulated: the suppression of immune response against nephritogenic streptococcal strains due to early antibiotic therapy (Roy et al., 1969; Sanjad et al., 1977); an absence of natural immune responses against nephritogenic streptococcal components without antibiotic therapy (Watanabe & Yoshizawa, 2001), and; a failure to exclude microbial agents through the digestive and respiratory tract due to IgA deficiency (Casquero et al., 2006).

Sanjado et al. suggested that reinfection with the same type of *Streptococcus* would occur if the patient lacked antibodies against that particular type, and penicillin therapy given in the first ten days after a streptococcal infection suppressed the formation of type-specific immunity conferring antibodies, which might increase the chances of re-infection with the same nephritogenic strain responsible for the initial episode of APSGN (Sanjad et al., 1977).

Recently, Yoshizawa et al. identified a new nephritogenic streptococcal antigen and termed it nephritis-associated plasmin receptor (NAPlr) (Yamakami et al., 2000; Yoshizawa et al., 2004). They demonstrated that most patients with APSGN had high titers of long-lasting antibody against NAPlr and that it was present in glomeruli in 100% of patients with APSGN early in the disease (Yoshizawa et al., 2004). Watanabe and Yoshizawa described an 8-year-old boy with recurrent ASPGN who did not have serum antibodies against NAPlr, even though NAPlr was detected in glomeruli of an early kidney biopsy specimen from the patient during the second attack of APSGN. These results indicated that recurrence of APSGN in some patients might be caused by an absence of a natural immune response to NAPlr (Watanabe & Yoshizawa, 2001).

Recently, Casquero et al. published a patient with selective IgA deficiency who experienced two episodes of APSGN (Casquero et al., 2006), suggesting that a failure of IgA defenses might also predispose to streptococcal re-infection and cause recurrent APSGN.

3. Conclusions

Patients with APSGN sometimes exhibit atypical or unusual clinical manifestations, which are divided into 3 categories: immune-mediated diseases (ARF, PSRA, vasculitis, ITP, AIHA, DAH and uveitis), non-immune mediated conditions (PRES, TMA and gallbladder wall thickening), and unusual clinical presentations or courses (minimal urinary abnormalities and recurrence).

Immune-mediated diseases seem to result from immune-complex formation between streptococcal antigens and their associated antibodies. Hypertension contributes to the development of PRES and TMA, while fluid retention results in PRES and gallbladder wall thickening. Recurrence of APSGN may be the consequence of suppressed immune responses against nephritogenic streptococcal strains caused by early antibiotic therapy, by the absence of natural immune responses against NAPlr, or by selective IgA deficiency.

Because atypical or unusual manifestations of APSGN may lead to diagnostic delays or misdiagnosis of the disorder, recognition of them is important in order to assure that the patient receives adequate treatment.

4. References

Ahn S., Ingulli E. (2008). Acute poststreptococcal glomerulonephritis: an update. *Current Opinion in Pediatrics,* Vol.20, No.2, (April 2008), pp. 157-162, ISSN 1040-8703

Akasheh M., al-Lozi M., Affarah H., Hajjiri F. al-Jitawi S. (1995). Rapidly progressive glomerulonephritis complicating acute rheumatic fever. *Postgraduate Medical Journal,* Vol.71, No.839, (September 1995), pp. 553-554, ISSN 0032-5473

Albert M., Leeming J. & Scaglione P. (1966). Acute glomerulonephritis without abnormality of the urine. *Journal of Pediatrics*, Vol.68, No.4, (April 1966), pp. 525-529, ISSN 0022-3476

al-Sheyyab M., Batieha A., el-Shanti H. & Daoud A. (1999). Henoch-Schönlein purpura and streptococcal infection: a prospective case-control study. *Annals of Tropical Paediatrics*, Vol.19, No.3, (September 1999), pp. 253-255, ISSN 0272-4936

Baldwin D., Gluck M., Schacht R. & Gallo G. (1974). The long-term course of poststreptococcal glomerulonephritis. *Annals of Internal Medicine*, Vol.80, No.3, (March 1974), pp. 342-358, ISSN 0003-4819

Barash J., Mashiach E., Navon-Elkan P., Berkun Y., Harel L., Tauber T., Padeh S., Hashkes P. & Uziel Y. (2008). Differentiation of post-streptococcal reactive arthritis from acute rheumatic fever. *Journal of Pediatrics*, Vol.153 No.5, (November 2008), pp. 696-699, ISSN 0022-1476

Bartynski W. (2008a). Posterior reversible encephalopathy syndrome, part 1: fundamental imaging and clinical features. *American Journal of Nueroradiology*, Vol.29, No.6, (June 2008), pp. 1036-1042, ISSN 0915-6108

Bartynski W. (2008b). Posterior reversible encephalopathy syndrome, part 2: controversies surrounding pathophysiology of vasogenic edema. *American Journal of Nueroradiology*, Vol.29, No.6, (June 2008), pp. 1043-1049, ISSN 0915-6108

Batsford S., Mezzano S., Mihatsch M., Schiltz E. & Rodriguez-Iturbe B. (2005). Is the nephritogenic antigen in post-streptococcal glomerulonephritis pyogenic exotoxin B (SPE B) or GAPDH? *Kidney International*, Vol.68, No.3, (September 2005), pp. 1120-1129, ISSN 0085-2538

Ben-Dov I., Berry E. & Kopolovic J. (1985). Poststreptococcal nephritis and acute rheumatic fever in two adults. *Archives of Internal Medicine*, Vol.145, No.2, (February 1985), pp. 338-339, ISSN 0003-9926

Bernstein S. & Stillerman M. (1960). A study of the association of group A streptococci with acute glomerulonephritis. *Annals of Internal Medicine*, Vol.52, (May 1960), pp. 1026-1034, ISSN 0003-4819

Blau E., Morris R. & Yunis E. Polyarteritis nodosa in older children. *Pediatrics*, Vol.60, No.2, (August 1977), pp. 227-234, ISSN 0031-4005

Blumberg R. & Feldman D. (1962). Observations on acute glomerulonephritis associated with impetigo. *Journal of Pediatrics*, Vol.60, (May 1962), pp. 677-685, ISSN 0022-3476

Bodaghi E., Kheradpir K. & Maddah M. (1987). Vasculitis in acute streptococcal glomerulonephritis. *International Journal of Pediatric Nephrology*, Vol.8, No.2, (April-June 1987), pp. 69-74, ISSN 0391-6510

Broyer M. (1995). Commentary. *Pediatric Nephrology*, Vol.9, No.3, (June 1995), pp. 392-394, ISSN 0931-041X

Cachat F., Dunsmore K. & Tufro A. (2003). Concomitant anuric post-streptococcal glomerulonephritis and autoimmune hemolytic anemia. *European Journal of Pediatrics*, Vol.162, No.7-8, (July 2003), pp. 552-553, ISSN 0340-6199ah

Carapetis J., Steer A., Mulholland E., & Weber M. (2005). The global burden of group A streptococcal diseases. *Lancet Infectious Disease*, Vol.5, No.11, (November 2005), pp. 685-694, ISSN 1473-3099

Carapetis J., McDonald M. & Wilson N. (2005). Acute rheumatic fever. *Lancet*, Vol. 366, No. 9480, (July 2005), pp. 155-168, ISSN 0140-6736

Casquero A., Ramos A., Barat A., Mampaso F., Caramelo C., Egido J. & Oriz A. (2006). Recurrent acute postinfectious glomerulonephritis, *Clinical Nephrology*, Vol.66, No.1, (July 2006), pp. 51-53, ISSN 0301-0430

Castillejos G., Padilla L., Lerma A., González S. & Reyes P. (1985). Coincidence of acute rheumatic fever and acute post streptococcal glomerulonephritis. *Journal of Rheumatology*, Vol.12, No.3, (June 1985), pp. 587-589, ISSN 0263-7103

Chalkias S., Samson S., Tiniakou E. & Sofair S. (2010). Poststreptococcal cutaneous leukocytoclastic vasculitis: a case report. *Connecticut Medicine*, Vol.74, No.7, (August 2010), pp. 399-402, ISSN 0010-6178

Chugh K., Gupta V., Singhal P. & Sehgal S. (1981). Case report: poststreptococcal crescentic glomerulonephritis and pulmonary hemorrhage simulating Goodpasture's syndrome. *Annals of Allergy*, Vol.47, No.2, (August 1981), pp. 104-106, ISSN 0003-4738

Cohen J. & Levitt M. (1963). Acute glomerulonephritis with few urinary abnormalities. Report of two cases proved by renal biopsy. *New England Journal of Medicine*, Vol.268, (April 1963), pp. 749-753, ISSN 0028-4793

Cokingtin C. & Han D. (1991). Bilateral nongranulomatous uveitis and a poststreptococcal syndrome. *American Journal of Ophthalmology*, Vol.112, No.5, (November 1991), pp. 595-596, ISSN 0002-9394

Cooper N. & Bussel J. (2006). The pathogenesis of immune thrombocytopenic purpura. *British Journal of Haematology*, Vol.133, No.4, (May 2006), pp. 364-374, ISSN 0007-1048

Copelovitch L. & Kaplan B. (2008). The thrombotic microangiopathies. *Pediatric Nephrology*, Vol.23, No.10, (October 2008), pp. 1761-1767, ISSN 0931-041X

David J., Ansell B. & Woo P. (1993). Polyarteritis nodosa associated with streptococcus. *Archives of Disease in Childhood*, Vol.69, No.6, (December 1993), pp. 685-688, ISSN 0003-9888

Dedeoglu F. & Sundel R. (2007). Vasculitis in children. *Rheumatic Diseases Clinics of North America*, Vol.33, No.3, (August 2007), pp. 555-583, ISSN 6889-857X

Derakhshan A. (2002). Another case of acute poststreptococcal glomerulonephritis with recurrence. *Pediatric Nephrology*, Vol.17, No.6, (June 2002), pp. 462, ISSN 0931-041X

Dillon M., Eleftheriou D. & Brogan P. (2010). Medium-size-vessel vasculitis. *Pediatric Nephrology*, Vol.25, No.9, (September 2010), pp. 1641-1652, ISSN 0931-041X

Dodge W., Spargo B., Basss J. & Travis L. (1968). The relationship between the clinical and pathologic features of poststreptococcal glomerulonephritis. A study of the early natural history. *Medicine*, Vol.47, No.3, pp. 227-267, ISSN 0025-7974

Dunn M. (1967). Acute glomerulonephritis with normal results from urinalyses. A report of two cases and comments on four additional cases with atypical findings from urinalyses. *Journal of the American Medical Association*, Vol. 201, No.12, (September, 1967), pp. 933-937, ISSN 0098-7484

Dursun I., Gunduz Z., Poyrazoglu H., Gumus H., Yilkilmaz A. & Dusunsel R. (2008). Cerebral vasculitis and unilateral sixth-nerve palsy in acute post-streptococcal glomerulonephritis. Annals of Tropical Paediatrics, Vol.28, No.2, (June 2008), pp. 155-159, ISSN 0272-4936

Duvic C., Desramé J., Hérody M. & Nédélec G. (2000). Acute poststreptococcal glomerulonephritis associated with thrombotic microangiopathy in an adult. *Clinical Nephrology*, Vol.54, No.2, (August 2000), pp. 169-173, ISSN 0301-0430

Eison T., Ault B., Jones D., Chesney R., & Wyatt R. (2011). Post-streptococcal acute glomerulonephritis in children: clinical features and pathogenesis. *Pediatric Nephrology*, Vol.26, No.2 (February 2011), pp. 165-180, ISSN 0931-041X

Feldon M., Dorfman L., Tauber T., Morad Y., Bistritzer T. & Goldman M. (2010). Post-streptococcal glomerulonephritis and uveitis - a case report. *Pediatric Nephrology*, Vol.25, No.11, (November 2010), pp. 2351-2353, ISSN 0931-041X

Fordham C. III, Epstein F., Huffines W. & Harrington J. (1964). Polyarteritis and acute post-streptococcal glomerulonephritis. *Annals of Internal Medicine*, Vol.61, (July 1964), pp. 89-97, ISSN 0003-4819

Froehlich T., Sandifer S., Varma P. & Testa F. (1999). Two cases of hypertension-induced reversible posterior leukoencephalopathy syndrome secondary to glomerulonephritis. *Current Opinion in Pediatrics*, Vol.11, No.6, (December 1999), pp. 512-518, ISSN 1040-8703

Fujinaga S., Ohtomo Y., Umino D., Mochizuki H., Takemoto M., Shimizu T., Yamashiro Y. & Kaneko K. (2007). Pulmonary edema in a boy with biopsy-proven poststreptococcal glomerulonephritis without urinary abnormalities. *Pediatric Nephrology*, Vol.22, No.1, (January 2007), pp. 154-155, ISSN 0931-041X

Fux C., Bianchetti M., Jakob S. & Remonda L. (2006). Reversible encephalopathy complicating post-streptococcal glomerulonephritis. *Pediatric Infectious Disease Journal*, Vol.25, No.1, (January 2006), pp. 85-87, ISSN 0891-3668

Garg R. (2001). Posterior leukoencephalopathy syndrome. *Postgraduate Medical Journal*, Vol.77, No.903, (January 2001), pp. 24-28, ISSN 0032-5473

Garrett P., Bass P., Atchley J., Theaker J. & Dathan J. (1993). Wegener's granulomatosis and acute poststreptococcal glomerulonephritis. *Nephrology Dialysis and Transplantation*, Vol.8, No.5, pp. 454-455, ISSN 0931-0509

Geber M. (2007). Group A streptococcus, In: *Nelson Textbook of Pediatrics*, M.A. Greber, R.M. Kiegman, R.E. Behrman, H.B. Jenson & B.F. Stanton, (Ed.), pp. 1135-1145, Saunders, ISBN 918-1-4160-2450-7, Philadelphia, USA

Gehrs B. & Friedberg R. (2002). Autoimmune hemolytic anemia. *American Journal of Hematology*, Vol.69, No.4, (April 2002), pp. 258-271, ISSN 0361-8609

Gibney R., Reineck H., Bannayan G. & Stein J. (1981). Renal lesions in acute rheumatic fever. *Annals of Internal Medicine*, Vol.94, No.3, (March 1981), pp. 322-326, ISSN 0003-4819

Gilboa N., McIntire S., Hopp L. & Ellis D. (1993). Acute noncrescentic poststreptococcal glomerulonephritis presenting with pulmonary hemorrhage. *Pediatric Nephrology*, Vol.7, No.2, (April 1993), pp. 147-150, ISSN 0931-041X

Glozt D., Jouvin M., Nochy D., Druet P. & Bariety J. (1991). Recurrent acute glomerulonephritis. *American Journal of Kidney Diseases*, Vol.17, No.2, (February 1991), pp. 228-230, ISSN 0272-6386

Goodyer P., de Chadarevian J. & Kaplan B. (1978). Acute poststreptococcal glomerulonephritis mimicking Henoch-Schönlein purpura. *Journal of Pediatrics*, Vol.93, No.3, (September 1978), pp. 412-415, ISSN 0022-3476

Goorno W., Ashworth C., & Carter N. (1967). Acute glomerulonephritis with absence of abnormal urinary findings. Diagnosis by light and electron microscopy. *Annals of Internal Medicine*, Vol.66, No.2, (February 1967), pp. 345-353, ISSN 0003-4819

Greenbaum L., Kerlin B., Why S., Punzalan R., Trost B., Pan C. & Scott J. (2003). Concurrent poststreptococcal glomerulonephritis and autoimmune hemolytic anemia. *Pediatric Nephrology*, Vol.18, No.12, (December 2003), pp. 1301-1303, ISSN 0931-041X

Grossman A., Ramanathan K. & Fresco R. (1973). Acute glomerulonephritis with minimal urinary abnormalities presenting as hypertension. *Clinical Pediatrics*, Vol.12, No.4, (April 1973), pp. 250-254, ISSN 0009-9228

Gupta S., Goyal V. & Talukdar B. (2010). Reversible posterior leukoencephalopathy syndrome in post streptococcal glomerulonephritis. *Indian Pediatrics*, Vol.47, No. 3, (March 2010), pp. 274-276, ISSN 0019-6061

Hinchey J., Chaves C., Appingnani B., Breen J., Pao L., Wang A., Pessin M., Lamy C., Mas J. & Caplan L. (1996). A reversible posterior leukoencephalopathy syndrome. *New England Journal of Medicine*, Vol.334, No.8, (February 1996), pp. 494-500, ISSN 0028-4793

Hoyer J., Michael A., Fish A. & Good R. (1967). Acute poststreptococcal glomerulonephritis presenting as hypertensive encephalopathy with minimal urinary abnormalities. *Pediatrics*, Vol.39, No.3, (March 1967), pp. 412-417, ISSN 0031-4005

Imanaka H., Eto S., Takei S., Yoshinaga M., Hokonohara A. & Miyata K. (1995). Acute rheumatic fever and poststreptococcal acute glomerulonephritis caused by T serotype 12 Streptococcus. *Acta Paediatrica Japonica*, Vol.37, No.3, (June 1995), pp. 381-383, ISSN 0374-5600

Ingelfinger J., McCluskey R., Schneeberger E. & Grupe W. (1977). Necrotizing arteritis in acute poststreptococcal glomerulonephritis. *Journal of Pediatrics*, Vol.91, No.2, (August 1997), pp. 228-232, ISSN 0022-3476

Izumi T., Hyodo T., Kikuchi Y., Imakiire T., Ikenoue T., Suzuki S., Yoshizawa N. & Miura S. (2005). An adult with acute poststreptococcal glomerulonephritis complicated by hemolytic uremic syndrome and nephrotic syndrome. *American Journal of Kidney Diseases*, Vol.46, No.4, (October 2005), pp. E59-E63, ISSN 0272-6386

Kasahara T., Hayakawa H., Okubo S., Okugawa T., Kabuki N., Tomizawa S., & Uchiyama M. (2001). Prognosis of acute poststreptococcal glomerulonephritis (APSGN) is excellent in children, when adequately diagnosed. *Pediatrics International*, Vol.43, No.4, (August 2001), pp. 364-367, ISSN 1442-200X

Kakkera D., Khan A., Bastawros M., Lao J. & Nudel D. (1998). Acute rheumatic pancarditis associated with poststreptococcal acute glomerulonephritis: a patient report. *Clinical Pediatrics*, Vol.37, No.9, (September 1998), pp. 569-572, ISSN 0009-9228

Kandall S., Edelmann C. Jr & Bernstein J. (1969). Acute poststreptococcal glomerulonephritis. A case with minimal urinary abnormalities. *American journal of Diseases of Children*, Vol.118, No.3, (September 1969), pp. 462-430, ISSN 0002-922X

Kaplan B. & Esseltine D. (1978). Thrombocytopenia in patients with acute post-streptococcal glomerulonephritis. *Journal of Pediatrics*, Vol.93, No.6, (December 1978), pp. 974-976, ISSN 0022-3476

Kaplan R., Zwick D., Hellerstein S., Warady B. & Alon U. (1993). Cerebral vasculitis in acute post-streptococcal glomerulonephritis. *Pediatric Nephrology*, Vol.7, No.2, (April 1993), pp. 194-195, ISSN 0931-041X

Keir L. & Coward R. (2011). Advances in our understanding of the pathogenesis of glomerular thrombotic microangiopathy. *Pediatric Nephrology*, Vol.26, No.4, (April 2011), pp. 523-533, ISSN 0931-041X

Kim P., Park S., Deung Y. & Choi I. (1979). Second attack of acute poststreptococcal glomerulonephritis; reports of two cases. *Yonsei Medical Journal*, Vol.20, No.1, pp. 61-68, ISSN 0513-5796

Kobayashi O. Wada H. & Okawa K. (1971). Extrarenal symptomatic glomerulonephritis in children. *Acta Medica et Biologica*, Vol.19, No.1, (June 1971), pp. 63-74, ISSN 0567-7734

Kujala G., Doshi H. & Brick J. (1989). Rheumatic fever and poststreptococcal glomerulonephritis: a case report. *Arthritis and Rheumatism*, Vol.32, No.2, (February 1989), pp. 236-239, ISSN 0004-3591

Kula S., Saygili A., Tunaoğlu F. & Olguntürk R. (2003). Acute poststreptococcal glomerulonephritis and acute rheumatic fever in the same patient: a case report and review of the literature. *Anadolu Kardiyoloji Dergisi*, Vol.3, No.3, (September 2003), pp. 272-274, ISSN 1302-8723

Kwong Y., Chan K. & Chan M. (1987). Acute post-streptococcal glomerulonephritis followed shortly by acute rheumatic fever. *Postgraduate Medical Journal*, Vol.63, No.737, (March 1087), pp. 209-210, ISSN 0032-5473

Laube G., Sarkissian A., Hailemariam S., Neuhaus T. & Leumann E. (2001). Simultaneous occurrence of the haemolytic uraemic syndrome and acute post-infectious glomerulonephritis. *European Journal of Pediatrics*, Vol.160, No.3, (March 2001), pp. 173-176, ISSN 0340-6199

Leiba H., Barash J. & Pollack A. (1998). Poststreptococcal uveitis. *American Journal of Ophthalmology*, Vol.126, No.2, (August 1998), pp. 317-318, ISSN 0002-9394

Lin W., Lo W. , Ou T. & Wang C. (2003). Haematuria, transient proteinuria, serpiginous-border skin rash, and cardiomegaly in a 10-year-old girl. *European Journal of Pediatrics*, Vol.162, No.9, (September 2003), pp. 655-657, ISSN 0340-6199

Lucus S. & Moxham J. (1978). Recurrent vasculitis associated with beta-haemolytic streptococcal infections. *British Medical Journal*, Vol.1. No.6123, (May 1978), pp. 1323, ISSN 0007-1447

Mackie S. & Keat A. (2004). Poststreptococcal reactive arthritis: what is it and how do we know? *Rheumatology*, Vol.43, No.8, (August 2004), pp. 949-954, ISSN 1462-0324

Maruyama K., Arai H., Ogawa T., Hoshino M., Tomizawa S. & Morikawa A. (1995). C9 deficiency in a patient with poststreptococcal glomerulonephritis. *Pediatric Nephrology*, Vol.9, No.6, (December 1995), pp. 746-748, ISSN 0931-041X

Masuda M, Nakanishi K., Yoshizawa N., Iijima K. & Yoshikawa N. (2003). Group A streptococcal antigen in the glomeruli of children with Henoch-Schönlein nephritis. *American Journal of Kidney Diseases*, Vol.41, No.2, (February 2003), pp. 366-370, ISSN 0272-6386

Matsell D., Baldree L., DiSessa T., Gaber L. & Stapleton F. (1990). Acute poststreptococcal glomerulonephritis and acute rheumatic fever: occurrence in the same patient. *Child Nephrology and Urology*, Vol.10, No.2, pp. 112-114, ISSN 1012-6694

Matsukura H., Ohtsuki A., Fuchizawa T. & Miyawaki T. (2003). Acute poststreptococcal glomerulonephritis mimicking Henoch-Schönlein purpura. *Clinical Nephrology*, Vol.59, No.1, (January 2003), pp. 64-65, ISSN 0301-0430

Medani C., Pearl P. & Hall-Craggs M. (1987). Acute renal failure, hemolytic anemia, and thrombocytopenia in poststreptococcal glomerulonephritis. *Southern Medical Journal*, Vol.80, No.3, (March 1987), pp. 370-373, ISSN 0038-4348

Muguruma T., Koyama T., Kanadani T., Furujo M., Shiraga H. & Ichiba Y. (2000). Acute thrombocytopenia associated with post-streptococcal acute glomerulonephritis. *Journal of Paediatrics and Child Health*, Vol.36, No.4, (August 2000), pp. 401-402, ISSN 1034-4810

Niewold T. & Ghosh A. (2003). Post-streptococcal reactive arthritis and glomerulonephritis in an adult. *Clinical Rheumatology*, Vol.22, No.4-5, (October 2003), pp. 350-352, ISSN 070-3198

Nordby J. (1997). Neurological presentation of poststreptococcal glomerulonephritis. *Clinical Pediatrics*, Vol.36, No.2, (February 1997), pp. 105-108, ISSN 0009-0228

Oda T., Yoshizawa N., Yamakami K., Tamura K., Kuroki A., Sugisaki T., Sawanobori E., Higashida K., Ohtomo Y., Hotta O., Kumagai H. & Miura S. (2010). Localization of nephritis-associated plasmin receptor in acute poststreptococcal glomerulonephritis. *Human Pathology*, Vol.41, No.9, (September 2010), pp. 1276-1285, ISSN 0046-8177

Öner A., Atalay S., Karademir S. and Pekuz O. (1993). Acute poststreptococcal glomerulonephritis followed by acute rheumatic carditis: an unusual case. *Pediatric Nephrology*, Vol.7, No.5, (October 1993), pp. 592-593, ISSN 0931-041X

Onisawa S., Morishima N. & Ichimura T. (1989). Concurrent poststreptococcal acute glomerulonephritis and Schönlein-Henoch purpura. *Acta Paediatrica Japonica*, Vol31, No.4, (August 1989), pp. 487-492, ISSN 0374-5600

Özcakar Z., Ekim M., Fitoz S., Teber S., Hizel S., Acar B., Yüksel S. & Yalcinkaya F. (2004). Hypertension induced reversible posterior leukoencephalopathy syndrome: a report of two cases. *European Journal of Pediatrics*, Vol.163, No.12, (December 2004), pp. 728-730, ISSN 0340-6199

Pais P., Kump T. & Greenbaum L. (2008). Delay in diagnosis in poststreptococcal glomerulonephritis. *Journal of Pediatrics*, Vol.153, No.4, (October 2008), pp. 560-564, ISSN 1687-9740

Papiris S., Manali E., Kalomenidis I., Kapotsis G., Karakatsani A. & Roussos C. (2007). Bench-to-bedside review: pulmonary-renal syndromes – an update for the intensivist. *Critical Care*, Vol.11, No.3, (May 2007), pp. 213, ISSN 1364-8535

Proesmans W. (1996). Haemolytic uremic syndrome superimposed on acute glomerulonephritis. *Pediatric Nephrology*, Vol.10, No.5, (October 1996), pp. 679, ISSN 0931-041X

Psaila B. & Bussel J. (2007). Immune thrombocytopenic purpura. *Hematology Oncology Clinics of North America*, Vol.21, No.4, (August 2007), pp. 743-759, ISSN 0889-8588

Ramberg R. (1947). The prognosis for acute nephritis. *Acta Medica Scandinavica*, Vol.127, No.4, (May 1947), pp. 396-423, ISSN 0001-6101

Ritt M., Campean V., Amann K., Heider A., Griesbach D. & Veelken R. (2006). Transient encephalopathy complicating poststreptococcal glomerulonephritis in an adult with diagnostic findings consistent with cerebral vasculitis. *American Journal of Kidney Diseases*, Vol.48, No.3, (September 2006), pp. 489-494, ISSN 0272-6386

Rizkallah M., Ghandour M., Sabbah R. & Akhtar M. (1984). Acute thrombocytopenic purpura and poststreptococcal acute glomerulonephritis in a child. *Clinical Pediatrics*, Vol.23, No.10, (October 1984), pp. 581-583, ISSN 0009-9228

Robson W. & Leung A. (1994). Henoch-Schönlein purpura. *Advances in Pediatrics*, Vol.41, pp. 163-194, ISSN 0065-3101

Rodriguez-Iturbe B. & Musser J. (2008). The current state of poststreptococcal glomerulonephritis. *Journal of the American Society of Nephrology*, Vol.19, No.10, (October 2008), pp. 1855-1864, ISSN 1046-6673

Rodriguez-Iturbe B. & Mezzani S. (2009). Acute postinfectious glomerulonephritis, In: *Pediatric Nephrology*, Avner E., Harman W., Niaudet P., Yoshikawa N., (Ed.), pp. 743-755, Springer Verlag, ISBN 978-3-540-76327-7, Berlin

Rosenberg H., Donoso P., Vial S., Carranza S. & Romero P. (1984). Clinical and morphological recovery between two episodes of acute glomerulonephritis: a light and electron microscopic study with immunofluorescence. *Clinical Nephrology*, Vol.21, No.6, (June 1984), pp. 350-354, ISSN 0301-0430

Rovang R., Zawada E. Jr, Santella R., Jaqua R., Boice J. & Welter R. (1997). Cerebral vasculitis associated with acute post-streptococcal glomerulonephritis. *American Journal of Nephrology*, Vol.17. No.1, pp. 89-92, ISSN 0250-8095

Roy S. III, Wall H. & Etteldorf J. (1969). Second attacks of acute glomerulonephritis. *Journal of Pediatrics*, Vol.75, No.5, (November 1969), pp. 758-767, ISSN 0022-3476

Said R., Hussein M. & Hassan A. (1986). Simultaneous occurrence of acute poststreptococcal glomerulonephritis and acute rheumatic fever. American Journal of Nephrology, Vol.6, No.2, pp. 146-148, ISSN 0250-8095

Sanjad S., Tolaymat A. & Levin S. (1977). Acute glomerulonephritis in children: a review of 153 cases. *Southern Medical Journal*, Vol.70, No.10, (October 1977), pp. 1202-1206, ISSN 0038-4348

Siebels M., Andrassy K., Waldherr R. & Ritz E. (1995). Hemolytic uremic syndrome complicating postinfectious glomerulonephritis in the adult. *American Journal of Kidney Diseases*, Vol.25, No.2, (February 1995), pp. 336-339, ISSN 0272-6386

Sieck J., Awad M., Saour J., Ali H., Qunibi W. & Mercer E. (1992). Concurrent post-streptococcal carditis and glomerulonephritis: serial echocardiographic diagnosis and follow-up. *European Heart Journal*, Vol.13, No.12, (December 1992), pp. 1720-1723, ISSN 0195-668X

Sinha R., Al-Alsheikh K., Prediville J., Magil A. & Matsell D. (2007). Acute rheumatic fever with concomitant poststreptococcal glomerulonephritis. *American Journal of Kidney Diseases*, Vol.50, No.1, (July 2007), pp. A33-A35, ISSN 0272-6386

Soylu A., Kavukçu S., Türkmen M. & Akbaş Y. (2001). Posterior leukoencephalopathy syndrome in poststreptococcal acute glomerulonephritis. *Pediatric Nephrology*, Vol.16, No.7, (July 2001), pp. 601-603, ISSN 0931-041X

Steer A. & Carapetis J. (2009). Acute rheumatic fever and rheumatic heart disease in indigenous populations. *Pediatric Clinics of North America*, Vol. 56, No.6, (December 2009), pp. 1410-1419, ISSN 0031-3955

Sugimoto T., Takeda N., Sakaguchi M., Koyama T., Isoya E., Yagi Y., Uzu T. & Kashiwagi A. (2008). A case of post-streptococcal reactive arthritis and acute nephritis after bacterial endophthalmitis due to *Streptococcus pyogenes*. *Rheumatology International*, Vol.28, No.12, (October 2008), pp. 1285-1286, ISSN 0172-8172

Sung H., Lim C., Shin M., Kim B., Kim Y., Song H., Kim S.,Choi E., Chang Y. & Bang B. (2007). A case of post-streptococcal glomerulonephritis with diffuse alveolar hemorrhage. *Journal of Korean Medical Science*, Vol. 22, No.6, (December 2007), pp. 1074-1078, ISSN 1011-8934

Talarico H. & Rubens D. (1990). Gallbladder wall thickening in acute pyelonephritis. *Journal of Clinical Ultrasound*, Vol.18, No.8, (October 1990), pp. 653-657, ISSN 0091-2751

Tan P., Yadin O., Kleinman K., Gura V. & Cohen A. (1998). Simultaneous postinfectious glomerulonephritis and thrombotic microangiopathy: a renal biopsy study. *American Journal of Kidney Diseases*, Vol.31, No.3, (March 1998), pp. 513-520, ISSN 0272-6386

Tasic V. & Polenakovic M. (2003). Thrombocytopenia during the course of acute poststreptococcal glomerulonephritis. *Turkish Journal of Pediatrics*, Vol.45, No.2, (April-June 2003), pp. 148-151, ISSN 0041-4301

Tokura T., Morita Y., Yorimitsu D., Horike H., Sasaki T. & Kashihara N. (2008). Co-occurrence of poststreptococcal reactive arthritis and acute glomerulonephritis. *Modern Rheumatology*, Vol.18, No.5, (October 2008), pp. 526-528, ISSN 1439-7595

Traverso F., Martini F., Banchi L., Maritato F. & Fazio B. (1997). Vasculitic neuropathy associated with beta-haemolytic streptococcal infection: a case report. *Italian Journal of Neurological Sciences*, Vol.18, No.2, pp. 105-107, ISSN 0392-0461

Ur Rehman S., Anand S., Reddy A., Backhous O., Mohamed M., Mahomed I., Atkins A. & James T. (2006). Poststreptococcal syndrome uveitis: a descriptive case series and literature review. *Ophthalmology*, Vol.113, No.4, (April 2006), pp. 701-706, ISSN 0161-6420

van Breda Vriesman A., Engelbrecht M., Smithuis R. & Puylaert J. (2007). Diffuse gallbladder wall thickening: differential diagnosis. *American Journal of Roentogenology*, Vol.188, No.2, (February 2007), pp. 459-501, ISSN 0361-803X

van der Helm-van Mil A. (2010). Acute rheumatic fever and poststreptococcal reactive arthritis reconsidered. *Current Opinion in Rheumatology*, Vol.22, No.4, (July 2010), pp. 437-442, ISSN 1040-8711

Velhote V., Saldanha L., Malheiro P., Praxedes J., Penna D., Marcondes M. & Sabbaga E. (1986). Acute glomerulonephritis: three episodes demonstrated by light and electron microscopy, and immunofluorescence studies – a case report. *Clinical Nephrology*, Vol.26, No.6, (December 1986), pp. 307-310, ISSN 0301-0430

Watanabe T. & Baba Y. (2009). Gallbladder wall thickening in a patient with acute poststreptococcal glomerulonephritis. *European Journal of Pediatrics*, Vol.168, No.6, (June 2009), pp. 717-719, ISSN 0340-6199

Watanabe T. & Yoshizawa N. (2001). Recurrence of acute poststreptococcal glomerulonephritis. *Pediatric Nephrology*, Vol.16, No.7, (July 2001), pp. 598-600, ISSN 0931-041X

Wong W. & Morris M. (2001). Cerebral vasculitis in a child following post-streptococcal glomerulonephritis. *Journal of Paediatrics and Child Health*, Vol.37, No. 6, pp. 597-599, ISSN 1034-4810

Yamakami K., Yoshizawa N., Wakabayashi K., Takeuchi A., Tadakuma T. & Boyle M. (2000). The potential role for nephritis-associated plasmin receptor in acute poststreptococcal glomerulonephritis. *Methods*, Vol.21, No.2, (June 2000), pp. 185-197, ISSN 1046-2023

Yoshizawa N. (2000). Acute glomerulonephritis. *Internal Medicine*, Vol.39, No.9, (September 2000), pp. 687-694, ISSN 0918-2918

Yoshizawa N., Yamakami K., Fujino M., Oda T., Tamura K., Matsumoto K., Sugisaki T., & Boyle M. (2004). Nephritis-associated plasmin receptor and acute poststreptococcal glomerulonephritis: characterization of the antigen and associated immune response. *Journal of the American Society of Nephrology*, Vol.15, No.7, (July 2004), pp. 1785-1793, ISSN 1046-66

10

Hepatitis C Virus Associated Glomerulonephritis

Vincent Ho[1] and Jason Chen[2]

[1]Department of Medicine, Campbelltown Hospital and School of Medicine,
University of Western Sydney, Sydney,
[2]Department of Anatomical Pathology, Royal North Shore Hospital, Sydney,
Australia

1. Introduction

Approximately 170 million persons worldwide are infected with the hepatitis C (HCV) virus. The incidence of glomerulonephritis in HCV-infected patients is unknown due to a lack of large-scale cross sectional surveys however subclinical renal involvement is believed to be highly prevalent among patients with HCV hepatitis. The most common HCV-associated glomerulonephritis is membranoproliferative glomerulonephritis (MPGN) type 1 with or without cryoglobulinaemia. MPGN typically presents several years, and often decades, after initial infection with HCV. Most patients have laboratory evidence of hypocomplementaemia, circulating rheumatoid factors, and cryoglobulinaemia. Other uncommon forms of glomerular disease that have been reported to be associated with HCV infection include membranous nephropathy, IgA nephropathy, focal segmental glomerulosclerosis, fibrillary glomerulonephritis/immunotactoid glomerulopathy, pauci-immune glomerulonephritis, and thrombotic microangiopathy.

The principal clinical manifestations of glomerular disease in HCV patients are the presence of proteinuria and microscopic haematuria with or without impaired kidney function. The clinical course of these HCV-associated glomerulopathies is generally characterised by remission and relapsing phases. The overall prognosis for HCV-associated glomerulonephritis remains poor, not only because of renal disease progression but because of the high incidence of cardiovascular disease, infection and hepatic failure.

The exact pathogenic sequence of injury that results in glomerulonephritis is not known. The prevailing theory is that glomerular injury results from deposition of circulating immune complexes that contain HCV antigens and anti-HCV antibody. Involvement of the innate immune system in HCV-associated MPGN has been suggested with demonstration of upregulation of Toll-like receptor 3.

In establishing a link between HCV infection and the immune response targeting the glomerulus, antiviral, plasma exchange and immunosuppressive therapies have been used in patients. The use of antiviral therapy in HCV-positive patients with glomerulonephritis is targeted at eliminating the virus and reducing the generation of HCV-related antibodies and immune complexes. The data to support antiviral treatment for HCV-associated glomerulonephritis is limited, however interferon therapy may be superior to immunosuppressive agents in HCV-associated cryoglobulinaemic glomerulonephritis in lowering proteinuria. Agents such as rituximab have also been shown to be efficacious in the treatment of HCV-associated cryoglobulinaemic glomerulonephritis.

This chapter provides the reader with an overview of hepatitis C-associated glomerulonephritis that covers epidemiology, clinical manifestations, natural history, immunopathophysiology, and a review of the evidence underpinning current therapeutic approaches.

Hepatitis C virus (HCV) is a leading cause of chronic liver disease in the world. The World Health Organization estimates that there are 170 million individuals with HCV infection and an incidence of 3–4 million new cases per year (WHO, 2000). HCV infection leads to chronic liver disease, but also to extra-hepatic manifestations. These include mixed cryoglobulinaemia, lymphoproliferative disorders and renal disease. HCV infection has been reported in association with distinct histological patterns of glomerulonephritis.

In this review, we will canvass the epidemiology, clinical manifestations, natural history, immunopathophysiology, and current therapies of HCV-associated glomerulonephritis, as well as cover issues around renal transplantation.

2. Immunopathogenesis

HCV is a single-stranded enveloped RNA virus. Its genome codes for a nucleocapsid core protein, envelope proteins, and a number of non-structural proteins. Glomerular injury due to HCV occurs as a result of the direct interaction of viral RNA and proteins with glomerular cells, as well as indirectly through immunological mediators such as immune complex deposition.

The adaptive immune response to HCV infection includes both cellular and humoral pathways. Unlike the overt cytotoxic cellular T-cell response to infected hepatocytes in the liver, the mechanism of injury in glomerulonephritis appears predominantly due to circulating immune complex deposition. This humoral response to HCV infection includes the production of various antibodies against HCV protein antigens. To evade this, HCV displays antigenic variability resulting from lack of proofreading activity in the HCV RNA polymerase. Hypervariable regions are present particularly in the envelope protein E2 sequence. Combined with a high replication rate, this antigenic variability allows mutant virus strains to escape antibody binding. Thus in chronic HCV infection, HCV RNA persists in serum despite the presence of anti-HCV antibodies. The chronic simultaneous presence of both HCV antigens and anti-HCV antibodies is a fertile setting for the formation of circulating immune complexes. In addition, HCV-induced liver injury decreases the hepatic clearance of circulating immune complexes, prolonging their survival in the circulation.

Often the anti-HCV antibodies have the properties of cryoglobulins, that is they precipitate at low temperatures. Serum cryoglobulins are present at low levels in up to 50% of chronic HCV infected patients, however symptomatic cryoglobulinaemia occurs in 1% or less of patients and usually only after years of chronic infection (Meyers et al., 2003). In HCV infection, the cryoglobulins are almost always of mixed type, with type 2 (monoclonal rheumatoid factor usually IgM kappa) more common than type 3 (polyclonal rheumatoid factor) (Miller and Howell, 2000). Possibly, IgM directed against epitopes of the HCV envelope cross-reacts with IgG, forming the rheumatoid factor (Alpers and Kowulewska, 2007). Thus, the cryoglobulins in HCV infection are composed of HCV RNA and/or proteins, complexed with anti-HCV IgG, in turn complexed to IgM rheumatoid factor. The concentration of HCV RNA in cryoprecipitates has been found to be around 1,000 times higher than in serum (Kamar et al., 2008). While symptomatic cryoglobulinaemia is relatively rare in HCV infected patients, conversely the vast majority (over 80%) of patients with mixed cryoglobulins have evidence of HCV infection (Kamar et al., 2008).

Circulating immune complexes, including cryoglobulins, deposit in glomeruli along the capillary walls and in the mesangium. IgM kappa rheumatoid factor has a particular affinity for cellular fibronectin in the mesangial matrix (Perico et al., 2009). While immunoglobulins are readily and routinely identified in glomerular tissues, the demonstration of HCV antigens in glomeruli is controversial and limited to relatively small numbers of studies. For example, Sansonno and colleagues (2005) used laser capture microdissection combined with PCR to identify HCV RNA in glomeruli, as well as immunohistochemistry to identify HCV core protein in glomeruli. Virus-like particles have been identified by electron microscopy in renal biopsies of patients with HCV infection (Sabry, 2002).

While much work has focused on humoral immunity and immune complex deposition, there has also been research on the innate immune response of the glomerulus to HCV. This innate immune response to microbes involves Toll-like receptors (TLRs), transmembrane proteins that recognise microbial antigens. Dolganiuc and colleagues (2004), using a variety of human and mouse cell types, found that HCV core protein and HCV non-structural protein 3 act via Toll-like receptor 2 (TLR2) to trigger inflammatory pathways. In the kidney, it is also hypothesized that HCV RNA is recognised by Toll-like receptor 3 (TLR3) expressed on mesangial cells. Using a microdissection technique, increased TLR3 mRNA expression has been demonstrated in glomeruli with HCV-associated glomerulonephritis, compared to glomeruli with non-HCV-associated glomerulonephritis (Wornle et al., 2006). Recognition of HCV by TLR3 with subsequent intracellular signalling activates mesangial cells to produce pro-inflammatory cytokines and growth factors. The cytokines involved include TNFalpha and the chemokine IP-10 (interferon gamma inducible protein-10), both of which are upregulated in HCV-associated glomerulonephritis (Merkle et al., 2011).

The innate immune response, together with the trapping and deposition of immune complexes, both contribute to generate activation of local inflammatory and complement cascades in glomeruli. These cascades induce glomerular cell proliferation and matrix production as well as the recruitment of inflammatory cells, which can be seen morphologically as the characteristic histological patterns of glomerulonephritis. While some morphological patterns are characteristic of HCV, none is specific, and the diagnosis of HCV-associated glomerulonephritis relies on correlation with clinical findings as well as the presence of serum anti-HCV antibody and HCV RNA. Evidence of HCV RNA and/or core protein in glomeruli has been identified irrespective of the histological pattern of glomerulonephritis (Sansonno et al., 2005).

Membranoproliferative glomerulonephritis (MPGN) type 1 with or without cryoglobulinaemia is the most characteristic pattern, comprising the large majority (roughly 80%) of all HCV-associated glomerulonephritis. Conversely, HCV is perhaps the most important cause of secondary MPGN. Histologically, the glomeruli have a membranoproliferative pattern with accentuated lobularity, mesangial hypercellularity, and mesangial interpositioning causing double contouring of the capillary walls. The glomeruli may have prominent inflammatory cell infiltration, particularly of monocytes (Alpers and Kowaleska, 2007). See Figure 1

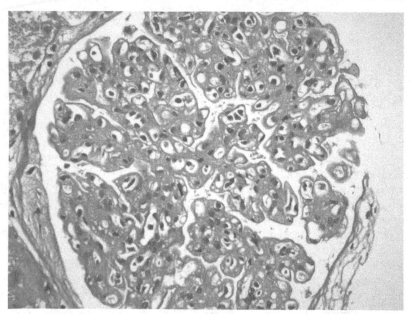

Fig. 1a. Membranoproliferative glomerulonephritis in a HCV-infected patient, with accentuated lobularity, mesangial hypercellularity and intracapillary mononuclear inflammatory cells (H&E, 400x).

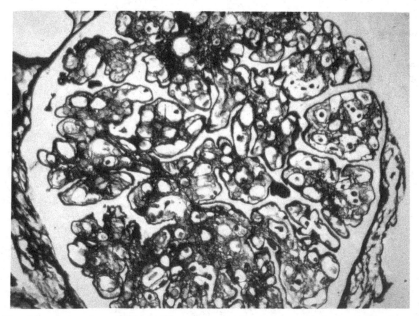

Fig. 1b. Double contouring of the capillary basement membranes is more evident on silver staining (Modified Wilder's silver stain, 400x).

Immunofluorescence staining highlights granular deposits of C3 and immunoglobulins (usually IgG and IgM) along capillary walls and in the mesangium, and electron microscopy confirms electron-dense immune complex deposits in subendothelial and mesangial locations. Cryoglobulin deposits themselves also produce a membranoproliferative pattern of injury. In these cases with cryoglobulinaemia, the deposits themselves may be seen histologically as eosinophilic glomerular capillary 'hyaline thrombi'. See Figure 2

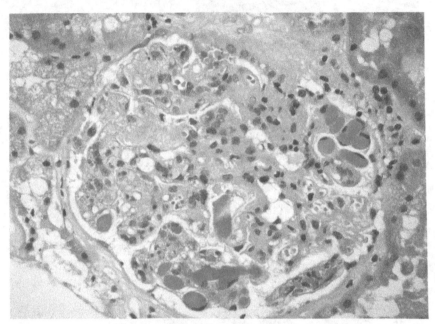

Fig. 2. Cryoglobulinaemic glomerulonephritis, with prominent intracapillary hyaline thrombi (H&E, 400x).

In a minority of cases, vasculitis of small vessels can also be seen on biopsy. Immunofluorescence staining reflects the composition of the usually mixed-type cryoglobulin precipitate, with strong staining for IgG, IgM and C3 as well as frequent kappa predominance. The cryoglobulin deposits by electron microscopy have variable morphology, but classically are seen as microtubular and/or annular organised structures (Iskanda and Herrera, 2002) . See Figure 3

MPGN type 3 has overlapping features of both MPGN type 1 in combination with membranous nephropathy, and has also been described as a pattern of HCV-associated glomerulonephritis.

The remaining patterns of glomerulonephritis are relatively uncommon and have been reported as small series and case reports, with varying degrees of strength in their association with HCV. Of these relatively uncommon forms of HCV-associated glomerulonephritis, membranous nephropathy is the most often quoted. In a study by Yamabe and colleagues (1995), 2 of 24 patients (8.3%) with membranous nephropathy had evidence of HCV infection. A separate Japanese study of 2 patients with membranous nephropathy demonstrated pathogenic linkage to HCV by detecting HCV core protein in the affected glomeruli using immunofluorescence (Okada et al., 1996). In contrast to HCV-associated MPGN, HCV-associated membranous nephropathy does not appear associated with cryoglobulinaemia, rheumatoid factor or hypocomplementaemia (Uchiyama-Tanaka et al., 2004).

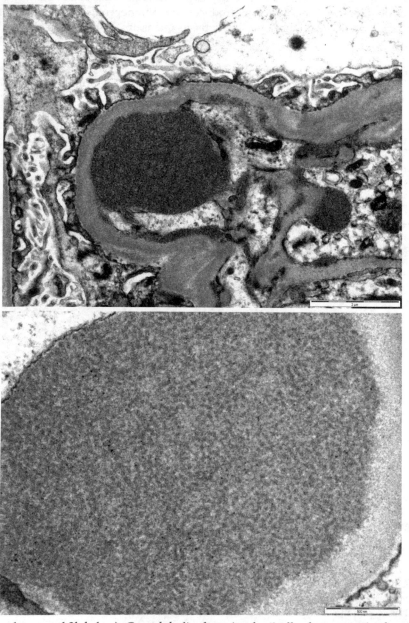

Fig. 3. (3a above and 3b below). Cryoglobulin deposits classically show organised substructure such as microtubular aggregates (EM; photos courtesy of Mr Paul Kirwan, EM unit Concord Repatriation General Hospital Sydney Australia).

A case series from the University of Alabama at Birmingham examined the kidney biopsies of 30 patients receiving liver transplants for HCV-induced cirrhosis at the time of liver engraftment (McGuire et al., 2006). Three types of disease were observed: membranoproliferative glomerulonephritis type 1, IgA nephropathy, and "mesangial glomerulonephritis". Cryoglobulins were not detected, even in rheumatoid factor-positive patients with urinary abnormalities.

Other rare, somewhat speculative, reported associations with HCV include focal segmental glomerulosclerosis (Stehman-Breen et al., 1999), fibrillary glomerulonephritis/immunotactoid glomerulopathy (Markowitz et al., 1998), pauci-immune glomerulonephritis (Usalan et al., 1998), and thrombotic microangiopathy (Herzenberg et al., 1998).

Lastly, it should be noted that the development of de novo immune complex glomerulonephritis in the transplanted kidney is one mechanism leading to the increased graft failure seen in HCV-infected renal transplant recipients (Scott et al., 2010).

3. Clinical manifestations

Glomerulonephritis can develop several years or even decades after initial infection with HCV. As described previously the principal renal manifestation of HCV infection is membranoproliferative glomerulonephritis (MPGN). This is usually accompanied by cryoglobulinaemia. Classically, HCV-associated MPGN is found in persons with long-standing infection and patients most often display mild subclinical liver disease. MPGN is rarely found in children. Clinically, patients may exhibit symptoms of cryoglobulinaemia, including palpable purpura, arthralgias, myalgias, neuropathy, and fatigue. The triad of purpura, peripheral neuropathy and arthralgia is evident in nearly 30% of cases (Monti et al., 1995). The majority of cryoglobulinaemic HCV-infected patients however have either no symptoms or nonspecific clinical manifestations. Cryoglobulins, or immunoglobulins (Igs) that precipitate at cold temperature, are detected in approximately 50–70% of patients. Cryoglobulinaemic vasculitis, predominantly involving the small vessels, is observed in less than 10% of patients (Lamprecht et al., 1999). The most frequently affected tissues/organs are skin, nerves, and kidney. Renal involvement has been reported in about one-third of cryoglobulinaemic patients (Meyers et al., 2003), but the predilection for renal involvement in certain patients is unclear. Renal signs of cryoglobulinaemia include nephrotic or non-nephrotic proteinuria and microscopic haematuria with mild to moderate renal insufficiency (Baid et al., 2000; Johnson et al., 1993; Markowitz et al., 1998). Glomerular disease may manifest acutely as oliguric acute renal failure in 5% of cases (Meyers et al., 2003). Around 80% of patients develop hypertension (Tarantino et al., 1995) which can be severe and difficult to control.

Usually, the diagnosis of HCV-associated MPGN is made by positive tests for serum HCV antibodies and HCV RNA. However patients with HCV-associated glomerulonephritis in whom HCV RNA were not detected in the blood have been reported (Yamabe et al., 2010). Serum aminotransferase levels are increased in the majority of patients and often low serum concentrations of complement components (C1q, C4, and C3) are found (Meyers et al., 2003). Elevated levels of serum cryoglobulins can be divided by the Brouet classification into three types (Brouet et al., 1974). Type 2 and 3 cryoglobulins which are strongly associated with hepatitis C, have rheumatoid factor activity and bind to polyclonal immunoglobulins (Ferri et al., 2002). These two types are known as mixed cryoglobulinaemia.

4. Natural history

A large prospective cohort study conducted in Northern Norway on 1010 HCV-positive patients found elevated alanine aminotransferases in 27.4%, decompensated liver disease in 2.9%, hepatocellular carcinoma in 0.4% but only 2 patients (or 0.2%) with end-stage renal failure caused by membranoproliferative glomerulonephritis (Kristiansen et al., 2010). The median observation period from estimated acquisition of the disease to follow-up in these patients was 26 years.

The long-term outcome of HCV-associated nephropathies is nebulous. A retrospective cohort study of 474,369 adult veterans in the United States (Tsui et al., 2007) found that patients with HCV infection were more likely to develop end-stage renal disease (4.3 per 1000 person year) than HCV-seronegative patients (3.1 per 1000 person year). For patients aged 18 to 70 years with an estimated glomerular filtration rate of at least 30 mL/min per 1.73 m2, HCV seropositivity was associated with a nearly threefold higher risk of developing ESRD (adjusted hazard rate, 2.80; 95% confidence interval, 2.43-3.23).

Another cross-sectional study (Dalrymple et al., 2007) showed that HCV-positive veterans after adjustment for age, race, gender, diabetes and hypertension, had 40% higher odds for renal insufficiency (odds ratio 1.40; 95% confidence interval 1.11 to 1.76) as compared with HCV-negative veterans.

An early literature review of patients with essential mixed cryoglobulinaemia (Ponticelli et al., 1986) found that of 11 patients with nephrotic syndrome and renal dysfunction who received supportive treatment alone, 4 patients (36%) died or exhibited progressive renal failure, 2 patients (18%) had stable renal disease, and spontaneous improvement occurred in the other 5 patients (45%).

Finally Tarantino and colleagues (1995) reported the overall poor clinical outcome of 105 essential mixed cryoglobulinaemia patients with renal involvement collected throughout 25 years in three renal units in Milan. Patient survival was 49% at 10 years after renal biopsy. Forty-two patients died primarily from cardiovascular disease, liver disease or infection, whereas 15 patients developed chronic renal failure. Two patients had a complete remission of the disease while 15 had a remission only of renal manifestations. Thirty-one patients were alive at the end of the study with persistent renal and extrarenal manifestations. Thus only a minority of patients eventually developed renal failure because most patients died from cardiovascular disease, liver disease or infection.

5. Therapy

5.1 Renoprotective therapies

As hypertension, proteinuria, and progressive renal failure are the main clinical manifestations of HCV-associated chronic renal disease, it is essential that renoprotective therapies be instituted. Diuretics, renin–angiotensin system inhibitors (angiotensin-converting enzyme inhibitors or angiotensin II receptor blockers), and lipid-lowering agents, have been proven to be beneficial in HCV patients with chronic renal disease (Chadban and Atkins, 2005; Ruggenenti et al., 2001; Ruggenenti et al., 2004).

5.2 Immunosuppressive therapy

High-dose methylprednisolone has been used to treat exacerbations of mixed cryoglobulinaemia for over 30 years (Tarantino et al., 1981; De Vecchi et al., 1983). In one of the earlier studies (De Vecchi et al., 1983), 3 pulses of intravenous methylprednisolone (0.5-1 gm each) was given for 3 consecutive days during episodes of acute renal function deterioration in 16 patients with essential mixed cryoglobulinaemia. The intravenous administration was followed by oral prednisone 0.5 mg/kg per day with a slow taper until withdrawal of steroids after 4-6 months. Intravenous methylprednisolone pulse therapy did have a dramatic effect on renal function with cumulative mean plasma creatinine values decreasing from 3.3 ± 1.3 mg/dL to 2.2 ± 0.7 mg/dL (p<0.001). Proteinuria levels were not found to be significantly changed as a result of therapy. The basal cryocrit level decreased after pulse therapy, however again this was not found to be significant.

In one case report of rapidly progressive MPGN type 1 with HCV and nephritic syndrome, intravenous pulsed methylprednisolone appeared to be useful in establishing rapid remission but as antiviral therapy was used concurrently it is impossible to ascertain the effect of methylprednisolone alone (Ahmed et al., 2008).

Unlike intravenous pulse steroid therapy, oral steroids however have not been found to be effective in the acute setting. Ponticelli and colleagues (1986) reported 27 patients with mixed cryoglobulinaemia and acute renal disease that were treated with oral corticosteroids alone or in combination with other cytotoxic agents. 10 patients (37%) died or showed progressively worsening renal function, 4 patients continued to have stable renal disease, and the other 13 patients (48%) had improved renal function. This does not appear to differ markedly from their reporting of the natural outcomes of such patients with supportive treatments alone.

Indeed there are conflicting results on the use of oral steroids for HCV-associated MPGN. A Japanese study (Komatsuda et al., 1996) found that only 2 out of 6 patients with MPGN responded to steroids but paradoxically found that the serum titre of HCV RNA decreased in 5 out of 7 treated patients.

Other studies have subsequently confirmed that HCV RNA levels increase with steroid exposure (Fong et al., 1994; Lake, 2003; McHutchinson et al., 1993).

Cyclophosphamide has been used successfully in the treatment of HCV-infected patients with cryoglobulinaemia and progressive loss of kidney function due to MPGN. In one case report a patient with HCV-associated MPGN and progressive renal failure displayed disappearance of serum cryoglobulins and a marked improvement in creatinine clearance with the institution of cyclophosphamide (Quigg et al., 1995). However cyclophosphamide treatment similar to steroids produces a rise in HCV RNA levels.

It is generally agreed that immunosuppressive medications do increase HCV RNA levels but their selective use does not appear to worsen the underlying hepatic disease (D'Amico and Fornaserieri, 2003). A review by D'Amico (1998) reported no evidence of acute liver damage in more than 100 treatment courses (steroids, cyclophosphamide, plasma exchange) in Italian patients with HCV-associated cryoglobulinaemic glomerulonephritis.

The expert consensus currently is that in patients with HCV-associated renal disease, treatment of acute flares does require immunosuppressive therapy to preserve renal function however prolonged therapy does not confer any additional benefit (Campise and Tarantino, 1999).

5.3 Antiviral therapy

Antiviral therapy in the form of alpha interferon was first used in a small pilot study of 7 patients with cryoglobulinaemic vasculitis in 1987, before the discovery of the critical role of HCV in its pathogenesis (Bonomo et al., 1987).

After a link was established between HCV infection and the occurrence of cryoglobulinaemic MPGN, a number of studies have examined the efficacy of antiviral treatment to achieve both sustained virological response (clearance of HCV from the serum for at least 6 months after completing an antiviral course) and to improve renal injury. The use of antiviral therapy in HCV-positive patients with glomerulonephritis is targeted at eliminating the virus and reducing the generation of HCV-related antibodies and immune complexes.

In the early 1990s, standard recombinant alpha interferon (α-IFN) was used by itself. The first prospective randomised controlled trial by Misiani and colleagues (1994) reported that 15 out of 25 patients with HCV-associated type II cryoglobulinaemia receiving recombinant alpha-interferon had a complete clearance of hepatitis C viral RNA and that all these patients reported improvements in cutaneous vasculitis and renal function. There was no effect on proteinuria. Unfortunately after treatment with interferon alpha-2a was discontinued, viraemia and cryoglobulinaemia recurred in all 15 HCV RNA-negative patients.

Johnson and colleagues (1994) reported the results of a prospective uncontrolled trial of fourteen patients receiving interferon alpha for 6 to 12 months. There was a significant reduction in proteinuria but no improvement in renal function. Although a good clinical response correlated with disappearance of HCV RNA from the serum during treatment, relapse of viraemia and renal disease was common after the completion of therapy.

It was clear at this stage that alpha-interferon was useful but the optimal treatment strategy was yet to be defined.

An advance came with the discovery that ribavirin played a synergistic role with an interferon-based regimen to increase the possibility that an on-treatment responder would become a sustained responder. Ribavirin monotherapy itself was found to be disappointing (Pham et al., 1998) although one case report referenced a patient with refractory nephritic syndrome secondary to HCV-associated membranous nephropathy who had a complete remission following the initiation of ribavirin monotherapy (Hu and Jaber, 2005).

Small scale studies examined the combination of standard interferon plus ribavirin for HCV-associated cryoglobulinaemic glomerulonephritis. Rossi and colleagues (2003) treated 3 patients with HCV-associated cryoglobulinaemic glomerulonephritis with standard interferon and ribavirin for 12 months and showed that all had sustained virological response, with reductions in daily proteinuria and rheumatoid factor at the end of follow-up. Brucheld and colleagues (2003) treated 7 patients with HCV and renal insufficiency (2 patients with cryoglobulinaemic vasculitis, 4 patients with MPGN, 1 patient with focal segmental glomerulosclerosis) with a combination of interferon and ribavirin. 4 of the 7 patients had maintained virological and renal remission. The frequency of haematuria and amount of proteinuria decreased after the course of antiviral treatment.

The next important clinical breakthrough was the introduction of a polyethylene glycol side chain (pegylation) to the interferon to give it a much longer bioavailability, allowing for weekly injections rather than three injections per week. Pegylated interferon was shown to double the sustained viral response rate in hepatitis C treatment (Lindsay et al., 2001).

Saadoun and colleagues (2006) carried out a study on 72 consecutive patients with HCV-associated mixed cryoglobulinaemic vasculitis receiving recombinant interferon or pegylated interferon, both in combination with oral ribavirin. A complete clinical response of the cryoglobulinaemic vasculitis occurred in 45 patients, a sustained virologic response occurred in 42 patients, and cryoglobulins cleared in 33 patients. Compared with patients treated with IFN alpha-2b plus ribavirin, those receiving PEG-IFN alpha-2b plus ribavirin had a higher sustained clinical (67.5% versus 56.3%), virologic (62.5% versus 53.1%), and immunologic (57.5% versus 31.3%) response, regardless of HCV genotype and viral load.

Fabrizi and colleagues (2007) then undertook a meta-analysis looking at clinical controlled trials of the 2 treatments (antiviral versus immunosuppressive) for HCV-associated glomerulonephritis. Six studies involving 145 patients with HCV-associated glomerulonephritis were identified (Alric et al., 2004; Beddhu et al., 2002; Johnson et al., 1994; Komatsuda et al., 1996; Mazzaro et al., 2000; Misiani et al., 1994). The primary endpoint was the frequency of patients with significant reduction in proteinuria (return of proteinuria to normal or decrease of >50%) at the conclusion of therapy. It was shown that standard interferon alpha therapy was more effective than immunosuppressive therapy in lowering proteinuria of patients with HCV-associated glomerulonephritis (OR 3.86, 95% CI 1.44-10.33; P=0.007). However renal dysfunction was not significantly improved with either therapy (Fabrizi et al., 2007).

This meta-analysis was methodologically flawed by the inclusion of studies where patients received immunosuppressive agents during antiviral treatment, making it difficult to ascertain the effect of each treatment alone.

A later meta-analysis (Feng et al., 2011) examined the results before and after stable regimens of antiviral therapy in subjects with HCV-associated glomerulonephritis and compared the results of those subjects who achieved sustained virological response (SVR) to those that did not. Improvement of proteinuria and serum creatinine levels after antiviral therapy were taken as the end points of interest. Eleven clinical trials involving 225 patients were included in the meta-analysis. At the end of antiviral therapy, the mean decrease in proteinuria was 2.71 g/24 h [95% confidence interval (CI) 1.38-4.04, P < 0.0001]. The pooled decrease in mean serum creatinine levels was 0.23 mg/dL (95% CI 0.02-0.44, P = 0.03). Comparison of nonsustained virological response (nonSVR) to SVR groups demonstrated a significant mean difference of proteinuria decrease in the SVR group of 1.04 g/24 h (95% CI 0.20-1.89, P = 0.02) but the serum creatinine decrease of 0.05 mg/dL was not significant (95% CI -0.33 to 0.43, P = 0.80).

A limitation of this meta-analysis is the small number of study subjects making it difficult to perform subgroup analysis on the basis of cryoglobulinaemia or baseline proteinuria. Another weakness is the lack of randomized controlled trials (RCTs) of interferon alpha-based therapy in HCV-associated glomerulonephritis. Indeed only 1 of the 11 studies in this analysis was an RCT (Misiani et al., 1994).

Thus antiviral therapy based on interferon alpha can significantly decrease proteinuria and hence should be undertaken in patients with HCV-associated glomerulonephritis.

It should be acknowledged that currently there are no long-term follow-up studies of antiviral therapy on HCV-associated glomerulonephritis patients. It is important to ascertain whether interferon alpha-based treatments can delay or halt the progression of chronic renal disease in the long term. This will require investment in large RCTs with longer durations of follow-up.

5.4 Rituximab

Treatment with interferon alpha in combination with ribavirin can suppress HCV RNA in 50-60% of patients with a subsequent decrease in cryoglobulins. Many patients however fail to respond to interferon therapy and half the responders relapse.

Rituximab is a monoclonal antibody against the CD20 antigen on the cell surface of B lymphocytes. Rituximab can thus reduce rheumatoid factor-producing B lymphocytes, resulting in a reduction in cryoglobulin production. In recent years the concept of anti-CD20 for mixed-type cryoglobulinaemia has emerged as an effective and safe treatment, inducing a rapid remission of disease activity (Sansonno et al., 2003; Zaja et al., 2003).

One study examined 20 HCV-positive patients with mixed-type cryoglobulinaemia (who were refractory to interferon therapy) that were treated with rituximab 375 mg/m² weekly for 4 weeks (Sansonno et al., 2003). Patients had a follow-up period of 12 months. Sixteen patients (80%) had a complete response defined as a 75% or greater reduction in cryoglobulins and resolution of at least 2 major clinical signs and symptoms. In these patients, rituximab treatment resulted in a reduction in both the IgM and IgG components of the cryoglobulin. Only 1 of the 20 patients had nephritis that did not respond to treatment.

Another study looked at the treatment of 15 patients with rituximab with a follow-up period of 9 to 31 months (Zaja et al., 2003). 12 patients were HCV-infected and 3 patients had mixed cryoglobulinaemia unrelated to HCV. All patients had early improvement in their cutaneous manifestations with rituximab however only 1 patient had complete resolution of the cryoglobulin at 6 months and only 3 lost their rheumatoid factor. It is worthwhile noting that in 7 of 8 patients, maintenance corticosteroids were successfully withdrawn by the second post-treatment month.

Quartuccio and colleagues (2006) carried out a study where 5 patients with HCV-associated mixed cryoglobulinaemia were treated with 4 weekly infusions of rituximab 375mg/m² without accompanying steroids. Renal function improved within 2 months in all 5 cases treated. There were no relevant short-term or delayed side effects reported. However 3 out of 5 patients showed a recurrence of disease at 5, 7 and 12 months. A repeated cycle of rituximab infusion induced rapid remission of disease activity in 2 of these patients. Only one patient achieved persistent remission after a single cycle and thus the results of the study suggest the need for repeated rituximab administrations for adequate control of nephritis. The optimal dosage and frequency of rituximab administrations in HCV-associated mixed cryoglobulinaemia remains unclear as all studies to date have been based on the rituximab prescribing regimen used in non-Hodgkin lymphoma (Coiffier et al., 1998).

6. Renal transplantation and HCV-related renal disease

It should be recognised that the most common cause of proteinuria and renal insufficiency after kidney transplantation in HCV-positive patients is not HCV-related damage but chronic allograft nephropathy (Cosio et al., 1996; Nampoory et al., 2001). Renal diseases that have been reported in HCV-infected patients after kidney transplantation include recurrent or *de novo* MPGN, membranous nephropathy, minimal change disease, thrombotic microangiopathy, acute transplant glomerulopathy, and chronic transplant glomerulopathy (Baid et al., 2000; Cruzado et al., 2001; Gallay et al., 1995; Gloor et al., 2007; Hammoud et al., 1996; Morales et al., 1997; Roth et al., 1995).

MPGN is the most commonly reported, with an incidence as high as 54% in HCV-positive renal transplant recipients (Cruzado et al., 2001; Hammoud et al., 1996; Roth et al., 1995). In these patients proteinuria or nephrotic syndrome is the commonest clinical presentation (Cruzado et al., 2001; Nampoory et al., 2001; Virgilio et al., 2001). Serum cryoglobulins are very often detected (Roth et al., 1995).

Early studies on patient and graft survival in HCV-positive renal transplant recipients have concentrated on recurrent liver disease as causes of morbidity and mortality rather than examining recurrent renal disease or graft loss (Batty et al., 2001; Meier-Kriesche, 2001; Pereira and Levy, 1997). Small single centre studies have shown that both graft and patient survival are lower for HCV-positive than HCV-negative patients (Batty et al., 2001; Pereira and Levy, 1997).

More recently two large population based studies have published long term results of patient and graft survival (Morales et al., 2010; Scott et al., 2010).

The outcomes of a large cohort of renal transplant patients was reviewed recently using the Australian and New Zealand Dialysis and Transplant registry (Scott et al., 2010). Survival outcomes, causes of mortality, and causes of graft failure were examined. 140 (1.8%) patients were HCV antibody positive. Patient survival among HCV antibody positive and HCV antibody negative groups was 77% versus 90% and 50% versus 79% at 5 and 10 years respectively. The adjusted hazard ratio for patient death was 2.38 (95% CI 1.69-3.37). Higher rates of death due to cardiovascular disease (adjusted hazard ratio 2.74), malignancy (adjusted hazard ratio 2.52) and hepatic failure (adjusted hazard ratio 22.1) were observed.

A large national study in Spain used data on 4304 renal transplant recipients, 587 of them with HCV antibody collected over a long period (1990-2002), to estimate graft and patient survival at 4 years (Morales et al., 2010). 4-year graft survival was found to be significantly better in HCV-negative versus HCV-positive patients (94.4% versus 89.5%, P < 0.005). Patient survival was 96.3% in the entire group with a demonstrable difference between HCV-negative and HCV-positive patients (96.6% vs 94.5%, P < 0.05). HCV-positive patients were characterised as having more episodes of acute rejection, a higher degree of proteinuria with impaired renal function and a greater need for renal graft biopsies. In particular de novo glomerulonephritis and transplant glomerulopathy rates in HCV-positive and HCV-negative renal graft biopsies was 9.3% versus 5.2% and 11.4% versus 5.0% respectively.

6.1 Hepatitis C treatment implications in renal transplantation

A meta-analysis of 12 trials of interferon alpha-based therapy in 102 kidney transplant patients showed that sustained virological response is extremely variable ranging from 0-50% with a variable and often extremely high drop-out rate (0% to 100%) (Fabrizi et al., 2006). HCV genotype is an important determinant of sustained virological response with genotype 1 being the most resistant (Lock et al., 1999). Any conferred benefit on the underlying disease is mitigated by a 15-60% increased risk of acute cellular or vascular rejection (Baid et al., 2003; Fabrizi et al., 2006; Weclawiack et al., 2008). Unfortunately graft rejection is often severe and resistant to steroid therapy (Fabrizi et al., 2006).

Cessation of standard interferon therapy leads to a surge in hepatitis C viral load (104,105). Avoidance of interferon in HCV-positive renal transplant patients has been recommended because of the potential to precipitate acute graft rejection. However combined therapy with ribavirin and pegylated interferon achieved sustained virological response in 5 out of 8 patients (62%) without unduly affecting renal function (Montalbano et al., 2007; Mukherjee and Ariyarantha, 2007; Schmitz et al., 2007). This suggests a therapeutic role in certain settings albeit with an appreciable risk of graft dysfunction.

Rituximab appeared to be safe in one study of 7 HCV RNA-positive kidney transplant patients with de novo cryoglobulinaemia-related MPGN. HCV infection remained stable during and after rituximab therapy (Kamar et al., 2007). Larger long-term studies will be necessary to establish efficacy.

7. References

Ahmed, M.S.; Wong, C.F., Shawki, H., Kapoor, N. and Pandya, B.K. (2008). Rapidly deteriorating renal function with membranoproliferative glomerulonephritis Type 1 associated with hepatitis C treated successfully with steroids and antiviral therapy: a case report and review of literature. *Clin Nephrol,* Vol. 69, No. 4, pp. 298-301.

Alpers, C.E. and Kowalewska, J. (2007). Emerging paradigms in the renal pathology of viral diseases. *Clin J Am Soc Nephrol,* Vol. 2, Suppl 1, S6-12.

Alric, L.; Plaisier, E., Thebault, S., Peron, J.M., Rostaing, L. and Pourrat, J. et al. (2004). Influence of antiviral therapy in hepatitis C virus-associated cryoglobulinaemic membranoproliferative glomerulonephritis. *Am J Kidney Dis,* Vol. 43, No. 4, pp. 617-623.

Baid, S.; Cosimi, A.B., Tolkoff-Rubin, N., Colvin, R.B. Williams, W.W. Jr. and Pascual, M. (2000). Renal disease associated with hepatitis C infection after kidney and liver transplantation. *Transplantation,* Vol. 70, No. 2, pp. 255-261.

Baid, S.; Tolkoff-Rubin, N., Saidman, S., Chung, R., Williams, W.W., Auchincloss, H. et al. (2003). Acute humoral rejection in hepatitis C infected renal transplant recipients receiving antiviral therapy. *Am J Transplant,* Vol. 3, No. 1, pp. 74-78.

Batty, D.S. Jr.; Swanson, S.J., Kirk, A.D., Ko, C.W., Agodoa, L.Y., and Abbott, K.C. (2001). Hepatitis C virus seropositivity at the time of renal transplantation in the United States: Associated factors and patient survival. *Am J Transplant,* Vol. 1, No. 2, pp. 179-184.

Beddhu, S.; Bastacky, S. and Johnson, J.P. (2002). The clinical and morphologic spectrum of renal cryoglobulinemia. *Medicine,* Vol. 81, No.5, pp. 398–409.

Bonomo, L.; Casato, M., Afeltra, A. and Caccavo, D. (1987). Treatment of idiopathic mixed cryoglobulinemia with alpha interferon. *Am J Med,* Vol. 83, No.4, pp. 726-730.

Brouet, J.C.; Clauvel, J.P., Danon, F., Klein, M. and Seligmann, M. (1974). Biologic and clinical significance of cryoglobulins. A report of 86 cases. *Am J Med,* Vol. 57, No. 5, pp. 775-88.

Bruchfeld, A.; Lindahl, K., Stahle, L., Sodeberg, M. and Schvarcz. R. (2003). Interferon and ribavirin treatment in patients with hepatitis C-associated renal disease and renal insufficiency. *Nephrol Dial Transplant.* Vol. 18, No. 8, pp. 1573-1580.

Campise, M.R. and Tarantino, A. (1999). Glomerulonephritis in mixed cryoglobulinemia: what treatment? *Nephrol Dial Transplant,* Vol. 14, No.2, pp. 281-283.

Chadban, S.J. and Atkins, R.C. (2005). Glomerulonephritis. *Lancet,* Vol. 365, No. 9473, pp. 1797–1806.

Coiffier, B.; Haioun, C., Ketterer, N., Engert, A., Tilly, H., Ma, D. et al. (1998). Rituximab (anti-CD20 monoclonal antibody) for the treatment of patients with relapsing or refractory aggressive lymphoma: a multicenter phase II study. *Blood,* Vol. 92, No.6, pp. 1927-32.

Cosio, F.G.; Roche, Z., Agarwal, A., Falkenhain, M.E., Sedmak, D.D. and Ferguson, R.M. (1996). Prevalence of hepatitis C in patients with idiopathic glomerulopathies in native and transplant kidneys. *Am J Kidney Dis*, Vol. 28, No.5, pp. 752-758.

Cruzado, J.M.; Carrera, M., Torras, J. and Grinyo, J.M. (2001). Hepatitis C virus infection and de novo glomerular lesions in renal allografts. *Am J Transplant*, Vol.1, No.2, pp. 171-178.

Dalrymple, L.S.; Koepsell, T., Sampson, J., Louie, T., Dominitz, J.A., Young, B. et al. (2007). Hepatitis C virus infection and the prevalence of renal insufficiency. *Clin J Am Soc Nephrol*, Vol. 2, No.4, pp. 715-721.

D'Amico, G. (1998). Renal involvement in hepatitis C infection: cryoglobulinemic glomerulonephritis. *Kidney Int*, Vol. 54, No. 2, pp. 650-671.

D'Amico, G. and Fornasieri, A. (2003). Cryoglobulinemia. In: Brady, H.R. and Wilcox, C.S. eds. *Therapy in Nephrology and Hypertension.*, pp. 147-151, Saunders.

De Vecchi, A.; Montagnino, G., Pozzi, C., Tarantino, A., Locatelli, F. and Ponticelli, C. (1983). Intravenous methylprednisolone pulse therapy in essential mixed cryoglobulinemia nephropathy. Clin Nephrol, Vol 19, No. 5, pp. 221-227.

Dolganiuc, A.; Oak, S., Kodys, K., Golenbock, D.T., Finberg, R.W., Kurt-Jones, E. et al. (2004). Hepatitis C core and nonstructural 3 proteins trigger toll-like receptor 2-mediated pathways and inflammatory activation. *Gastroenterology*, Vol. 127, No. 5, pp. 1513-24.

Fabrizi, F.; Lunghi, G., Dixit, V. and Martin, P. (2006). Meta-analysis: anti-viral therapy of hepatitis C virus-related liver disease in renal transplant patients. *Aliment Pharmacol Ther*, Vol. 24. No. 10, pp. 1413-1422.

Fabrizi, F., Bruchfeld, A., Mangano, S., Dixit, V., Messa, P. and Martin, P. (2007). Interferon therapy for HCV associated glomerulonephritis: meta-analysis of controlled trials. *Int J Artif Organs*, Vol. 30, No.3, pp. 212-219.

Feng, B.; Eknoyan, G., Guo, Z., Jadoul, M., Rao, H., Zhang, W. et al. (2011). Effect of interferon-alpha-based antiviral therapy on hepatitis C virus-associated glomerulonephritis: a meta-analysis. *Nephrol. Dial. Transplant*, May 10. [Epub ahead of print]

Ferri, C.; Zignego, A.L. and Pileri, S.A. (2002). Cryoglobulins. *J Clin Pathol*, Vol. 55, No. 1, pp. 4-13.

Fong, T.L.; Valinluck, B., Govindarajan, S., Charboneau, F., Adkins, R.H. and Redeker, A.G. (1994). Short-term prednisone therapy affects aminotransferase activity and hepatitis C virus RNA levels in chronic hepatitis C. *Gastroenterology*, Vol. 107, No.1, pp. 196-199.

Gallay, B.J.; Alpers, C.E., Davis, C.L., Schultz, M.F. and Johnson, R.J. (1995). Glomerulonephritis in renal allografts associated with hepatitis C infection: A possible relationship with transplant glomerulopathy in two cases. *Am J Kidney Dis*, Vol. 26, No.4, pp. 662-667.

Gloor, J.; Sethi, S., Stegall, M.D., Park, W.D., Moore, S.B., DeGoey, S. et al. (2007). Transplant glomerulopathy subclinical incidence and association with alloantibody. *Am J Transplant*, Vol. 7, No.9, pp. 2124-2132.

Hammoud, H.; Haem, J.; Laurent, B., Alamartine, E., Diab, N., Defilippis, J.P. et al. (1996). Glomerular disease during HCV infection in renal transplantation. *Nephrol Dial Transplant*, Vol. 11, Suppl 4, S54-S55.

Herzenberg, A.M.; Telford, J.J., De Luca, L.G., Holden, J.K. and Magil, A.B. (1998). Thrombotic microangiopathy associated with cryoglobulinemic membranoproliferative glomerulonephritis and hepatitis C. *Am J Kidney Dis*, Vol. 31, No. 3, pp. 521-6.

Hu, S.L. and Jaber, B.L. (2005). Ribavirin monotherapy for hepatitis C virus-associated membranous nephropathy. *Clin Nephrol*, Vol. 63, No. 1, pp. 41-45.

Iskandar, S.S. and Herrera, G.A. (2002). Glomerulopathies with organized deposits. *Semin Diagn Pathol*, Vol. 19, No. 3, pp. 116-32.

Johnson, R.J.; Gretch, D.R., Yamabe, H., Hart, J., Bacchi, C.E., Hartwell, P. et al. (1993). Membranoproliferative glomerulonephritis associated with hepatitis C virus infection *N Engl J Med*, Vol. 328, No. 7, pp. 465-470.

Johnson, R.J.; Gretch, D.R., Couser, W.G., Alpers, C.E., Wilson, J., Chung, M. et al. (1994). Hepatitis C virus-associated glomerulonephritis. Effect of alpha-interferon therapy. *Kidney Int*, Vol. 46, No. 6, pp. 1700-1704.

Kamar, N.; Sandres-Saune, K. and Rostaing, L. (2007). Influence of rituximab therapy on hepatitis C virus RNA concentration in kidney-transplant patients. *Am J Transplant*, Vol. 7, No. 10, pp. 2440.

Kamar, N.; Izopet, J., Alric, L., Guilbeaud-Frugier, C. and Rostaing, L. (2008). Hepatitis C virus-related kidney disease: an overview. *Clin Nephrol*, Vol. 69, No. 3, pp. 149-60.

Komatsuda, A.; Imai, H., Wakui, H., Hamai, K., Ohtani, H., Kodama, T. et al. (1996). Clinicopathological Analysis and Therapy in Hepatitis C Virus-Associated Nephropathy. *Internal Medicine*, Vol.35, No.7 pp. 529-533.

Kristiansen, M.G.; Gutteberg, T.J., Mortensen, L., Berg, L.K., Goll, R. and Florholmen, J. (2010). Clinical outcomes in a prospective study of community-acquired hepatitis C virus infection in Northern Norway. *Scand J Gastroenterol*, Vol. 45, No. 6, pp. 746-51.

Lake, J.R. (2003). The role of immunosuppression in recurrence of hepatitis C. *Liver Transpl*, Vol. 9, Suppl 3, S63-S66.

Lamprecht, P.; Gause, A. and Gross, W.L. (1999). Cryoglobulinemic vasculitis. *Arthritis Rheum*, Vol. 42, No. 12, pp. 2507-2516.

Lindsay, K.L.; Trepo, C., Heintges, T., Shiffman, ML., Gordon, SC., Hoefs, J.C. et al. (2001). A randomized, double-blind trial comparing pegylated interferon alfa-2b to interferon alfa-2b as initial treatment for chronic hepatitis C. *Hepatology*, Vol. 34, No. 2, pp. 395-403.

Lock, G.; Reng, C.M., Graeb, C., Anthuber, M. and Wiedmann, K.H. (1999). Interferon-induced hepatic failure in a patient with hepatitis C. *Am J Gastroenterol*, Vol. 94, No. 9, pp. 2570-2571.

Markowitz, G.S.; Cheng, J.T., Colvin, R.B., Trebbin, W.M. and D'Agati, V.D. (1998). Hepatitis C viral infection is associated with fibrillary glomerulonephritis and immunotactoid glomerulopathy. *J Am Soc Nephrol*, Vol 9, No. 12, pp. 2244-52.

Mazzaro, C.; Panarello, G., Carniello, S., Faelli, A., Mazzi, G., Crovatto, M. et al. (2000). Interferon versus steroids in patients with hepatitis C virus-associated cryoglobulinaemic glomerulonephritis. *Digest Liver Dis,* Vol. 32, No. 8, pp. 708–715.

McGuire, BM.; Julian, B.A., Bynon, J.S., Cook, W.S., King, S.J., Curtis, J.J. et al. (2006). Brief communication: Glomerulonephritis in patients with hepatitis C cirrhosis undergoing liver transplantation. *Ann Intern Med,* Vol. 144, No.10, pp. 735–741.

McHutchison, J.G.; Wilkes, L.B., Pockros, P.J., Chan, C.S., Neuwald, P., Urdea, M. et al. (1993). Pulse corticosteroid therapy increases viremia in patients with chronic HCV infection. *Hepatology,* Vol. 18, 87A.

Meier-Kriesche, H.U.; Ojo, A.O., Hanson, J.A. and Kaplan, B. (2001). Hepatitis C antibody status and outcomes in renal transplant recipients. *Transplantation,* Vol. 72, pp. 241-244.

Merkle, M.; Ribeiro, A. and Wörnle, M. (2011). TLR3 dependent regulation of cytokines in human mesangial cells: a novel role for IP-10 and TNFa in hepatitis C associated glomerulonephritis. *Am J Physiol Renal Physiol,* Mar 30. [Epub ahead of print]

Meyers, C.M.; Seeff, L.B., Stehman-Breen, C.O. and Hoofnagle, J.H. (2003). Hepatitis C and renal disease: an update. *Am J Kidney Dis,* Vol 42, No. 4, pp. 631-57.

Miller, S.E. and Howell, D.N. (2000). Glomerular diseases associated with hepatitis C virus infection. *Saudi J Kidney Dis Transpl,* Vol. 11, No. 2, pp. 145-60.

Misiani, R. ; Bellavita, P., Fenili, D., Vicari, O., Marchesi, D., Sironi, P.L. et al. (1994). Interferon alfa-2a therapy in cryoglobulinemia associated with hepatitis C virus. *N Engl J Med,* Vol. 330, No. 11, pp. 751–756.

Montalbano, M.; Pasulo, L., Sonzogni, A., Remuzzi, G., Colledan, M. and Strazzabosco, M. (2007). Treatment with pegylated interferon and ribavirin for hepatitis C virus-associated severe cryoglobulinemia in a liver/kidney transplant recipient. *J Clin Gastroenterol,* Vol. 41, No. 2, pp. 216–220.

Monti, G.; Galli, M., Invernizzi, F., Pioltelli, P., Saccardo, F., Monteverde, A. et al. (1995). Cryoglobulinaemias: A multi-centre study of the early clinical and laboratory manifestations of primary and secondary disease. Italian Group for the Study of Cryoglobulinaemias. *QJM,* Vol. 88, No.2, pp. 115–126.

Morales, J.M.; Pascual-Capdevila, J., Campistol, J.M., Fernandez-Zatarain, G., Muñoz, M.A. Andres, A. et al. (1997). Membranous glomerulonephritis associated with hepatitis C virus infection in renal transplant patients. *Transplantation,* Vol. 63, No.11, pp. 1634-1639.

Morales, J.M.; Marcén, R., Andres, A., Domínguez-Gil, B., Campistol, J.M., Gallego, R. et al. (2010). Renal transplantation in patients with hepatitis C virus antibody. A long national experience. *NDT Plus,* Vol. 3, Suppl 2, ii41-ii46.

Mukherjee, S. and Ariyarantha, K. Successful hepatitis C eradication with preservation of renal function in a liver/kidney transplant recipient using pegylated interferon and ribavirin. (2007). *Transplantation,* Vol. 84, No. 10, pp. 1374–1375.

Nampoory, M.R.; Johny, K.V., Costandi, J.N., Said, T., Abraham, M., Gupta, R.K. et al. (2001). High incidence of proteinuria in hepatitis C virus-infected renal transplant recipients is associated with poor patient and graft outcome. *Transplant Proc,* Vol. 33, No. 5, pp. 2791-2795.

Okada, K.; Takishita, Y., Shimomura, H., Tsuji, T., Miyamura, T., Kuhara, T. et al. (1996). Detection of hepatitis C virus core protein in the glomeruli of patients with membranous glomerulonephritis. *Clin Nephrol*, Vol. 45, No. 2, pp. 71-6.

Pereira, B.J. and Levey, A.S. (1997). Hepatitis C virus infection in dialysis and renal transplantation. *Kidney Int*, Vol. 51, No.4, pp. 981-999.

Perico, N.; Cattaneo, D., Bikbov, B. and Remuzzi, G. (2009). Hepatitis C infection and chronic renal diseases. *Clin J Am Soc Nephrol*, Vol. 4, No. 1, pp. 207-20.

Pham, H.P. ; Feray, C., Samuel, D., Gigou, M., Azoulay, D., Paradis, V. et al. (1998). Effects of ribavirin on hepatitis C-associated nephrotic syndrome in four liver transplant recipients. *Kidney Int*, Vol. 54, No. 4, pp. 1311-1319.

Ponticelli, C.; Montagnino, G., Campise, M.R., Baldassari, A. and Tarantino, A. (1986). Treatment of renal disease in essential mixed cryoglobulinemia. In: Minetti, L. and D'Amico, G. eds. *Antiglobulins, cryoglobulins, and glomerulonephritis.*, pp. 265-272, Martinus Nijoff.

Quartuccio, L.; Soardo, G., Romano, G., Zaja, F., Scott, C.A., De Marche, G. et al. (2006). Rituximab treatment for glomerulonephritis in HCV-associated mixed cryoglobulinemia: efficacy and safety in the absence of steroids. *Rheumatology*, Vol. 45, No. 7, pp. 842-6.

Quigg, R.J.; Brathwaite, M., Gardner, D.F., Gretch, D.R. and Ruddy, S. (1995). Successful cyclophosphamide treatment of cryoglobulinemic membranoproliferative glomerulonephritis associated with hepatitis C virus infection. *Am J Kidney Dis*, Vol. 25, No.5, pp. 798–800.

Rossi, P. ; Bertani, T., Baio, P., Caldara, R., Luliri, P., Tengattini, F. et al. (2003). Hepatitis C virus-related cryoglobulinemic glomerulonephritis: long-term remission after antiviral therapy. *Kidney Int*. Vol. 63, No. 6, pp. 2236-2241.

Roth, D.; Cirocco, R., Zucker, K., Ruiz, P., Viciana, A., Burke, G. et al. (1995). De novo membranoproliferative glomerulonephritis in hepatitis C virus-infected renal allograft recipients. *Transplantation*, Vol. 59, No. 12, pp. 1676-1682.

Ruggenenti, P.; Schieppati, A. and Remuzzi, G. (2001). Progression, remission, regression of chronic renal diseases. *Lancet*, Vol. 357, No. 9268, pp. 1601–1608.

Ruggenenti, P.; Fassi, A., Ilieva, A.P., Bruno, S., Iliev, I.P., Brusegan, V. et al. (2004). Bergamo Nephrologic Diabetes Complications Trial (BENEDICT) Investigators: Preventing microalbuminuria in type 2 diabetes. *N Engl J Med*, Vol. 351, No.19, pp. 1941–1951.

Saadoun, P.; Resche-Rigon, M., Thibault, V., Piette, K.C. and Cacoub, P. (2006). Antiviral therapy for hepatitis C virus-associated mixed cryoglobulinemia vasculitis. *Arthritis Rheum*. Vol. 54, No. 11, pp. 3696-3706.

Sabry, A.A.; Sobh, M.A., Irving, W.L., Grabowska, A., Wagner, B.E., Fox, S. et al. (2002). A comprehensive study of the association between hepatitis C virus and glomerulopathy. *Nephrol Dial Transplant*, Vol. 17, No. 2, pp. 239-45.

Sansonno, D.; De Re, V., Lauletta, G., Tucci, F.A., Boiocchi, M. and Dammacco, F. (2003). Monoclonal antibody treatment of mixed cryoglobulinaemia resistant to interferon alfa with an anti-CD20. *Blood* Vol. 101, No. 10, pp. 3818-26.

Sansonno, D.; Lauletta, G., Montrone, M., Grandaliano, G., Schena. F.P. and Dammacco, F. (2005). Hepatitis C virus RNA and core protein in kidney glomerular and tubular structures isolated with laser capture microdissection. *Clin Exp Immunol,* Vol. 140, No. 3, pp. 498-506.

Schmitz, V.; Kiessling, A., Bahra, M., Puhl, G., Kahl, A., Berg, T. et al. (2007). Peginterferon alfa-2b plus ribavirin for the treatment of hepatitis C recurrence following combined liver and kidney transplantation. *Ann Transplant,* Vol. 12, No.3, pp. 22–27.

Scott, D.R.; Wong, J.K., Spicer, T.S., Dent, H., Mensah, F.K., McDonald, S. et al. (2010). Adverse impact of hepatitis C virus infection on renal replacement therapy and renal transplant patients in Australia and New Zealand. *Transplantation,* Vol. 90, No. 11, pp. 1165-71.

Stehman-Breen, C.; Alpers, C.E., Fleet, W.P. and Johnson, R.J. (1999). Focal segmental glomerular sclerosis among patients infected with hepatitis C virus. *Nephron,* Vol. 81, No. 1, pp. 37-40.

Tarantino, A.; De Vecchi, A., Montagnino, G., Imbasciati, E., Mihatsch, M.J. Zollinger, H.U. et al. (1981). Renal disease in essential mixed cryoglobulinemia nephropathy. *Q J Med,* Vol.50, No. 197, pp. 1-30.

Tarantino, A.; Campise, M., Banfi, G., Confalonieri, R., Bucci, A., Montoli, A. et al. (1995). Long-term predictors of survival in essential mixed cryoglobulinemic glomerulonephritis. *Kidney Int,* Vol. 47, No. 2, pp. 618–623.

Tsui, J.I.; Vittinghoff, E., Shlipak, M.G., Bertenthal, D., Inadomi, J., Rodriguez, R.A. et al. (2007). Association of hepatitis C seropositivity with increased risk for developing end-stage renal disease. *Arch Intern Med,* Vol. 167, No.12, pp. 1271-1276.

Uchiyama-Tanaka, Y.; Mori, Y., Kishimoto, N., Nose, A., Kijima, Y., Nagata, T. et al. (2004). Membranous glomerulonephritis associated with hepatitis C virus infection: case report and literature review. *Clin Nephrol,* Vol. 61, No. 2, pp. 144-50.

Usalan, C.; Erdem, Y., Altun, B., Nar, A., Yasavul, U, Turgan, C. et al. (1998). Rapidly progressive glomerulonephritis associated with hepatitis C virus infection. *Clin Nephrol,* Vol. 49, No. 2, pp. 129-31.

Virgilio, B.; Palminteri, G., Maresca, M.C., Brunello, A., Calconi, G. and Vianello, A. (2001). Proteinuria at five years after kidney transplantation: The role of anti-HCV-positive state. *Transplant Proc,* Vol. 33, No. 7-8, pp. 3639-3640.

Weclawiack, H.; Kamar, N., Mehrenberger, M., Guilbeau-Frugier, C., Modesto, A., Izopet, J. et al. (2008). Alpha-interferon therapy for chronic hepatitis C may induce acute allograft rejection in kidney transplant patients with failed allografts. *Nephrol Dial Transplant,* Vol. 23. No. 3, pp. 1043-1047.

WHO Health Organization. Weekly Epidemiological Record. No. 49,10 December 1999, WHO; Hepatitis C fact sheet N0. 164, October 2000 http://www.who.int/inf-fs/en/fact164.html (May 2011, date last accessed)

Wörnle, M.; Schmid, H., Banas, B., Merkle, M., Henger, A., Roeder, M. et al. (2006). Novel role of toll-like receptor 3 in hepatitis C-associated glomerulonephritis. *Am J Pathol,* Vol. 168, No. 2, pp. 370-85.

Yamabe, H.; Johnson, R.J., Gretch, D.R., Fukushi, K., Osawa, H., Miyata, M. et al. (1995). Hepatitis C virus infection and membranoproliferative glomerulonephritis in Japan. *J Am Soc Nephrol,* Vol. 6, No. 2, pp. 220-23.

Yamabe, H.; Nakamura, N., Shimada, M., Murakami, R., Fujita, T., Shimaya, Y. et al. (2010). Clinicopathological Study on Hepatitis C Virus-associated Glomerulonephritis without Hepatitis C Virus in the Blood. *Inter Med,* Vol. 49, No. 14, pp. 1321-1323.

Zaja, F.; De Vita, S., Mazzaro, C., Sacco, S., Damiani, D., De Marchi, G. et al. (2003). Efficacy and safety of rituximab in type II mixed cryoglobulinaemia. *Blood,* Vol. 101, No.10, pp. 3827-34.

11

Insights from Genomics on Post-Infectious Streptococcal Glomerulonephritis

W. Michael McShan and Roya Toloui
Department of Pharmaceutical Sciences
University of Oklahoma Health Sciences Center, Oklahoma City,
USA

1. Introduction

Acute post-streptococcal glomerulonephritis (APSGN) is one of the nonsuppurative sequelae that can occur following a group A streptococcal infection, the other common post-infection sequelae being rheumatic heart disease. Worldwide, it is estimated that approximately 470,000 cases of APSGN occur annually. Children and young adults most commonly are affected with males having twice the incidence as females. By the middle of the twentieth century, evidence was found that streptococcal skin infections were associated with APSGN, and these infections usually did not cause rheumatic fever, leading to the hypothesis that certain GAS strains were "rheumatogenic" while others were "nephritogenic." In contrast to the molecular and immunological details that have brought considerable insight into the pathogenesis of rheumatic heart disease, the bacterial and host factors that contribute to ASPGN remain poorly defined and at times controversial. Modern bacterial genome sequencing projects have now provided a rich genetic resource that includes complete sequences of nephritogenic group A streptococcus strain NZ131 (McShan et al., 2008) and nephritogenic group C streptococcus strain MGCS10565 (Beres et al., 2008) as well as other group A and C strains associated with rheumatic heart disease and other syndromes. A metagenomic analysis is presented and considers the contribution of genes previously associated with APSGN strains (such as streptokinase, protease SpeB, and M protein) as well as other potential genetic factors that may be found uniquely in these genomes including genes acquired by horizontal transfer and via mobile genetic elements. This analysis provides complementary information to the many published studies using nephritogenic *S. pyogenes* strain NZ131 and places them in a broader context, shedding light upon the genetic basis for the human disease caused by this and related streptococci.

2. Acute post-streptococcal glomerulonephritis

Streptococcus pyogenes (group A streptococcus) is a common bacterial pathogen of humans, causing a wide range of disease from uncomplicated pharyngitis to severe life-threatening infections like toxic shock syndrome or necrotizing fasciitis. Acute post-streptococcal glomerulonephritis (APSGN) is one of the two major post-infection sequelae that can follow acute streptococcal infections, the other being rheumatic heart disease. The typical causative agent of APSGN is the group A streptococcus although other Lancefield groups may occasionally trigger this disease. Worldwide, it is estimated that approximately 470,000 cases of APSGN occur annually (Carapetis et al., 2005). Children and young adults are the group that is most commonly presents with APSGN, and males have twice the incidence as females (Silva, 1998).

The link between group A streptococcal infections and the onset of nephritis was considered as early as 1917 by Ophuls (Ophuls, 1917). By the 1940s, a link had been found between streptococcal skin infections and the onset of APSGN, and since the associated strains usually did not cause rheumatic fever, the hypothesis was developed that certain *S. pyogenes* strains were "rheumatogenic" while others were "nephritogenic" (Futcher, 1940; Osman et al., 1933; Seegal and Earle, 1941). Additionally, it was observed that there were divergent seasonal patterns of peak incidence separating nephritogenic and rheumatogenic GAS, with skin infections and APSGN cases peaking in the late summer while throat infections and rheumatic fever had the highest incidence in October (Bisno et al., 1970). Cases of rheumatic fever were rare during the summer APSGN outbreaks, peaking instead during the autumn season. These observations lead to the development of the hypothesis that subpopulations of GAS exist that were adapted for colonization and infection of either the throat or the skin. These "throat specialists" and "skin specialists" were proposed to have specific sets of virulence factors that lead to the post-streptococcal sequelae of rheumatic heart disease or APSGN, respectively. This hypothesis has been refined over time to now define throat specialists, skin specialists and generalists using a classification scheme that relates the Mga regulon, the gene complement surrounding the major antiphagocytic protein M gene (*emm*), to preferred anatomical site of infection (Bessen et al., 1997; Enright et al., 2001; McGregor et al., 2004).

3. Comparative genomics of nephritogenic streptococcal strains

3.1 The nephritogenic streptococcal genomes

The role of streptococcal induced autoimmunity as the basis for the development of rheumatic heart disease has been supported by a number of detailed studies (Cunningham, 2000a; Cunningham et al., 1989; Ellis et al., 2010; Krisher and Cunningham, 1985). It is reasonable therefore to expect that a similar underlying source of antigenic cross-reactivity might be responsible for the development of APSGN, especially since the time of onset roughly follows the time required for the adaptive immune response. However, to date no definitive link has been found although a number of candidate streptococcal proteins have been proposed over the years, including streptokinase, protease SpeB, and the antiphagocytic M protein (reviewed by Cunningham (Cunningham, 2000b)). One of the goal's for genome sequencing of multiple streptococcal strains associated with different diseases was to use comparative genomics to gain insight into the genetic variations that underlie virulence. Several nephritogenic streptococcal isolates now have had their genome sequences determined, and this information will be crucial in understanding the pathogenic mechanisms underlying APSGN.

3.2 Physical chromosome characteristics

The genomes of nephritis-associated streptococcal isolates *S. pyogenes* NZ131 (group A) and *S. equi* subsp. *zooepidemicus* MGCS10565 (group C) were completely sequenced in independent efforts in 2008 (Beres et al., 2008; McShan et al., 2008). Both of these isolates were originally isolated from cases of human glomerulonephritis (Beres et al., 2008; McShan et al., 2008); additionally, NZ131 has been also studied intensively in over thirty published studies (McShan et al., 2008). Both genomes are single circular molecules of 1,815,783 bp and 2,024,171 bp for NZ131 and MGCS10565, respectively. Neither strain has been found to have naturally occurring plasmids or other episomes. Strain NZ131 has 1,699 predicted open reading frames (ORFs) that use 1,548,919 bases so that 85.3% of the genomic DNA is used as coding sequences. The base composition of the ORFs is 39.18% G+C while the composition of the total genome is 38.57%; both values are similar to the composition seen in the other completed GAS genomes (McShan et al., 2008). The MGCS10565 genome has a 42.59% G+C content, and its genome has 1,961 predicted ORFs, which require 85% of the genome (Beres et al., 2008). The physical parameters of both genomes are typical for the family streptococcaceae.

3.3 Prophages and mobile genetic elements
Strikingly, strain NZ131 carries three prophages in its genome while MGCS10565 carries none. Prophages are always prominent features in the group A streptococcal genomes, sometimes accounting for 10% of the total DNA, and are well-known as vectors for carrying virulence genes such as superantigens or other bioactive proteins. While MGCS10565 has genes that are homologous to prophage integrases or regulatory proteins as well as virulence factors that are often associated with prophages (two DNases and a phospholipase A2), no organized prophage genome exists (Beres et al., 2008). This lack of prophages is in contrast to the *S. equi* subsp. *zooepidemicus* animal pathogen strain NC_012470 that was recently described as having four endogenous prophages (Holden et al., 2009).

The naturally competent streptococci have the *com*CDE operon that is thought to be essential in genetic transformation (Cvitkovitch, 2001). Although a previous study had not found this operon in *S. equi* subsp. *zooepidemicus* strain NCTC 4676 (Havarstein et al., 1997), it is present in MGSA10565 (Beres et al., 2008). The genomes of the naturally competent streptococci (including *S. pneumoniae* and *S. mutans* (Ajdic et al., 2002; Hoskins et al., 2001; Tettelin et al., 2001)) contain *com*CDE and lack prophages, and it is often suggested that frequent DNA transformation events may disrupt the genomes of prophages; thus, their typical absence. The presence of *com*CDE in MGCS10565 suggests that this isolate also may be naturally competent for DNA transformation, and this phenotype may be responsible for the absence of prophages (Beres et al., 2008). Balancing that viewpoint is the fact that these genes appear in the genome of *S. equi* subsp. *zooepidemicus* strain NC_120470, which does carry prophages. Thus, there may be other factors controlling competence in this species.

The prophages of NZ131 carry the virulence genes streptococcal pyrogenic exotoxin H (*spe*H), a streptodornase (*spd*3) and the paratox gene (McShan et al., 2008). Prophage-associated virulence factors have not been linked to APSGN in the literature, and comparison of these two genomes would tend to confirm that non-association. Rather, it would seem that if a common genetic trait exists that leads to APSGN, it would be found among the bacterial genes. Further, the absence of prophages in MGCS10565 and its potential to be competent suggests that if it has acquired genetic material from group A streptococci, it may have occurred via uptake of DNA from the environment rather by bacteriophage mediated transduction. This scenario suggests that genetic transfer may be somewhat of a one-way street, flowing from *S. pyogenes* to this and similar *S. zooepidemicus* strains since group A streptococci have not been demonstrated to be naturally competent. Therefore, the lack of prophages in MGCS10565 argues that group A streptococci, which probably use transduction as a means for horizontal transfer, would be somewhat genetically isolated from these group C streptococcal strains.

3.4 The nephritogenic strains and diversity
The NZ131 and MGCS10565 genomes are not collinear with respect to gene order, but a great number of genes are shared between the two. The genome map of NZ131 is shown in

Fig. 1 with gene homology comparisons to strains MGCS10565 (circle 6) and MGAS2096 (circle 5). Strain MGAS2096 is a group A streptococcus M12 serotype strain that was also isolated from a case of APSGN (Beres et al., 2006) and provides an inter-species reference.

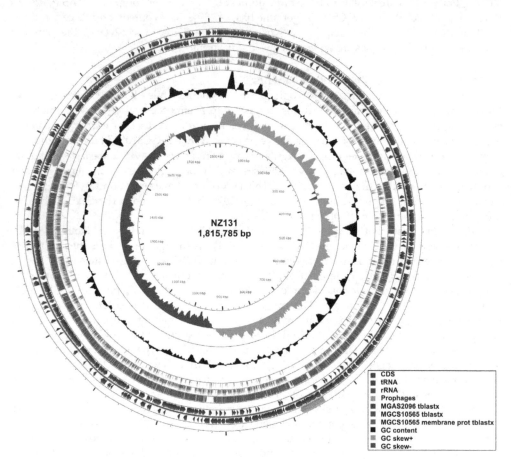

Fig. 1. **The genome map of M49 S. pyogenes strain NZ131.** The NZ131 genome map is shown with comparisons to the other two sequenced nephritogenic streptococcal genomes, S. pyogenes strain MGAS2096 and S. equi subsp. zooepidemicus strain MGCS10565. The outer circle and circle 4 indicate the positions of the three endogenous prophages in strain NZ131. The two circles they enclose (circles 2 and 3) show the location of the predicted NZ131 ORFs encoded by the two strands of DNA. The open reading frames were extracted from S. pyogenes strain MGAS2096 and S. equi subsp. zooepidemicus strain MGCS10565 and were compared to the genome of NZ131 using tblastx (circles 5 and 6). Circle 7 shows the specific tblastx hits of surface exposed proteins from MGCS10565. The innermost circles show the total G+C percentage of the NZ131 genomic DNA and the %G+C skew. The ribosomal RNA (rRNA) and tRNA (tRNA) genes were not included in the tblastx comparison. The figure was created using the online tools available at http://stothard.afns.ualberta.ca/cgview_server/index.html.

Overall, the main regions of divergence between the two *S. pyogenes* strains are in the endogenous prophages and other mobile genetic elements (MGE) carried by each (Fig. 1, circles 1 and 4), the genetic structures of the M protein gene region (Mga regulon) and streptococcal pilus region (circle 5), and by the presence the novel M49 and M82 specific NUDIX hydrolase operon in NZ131 (circle 5 (McShan et al., 2008)). NZ131 prophage NZ131.2 shares significant homology with a prophage from MGAS2096 (circle 5) but not including the crucial lysogeny module or virulence genes. Additionally, MGAS2096 has a deletion of a cluster of genes required for citrate metabolism (circle 5, about 925 kb on the map). To date, little evidence has been found to suggest that genes found on prophages or other MGE play a role in APSGN, and the lack of homology in these elements from the two group A streptococcal strains strengthens this idea. Thus, if a common mechanism for triggering APSGN exists, one would predict that bacterially encoded genes would be responsible, either in the form of unique nephritis-associated genes or gene alleles. A number of streptococcal proteins have been investigated as potential triggers of APSGN, and many of targets remain still largely unexplored. For example, circles 6 and 7 show the homology of MGCS10565 total genes and predicted membrane associated genes, respectively, to NZ131. While the homology is not as complete as was for the inter-species strain, many genes and particularly genes encoding cell-surface proteins are present in this intra-species streptococcus. Most of these proteins have not had their function or their potential immunogenicity identified. Thus, if genome comparisons tell us anything, it is that that many targets for future investigations remain. However, several genes have been considered to play a role in APSGN in previous work, and it is worthwhile to examine the variants found in each of these nephritogenic strains for possible shared features.

4. Genes associated with post-streptococcal glomerulonephritis

4.1 Streptokinase

Streptokinase is a plasminogen activator that is released as an extracellular protein by groups A, C, and G streptococci. It generates plasmin, which may promote bacterial spread through fibrinolysis and degradation of the extracellular matrix as well as induce inflammation via complement activation. This latter event may play a role in post-infection sequelae like APSGN (Nordstrand et al., 1999). It has been proposed that structural differences between alleles of streptokinase may be associated with diverse pathogenic outcomes, particularly in the variable βeta-domain (Lizano and Johnston, 2005). The role of streptokinase in the pathogenesis of APSGN has been supported by the use of a mouse model and derivatives of strain NZ131 with either nephritis- or non-nephritis-associated alleles of streptokinase (Nordstrand et al., 2000; Nordstrand et al., 1998).

The streptococcal streptokinase is composed of three domains, which are the highly conserved alpha and gamma domains and the variable βeta domain (Wang et al., 1998). The alpha and βeta domains are associated with plasminogen activation while the variable βeta domain is not required for this enzymatic activity (Lizano and Johnston, 2005). However, in the mouse model used by Nordstrand and her co-workers, the alleles that caused the onset of nephritis mapped their variations to the βeta domain (Nordstrand et al., 2000; Nordstrand et al., 1998). These studies, along with clinical observations (Johnston et al., 1992), have lead to a proposed role for streptokinase in APSGN, possibly in mediating complement deposition in the kidney.

One of the striking observations from the genome of the nephritis-associated group C MGCS10565 strain is the divergence of the encoded streptokinase when compared to those encoded by other group C and group A strains, whether nephritis-associated or not. Figure 2 shows a clustalw alignment of the amino acids from the streptokinase βeta regions from the group A genome strains M1, M2, M3, M4, M6, M12, M18, M28, and M49 as well as the group C strains H46 and GGS 124 (*S. dysgalactiae* subsp. *equisimilis*) and H70 and MGCS10565 (*S. equi* subsp. *zooepidemicus*). The βeta region from the two *zooepidemicus* strains is quite divergent from the other streptokinase proteins from both groups A and C subsp. *equisimilis* strains. Considerable divergence is also observed in the alpha and gamma domains (not shown). The βeta domain is required for docking to plasminogen via a kringle binding hairpin loop (Dhar et al., 2002; Wang et al., 1998), and the variation seen in this region suggests that a number of primary sequences are able to generate the needed secondary and tertiary protein structures.

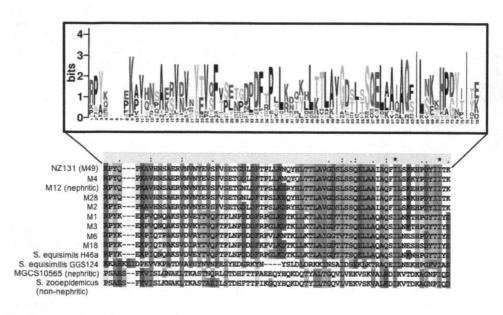

Fig. 2. **Analysis of the streptokinase gene *ska* βeta-region.** The variable βeta-region from the *ska* genes from GAS genome strains (NZ131 (M49, APSGN), MGAS10750 (M4), MGAS2096 (M12, APSGN), MGAS6180 (M28), MGAS10270 (M2), SF370 (M1), MGAS315 (M3), MGAS10394 (M6), and MGAS8232 (M18)) and GCS strains (*S. equisimilis* H46a, *S. equisimilis* GGS124, MGCS10565 (APSGN), and the non-nephritogenic *S. zooepidemicus* H70) was aligned using CLUSTALW (Thompson et al., 1994) and the resulting consensus analyzed using WebLogo (Crooks et al., 2004). The non-nephritogenic M12 *S. pyogenes* strain MGAS9429 was omitted from this analysis since its sequence is 100% identical to that of the nephritis-associated M12 strain MGAS2096. The primary descriptions of each of these genomes are found in the literature (Banks et al., 2004; Beres et al., 2006; Beres et al., 2008; Beres et al., 2002; Ferretti et al., 2001; Green et al., 2005; Holden et al., 2009; Holden et al., 2007; McShan et al., 2008; Shimomura et al., 2011; Smoot et al., 2002)

Further, it should be noted that a number of conserved neutral amino acid residues are positioned in the βeta domain, suggesting an essential contribution to function. Inspection of the primary sequence of the streptokinase proteins in this group shows additional conserved sequences in the two nephritogenic group A streptococcal isolates (NZ131 and MGAS2096) but not found in the nephritogenic group C strain. Protein folding of this domain may create similar structures in both groups that might contribute to APSGN, but such information is not available yet. Interestingly, the streptokinase gene from the non-nephritis M12 serotype strain MGAS9429 is 100% identical to the nephritogenic M12 strain. It is also possible that the mechanisms of pathogenesis that trigger nephritis following group A or group C infection may be different. Clearly, more detailed studies need to be done to address the possible role of streptokinase in APSGN.

4.2 Protease SpeB

Zabriskie and co-workers first observed that strains were associated with APSGN produced an extracellular protein not seen in non-nephritis strains, which was subsequently found to be bound to plasmin (Poon-King et al., 1993; Villarreal et al., 1979). This plasmin binding protein was discovered to be the major extracellular protease SpeB, and analysis of patient sera showed significantly higher levers of anti-SpeB antibodies in APSGN patients as compared to rheumatic fever patients or controls (Cu et al., 1998; Poon-King et al., 1993). Recent studies using a mouse tissue cage model have demonstrated that SpeB expression is inhibited in *S. pyogenes* strains that are maintained in the animal for extended periods, and this inhibition is inversely related to the increased expression of phage-encoded pyogenic exotoxins and DNases (Aziz et al., 2004). The strains studied were not associated with nephritis, suggesting that group A streptococci which cause APSGN may differentially express this protein when compared to non-nephritogenic strains. The lack of an identifiable homolog to SpeB in the group C strain MGCS10565 argues against the necessity of it in either the onset or progression of APSGN. However, the molecular mechanisms that underlie APSGN in the group C species may be different in some aspects from group A nephritogenic strains, and thus the absence of this protein in MGCS10565 may not be informative about group A APSGN disease. Further studies on this problem are clearly warranted.

4.3 Surface associated proteins
4.3.1 The Mga regulon genes

The molecular mimicry that underlies the onset of rheumatic heart disease results from the immune response to a prominent surface antigen of group A streptococci, the M protein. Therefore, such immunological cross-reactivity may be expected to contribute to APSGN, especially considering the time course of onset of symptoms. Particular M protein serotypes have been associated with APSGN, with M types 2, 49, 42, 56, 57, and 60 being associated with skin infections and APSGN while M types 1, 4, 12, and 25 being associated with throat infections and APSGN (Bessen et al., 1997; Bessen et al., 1996; Bisno, 1995; Enright et al., 2001; Kalia et al., 2002; Silva, 1998). As reported in the original description of the MGCS10565 genome, this group C contains a major deletion in much of the Mga regulon, including the genes for protease SpeB and the serum opacity factor (*sof*), although orthologs of many of these proteins including the M protein gene (*emm*) are found elsewhere in this genome (Beres et al., 2008). The genome of MGCS10565 revealed a large number of predicted extracellular collagen-like proteins, but none of these provided direct evidence of linkage to the nephritis-associated group A streptococcal serotypes. The linkage of serotype and disease in the streptococcal, while clearly observed, remains somewhat unclear from the genetic level in terms of gene linkage or evolutionary co-selection.

4.3.2 Glyceraldehyde phosphate dehydrogenase (GAPDH)

Surface associated glyceraldehyde phosphate dehydrogenase (GAPDH) from nephritogenic strains of group A streptococci have been implicated in APSGN, with the molecule often detected in renal biopsies and patient sera having elevated anti-GAPDH antibody titers (Lange et al., 1976; Yamakami et al., 2000; Yoshizawa et al., 1992; Yoshizawa et al., 2004). This protein, which also has been referred to in the literature as the nephritis associated plasmin receptor, shows >85% homology between *S. zooepidemicus* MGCS10565 and the group A genome strains, which are virtually identical in amino acid sequence (Beres et al., 2008). Thus, it seems that if GAPDH plays a role in APSGN it is not a specific trigger for the disease. Indeed, other investigators have failed to find an association between GAPDH and APSGN (Batsford et al., 2005), so its role remains somewhat in question.

4.3.3 Enolase

Another *S. pyogenes* surface associated protein that has been implicated in APSGN is enolase, which is a major plasminogen binding protein and may be involved in triggering APSGN (Fontan et al., 2000). The phylogenetic analysis of the enolase genes from the *S. pyogenes*, *S. zooepidemicus*, *S. equisimilis* subsp. *dysgalactiae*, *S. pneumoniae*, and *S. mutans* genomes is presented in Fig. 3. The two *S. zooepidemicus* genes form a separate branch that is quite distinct from the *S. pyogenes* genes and encode proteins that are 100% identical.

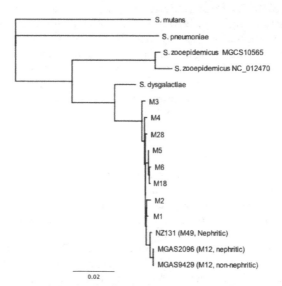

Fig. 3. **Phylogenetic analysis of streptococcal enolase genes.** The enolase genes from the group A streptococcal genomes (see Fig. 2 legend), now including the non-nephritogenic M12 strain MGAS2096, along with the genes from *S. zooepidemicus* strains MGCS10565 (nephritogenic) and NC_012470 (non-nephritogenic), *S. dysgalactiae* subsp. *equisimilis* GGS_124, *S. pneumoniae* TIGR4, and *S. mutans* UA159 were compared and a phylogenetic tree constructed using Geneious (Drummond et al., 2010).

Interestingly, the two nephritogenic group A streptococcal strains, NZ131 and MGAS2096, occupy a separate branch from the other *S. pyogenes* strains. However, this branch also includes the other M12 genome strain (MGAS9429) that was not nephritis associated. It may be that these closely related alleles of enolase play a role in the onset or development of APSGN in *S. pyogenes*, but the presence a non-nephritogenic strain argues that other factors must be required. Further, it would seem that enolase is probably not a common factor between groups A and C streptococci in the onset of APSGN.

4.3.4 Streptococcal pilus genes

Recent studies have demonstrated that group A streptococci and other Gram positive bacteria produce long, pili-like appendages that mediate binding to human fibronectin or collagen (Kang et al., 2007; Mora et al., 2005). These regions are identified by the presence of the genes encoding the pilus subunit proteins and their associated C sortases. A transcriptional regulator is included in the gene cluster of group A streptococci, and strains may be subdivided into two groups based upon whether the pilus region carries *rof*A or *nra* regulator genes. A recent classification scheme has described this region in *S. pyogenes* as belonging to one of six FCT groups (Kratovac et al., 2007). Strain NZ131 is a member of the *nra* group (FCT-3) that also includes the M3, M5, and M18 genome strains.

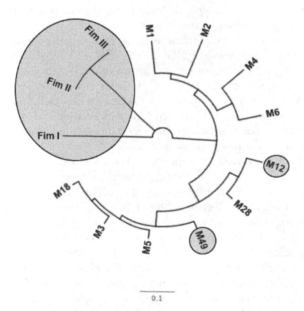

Fig. 4. **Phylogeny of the streptococcus pili regions.** The phylogenetic tree of the streptococcal pilus (fibronectin binding) regions from the *S. pyogenes* genome strains (see Fig. 2 legend) and from MGCS10565 is shown. The regions from the *S. pyogenes* genomes are indicated by the M protein serotype, and the nephritogenic group A streptococcal strains (NZ131 and MGCS2096) and group C strain (MGCS10565) are shaded.

Group C strain has three potential pilus (fibronectin binding protein) regions (Beres et al., 2008), which is in contrast to the one pilus (T antigen) cluster found in the group A streptococci (McShan et al., 2008). Two of the group C pilus regions have homology to the pilus regions from the M2 and M6 genomes but little match that genome location in either the NZ131 or MGAS2096 chromosomes. Sortases are Gram-positive transpeptidases that anchor pili and other surface proteins to the cell wall (Hae Joo Kang and Baker, 2011; Janulczyk and Rasmussen, 2001). Strain NZ131 encodes an alternate sortase in this region (*src*C2, Spy49_0116). Interestingly, the *rof*A gene in MGCS10565 is not included in this gene cluster, being encoded elsewhere on the genome. When a phylogenetic tree of the pilus regions from the *S. pyogenes* and *S. equi* subsp. *zooepidemicus* genomes is constructed (Figure 4), the three pili regions (FimI – FimIII) form a distinct out-group from the *S. pyogenes* regions. The regions from the two nephritogenic group A streptococcal strains, NZ131 and MGAS2096, also are not closely related to each other, and the diversity of this region again argues that this is not the genetic location where are located unique factors that define nephritogenic strains of streptococci.

5. Conclusions

Comparison of the genomes of nephritogenic strain NZ131 and MGCS10565 reveals many similarities and differences that reflect related genera but distinct species. It is difficult, however, to make a convincing argument that an obvious shared trait is responsible for APSGN in both strains; rather, it is the differences that seem the most obvious when comparing potential virulence mechanisms.

One striking finding from genome comparison is the level of diversity between the group A streptococcal genomes and the genome of MGCS10565. Indeed, no common link to APSGN is immediately evident from the examination of the potential genetic sources from previous studies to the genomes. Beres et al. (Beres et al., 2008), after considering the diversity between the group A and group C genomes, tended to discount potential roles for streptokinase and protease SpeB in APSGN. Indeed, these proteins may not be key in the onset or progression of the disease although there are a number of studies supporting both. However, this conclusion presumes that the mechanism of pathogenesis of APSGN is the same in both species, which it well may not be. Many diarrheal diseases present with similar symptoms even though the underlying bacterial infection may be quite different, and it is possible that streptococcal nephritis caused by different species may result from a different series of molecular events. Further, even if there is a common molecular trigger for APSGN, it may be also true that for some bacterial factors that may amplify or promote the disease the phenotype may be more important through their enzymatic activity than their antigenicity. Thus, the important message from genomics at this time is that many aspects of APSGN remain to be explored so to uncover the roles played by virulence factors both known and yet to be characterized. Additional genome sequences from nephritogenic streptococci would help increase our understanding. The genomic information that is already available provides a rich resource for future studies as well as providing a framework for understanding the previous efforts in this field of investigation.

6. Acknowledgments

This work was supported in part by NIH Grant R15 AI072718-02A1 to WMM. Its contents are solely the responsibility of the authors and do not necessarily represent the official views of NIH.

7. References

Ajdic, D., McShan, W., McLaughlin, R., Savic, G., Chang, J., Carson, M., Primeaux, C., Tian, R., Kenton, S., Jia, H., et al. (2002). Genome sequence of Streptococcus mutans UA159, a cariogenic dental pathogen. Proc Natl Acad Sci USA 99, 14434-14439.

Aziz, R.K., Pabst, M.J., Jeng, A., Kansal, R., Low, D.E., Nizet, V., and Kotb, M. (2004). Invasive M1T1 group A Streptococcus undergoes a phase-shift in vivo to prevent proteolytic degradation of multiple virulence factors by SpeB. Mol Microbiol 51, 123-134.

Banks, D.J., Porcella, S.F., Barbian, K.D., Beres, S.B., Philips, L.E., Voyich, J.M., DeLeo, F.R., Martin, J.M., Somerville, G.A., and Musser, J.M. (2004). Progress toward characterization of the group A Streptococcus metagenome: complete genome sequence of a macrolide-resistant serotype M6 strain. J Infect Dis 190, 727-738.

Batsford, S.R., Mezzano, S., Mihatsch, M., Schiltz, E., and Rodriguez-Iturbe, B. (2005). Is the nephritogenic antigen in post-streptococcal glomerulonephritis pyrogenic exotoxin B (SPE B) or GAPDH? Kidney international 68, 1120-1129.

Beres, S.B., Richter, E.W., Nagiec, M.J., Sumby, P., Porcella, S.F., Deleo, F.R., and Musser, J.M. (2006). Molecular genetic anatomy of inter- and intraserotype variation in the human bacterial pathogen group A Streptococcus. Proc Natl Acad Sci USA 103, 7059-7064.

Beres, S.B., Sesso, R., Pinto, S.W., Hoe, N.P., Porcella, S.F., Deleo, F.R., and Musser, J.M. (2008). Genome sequence of a Lancefield group C Streptococcus zooepidemicus strain causing epidemic nephritis: new information about an old disease. PLoS ONE 3, e3026.

Beres, S.B., Sylva, G.L., Barbian, K.D., Lei, B., Hoff, J.S., Mammarella, N.D., Liu, M.Y., Smoot, J.C., Porcella, S.F., Parkins, L.D., et al. (2002). Genome sequence of a serotype M3 strain of group A Streptococcus: phage-encoded toxins, the high-virulence phenotype, and clone emergence. Proc Natl Acad Sci USA 99, 10078-10083.

Bessen, D., Fiorentino, T., and Hollingshead, S. (1997). Molecular markers for throat and skin isolates of group A streptococci. Adv Exp Med Biol 418, 537-543.

Bessen, D., Sotir, C., Readdy, T., and Hollingshead, S. (1996). Genetic correlates of throat and skin isolates of group A streptococci. The Journal of infectious diseases 173, p896-900.

Bisno, A.L. (1995). Non-suppurative poststreptococcal sequelae: rheumatic fever and glomerulonephritis. In Principles and practice of infectious diseases, G.L. Mandell, J.E. Bennett, and R. Dolin, eds. (New York, N.Y., Churchill Livingstone), pp. 1799-1810.

Bisno, A.L., Pearce, I.A., Wall, H.P., Moody, M.D., and Stollerman, G.H. (1970). Contrasting epidemiology of acute rheumatic fever and acute glomerulonephritis. N Engl J Med 283, 561-565.

Carapetis, J.R., Steer, A.C., Mulholland, E.K., and Weber, M. (2005). The global burden of group A streptococcal diseases. Lancet Infect Dis 5, 685-694.

Crooks, G.E., Hon, G., Chandonia, J.M., and Brenner, S.E. (2004). WebLogo: a sequence logo generator. Genome Res 14, 1188-1190.

Cu, G.A., Mezzano, S., Bannan, J.D., and Zabriskie, J.B. (1998). Immunohistochemical and serological evidence for the role of streptococcal proteinase in acute post-streptococcal glomerulonephritis. Kidney international 54, 819-826.

Cunningham, M.W. (2000a). Cross-reactive antigens of group A streptococci. In Gram-Positive Pathogens, V.A. Fischetti, R.P. Novick, J.J. Ferretti, and J.I. Rood, eds. (Washington, D.C., ASM Press), pp. 66-77.

Cunningham, M.W. (2000b). Pathogenesis of group A streptococcal infections. Clin Microbiol Rev 13, 470-511.

Cunningham, M.W., McCormack, J.M., Fenderson, P.G., Ho, M.K., Beachey, E.H., and Dale, J.B. (1989). Human and murine antibodies cross-reactive with streptococcal M protein and myosin recognize the sequence GLN-LYS-SER-LYS-GLN in M protein. J Immunol 143, 2677-2683.

Cvitkovitch, D.G. (2001). Genetic competence and transformation in oral streptococci. Crit Rev Oral Biol Med 12, 217-243.

Dhar, J., Pande, A.H., Sundram, V., Nanda, J.S., Mande, S.C., and Sahni, G. (2002). Involvement of a nine-residue loop of streptokinase in the generation of macromolecular substrate specificity by the activator complex through interaction with substrate kringle domains. The Journal of biological chemistry 277, 13257-13267.

Drummond, A., Ashton, B., Buxton, S., Cheung, M., Cooper, A., Heled, J., Kearse, M., Moir, R., Stones-Havas, S., Sturrock, S., et al. (2010). Geneious v5.3 (Available from http://www.geneious.com).

Ellis, N.M., Kurahara, D.K., Vohra, H., Mascaro-Blanco, A., Erdem, G., Adderson, E.E., Veasy, L.G., Stoner, J.A., Tam, E., Hill, H.R., et al. (2010). Priming the immune system for heart disease: a perspective on group A streptococci. The Journal of infectious diseases 202, 1059-1067.

Enright, M.C., Spratt, B.G., Kalia, A., Cross, J.H., and Bessen, D.E. (2001). Multilocus sequence typing of Streptococcus pyogenes and the relationships between emm type and clone. Infect Immun 69, 2416-2427.

Ferretti, J.J., McShan, W.M., Ajdic, D., Savic, D.J., Savic, G., Lyon, K., Primeaux, C., Sezate, S., Suvorov, A.N., Kenton, S., et al. (2001). Complete Genome Sequence of an M1 Strain of Streptococcus pyogenes. Proc Natl Acad Sci USA 98, 4658-4663.

Fontan, P.A., Pancholi, V., Nociari, M.M., and Fischetti, V.A. (2000). Antibodies to streptococcal surface enolase react with human alpha-enolase: implications in poststreptococcal sequelae. The Journal of infectious diseases 182, 1712-1721.

Futcher, P.H. (1940). Glomerulonephritis following infections of the skin. Archives of Internal Medicine 65, 1192-1210.

Green, N.M., Zhang, S., Porcella, S.F., Nagiec, M.J., Barbian, K.D., Beres, S.B., Lefebvre, R.B., and Musser, J.M. (2005). Genome Sequence of a Serotype M28 Strain of Group A Streptococcus: Potential New Insights into Puerperal Sepsis and Bacterial Disease Specificity. J Infect Dis 192, 760-770.

Hae Joo Kang, F.C.T.P., and Baker, E.N. (2011). Crystal Structure of Spy0129, a Streptococcus pyogenes Class B Sortase Involved in Pilus Assembly. PLoS ONE 6.

Havarstein, L., Hakenbeck, R., and Gaustad, P. (1997). Natural competence in the genus Streptococcus: evidence that streptococci can change pherotype by interspecies recombinational exchanges. J Bacteriol 179, 6589-6594.

Holden, M.T., Heather, Z., Paillot, R., Steward, K.F., Webb, K., Ainslie, F., Jourdan, T., Bason, N.C., Holroyd, N.E., Mungall, K., et al. (2009). Genomic evidence for the evolution of Streptococcus equi: host restriction, increased virulence, and genetic exchange with human pathogens. PLoS pathogens 5, e1000346.

Holden, M.T., Scott, A., Cherevach, I., Chillingworth, T., Churcher, C., Cronin, A., Dowd, L., Feltwell, T., Hamlin, N., Holroyd, S., et al. (2007). Complete genome of acute rheumatic fever-associated serotype M5 *Streptococcus pyogenes* strain manfredo. J Bacteriol *189*, 1473-1477.

Hoskins, J., Alborn, W.E., Jr., Arnold, J., Blaszczak, L.C., Burgett, S., DeHoff, B.S., Estrem, S.T., Fritz, L., Fu, D.J., Fuller, W., *et al.* (2001). Genome of the bacterium *Streptococcus pneumoniae* strain R6. J Bacteriol *183*, 5709-5717.

Janulczyk, R., and Rasmussen, M. (2001). Improved pattern for genome-based screening identifies novel cell wall-attached proteins in gram-positive bacteria. Infect Immun *69*, 4019-4026.

Johnston, K.H., Chaiban, J.E., and Wheeler, R.C. (1992). Analysis of the variable domain of the streptokinase gene from streptococci associated with poststreptococcal glomerulonephritis. In New perspectives on streptococci and streptococcal infections Proceedings of the XI Lancefield International Symposium Zentralbl Bakteriol Suppl 22 G. Orefici, ed. (New York, NY, Gustav-Fischer-Verlag), p. 339.

Kalia, A., Spratt, B.G., Enright, M.C., and Bessen, D.E. (2002). Influence of recombination and niche separation on the population genetic structure of the pathogen *Streptococcus pyogenes*. Infect Immun *70*, 1971-1983.

Kang, H.J., Coulibaly, F., Clow, F., Proft, T., and Baker, E.N. (2007). Stabilizing isopeptide bonds revealed in gram-positive bacterial pilus structure. Science (New York, NY) *318*, 1625-1628.

Kratovac, Z., Manoharan, A., Luo, F., Lizano, S., and Bessen, D.E. (2007). Population genetics and linkage analysis of loci within the FCT region of *Streptococcus pyogenes*. J Bacteriol *189*, 1299-1310.

Krisher, K., and Cunningham, M.W. (1985). Myosin: a link between streptococci and heart. Science *227*, 413-415.

Lange, K., Ahmed, U., Kleinberger, H., and Treser, G. (1976). A hitherto unknown streptococcal antigen and its probable relation to acute poststreptococcal glomerulonephritis. Clinical nephrology *5*, 207-215.

Lizano, S., and Johnston, K.H. (2005). Structural diversity of streptokinase and activation of human plasminogen. Infect Immun *73*, 4451-4453.

McGregor, K.F., Spratt, B.G., Kalia, A., Bennett, A., Bilek, N., Beall, B., and Bessen, D.E. (2004). Multilocus sequence typing of *Streptococcus pyogenes* representing most known emm types and distinctions among subpopulation genetic structures. J Bacteriol *186*, 4285-4294.

McShan, W.M., Ferretti, J.J., Karasawa, T., Suvorov, A.N., Lin, S., Qin, B., Jia, H., Kenton, S., Najar, F., Wu, H., *et al.* (2008). Genome Sequence of a Nephritogenic and Highly Transformable M49 Strain of *Streptococcus pyogenes*. J Bacteriol *190*, 7773–7785.

Mora, M., Bensi, G., Capo, S., Falugi, F., Zingaretti, C., Manetti, A.G.O., Maggi, T., Taddei, A.R., Grandi, G., and Telford, J.L. (2005). Group A Streptococcus produce pilus-like structures containing protective antigens and Lancefield T antigens. Proc Natl Acad Sci USA *102*, 15641-15646.

Nordstrand, A., McShan, W.M., Ferretti, J.J., Holm, S.E., and Norgren, M. (2000). Allele Substitution of the Streptokinase Gene Reduces the Nephritogenic Capacity of Group A Streptococcal Strain NZ131. Infect Immun *68*, 1019-1025.

Nordstrand, A., Norgren, M., Ferretti, J.J., and Holm, S.E. (1998). Streptokinase as a mediator of acute post-streptococcal glomerulonephritis in an experimental mouse model. Infect Immun *66*, 315-321.

Nordstrand, A., Norgren, M., and Holm, S.E. (1999). Pathogenic mechanism of acute post-streptococcal glomerulonephritis. Scandinavian journal of infectious diseases *31*, 523-537.

Ophuls, W. (1917). The Etiology and Development of Nephritis. J Am Med Assoc *69*, 1223-1227.

Osman, A.A., Close, H.G., and Carter, H. (1933). Studies in Bright's disease. VIII. Observations on the aitiology of scarlatinal nephritis. Guy's Hosp Rep *83*, 360.

Poon-King, R., Bannan, J., Viteri, A., Cu, G., and Zabriskie, J.B. (1993). Identification of an extracellular plasmin binding protein from nephritogenic streptococci. The Journal of experimental medicine *178*, 759-763.

Seegal, D., and Earle, D.P. (1941). A consideration of certain biological differences between glomerulonephritis and rheumatic fever. American Journal of the Medical Sciences *201*, 528-529.

Shimomura, Y., Okumura, K., Murayama, S.Y., Yagi, J., Ubukata, K., Kirikae, T., and Miyoshi-Akiyama, T. (2011). Complete genome sequencing and analysis of a Lancefield group G Streptococcus dysgalactiae subsp. equisimilis strain causing streptococcal toxic shock syndrome (STSS). BMC Genomics *12*, 17.

Silva, F.G. (1998). Acute postinfectious glomerulonephritis and glomerulonephritis complicating persistent bacterial infection. In Hepinstall's pathology of the kidney, J.C. Jennette, J.L. Olson, M.M. Schwartz, and F.G. Silva, eds. (Philadelphia, Pa., Lippincott-Raven Publishers), pp. p. 389-453.

Smoot, J.C., Barbian, K.D., Van Gompel, J.J., Smoot, L.M., Chaussee, M.S., Sylva, G.L., Sturdevant, D.E., Ricklefs, S.M., Porcella, S.F., Parkins, L.D., et al. (2002). Genome sequence and comparative microarray analysis of serotype M18 group A Streptococcus strains associated with acute rheumatic fever outbreaks. Proc Natl Acad Sci USA *99*, 4668-4673.

Tettelin, H., Nelson, K.E., Paulsen, I.T., Eisen, J.A., Read, T.D., Peterson, S., Heidelberg, J., DeBoy, R.T., Haft, D.H., Dodson, R.J., et al. (2001). Complete genome sequence of a virulent isolate of *Streptococcus pneumoniae*. Science *293*, 498-506.

Thompson, J.D., Higgins, D.G., and Gibson, T.J. (1994). CLUSTAL W: improving the sensitivity of progressive multiple sequence alignment through sequence weighting, positions-specific gap penalties and weight matrix choice. Nucleic Acids Res *22*, 4673-4680.

Villarreal, H., Jr., Fischetti, V.A., van de Rijn, I., and Zabriskie, J.B. (1979). The occurrence of a protein in the extracellular products of streptococci isolated from patients with acute glomerulonephritis. The Journal of experimental medicine *149*, 459-472.

Wang, X., Lin, X., Loy, J.A., Tang, J., and Zhang, X.C. (1998). Crystal structure of the catalytic domain of human plasmin complexed with streptokinase. Science *281*, 1662-1665.

Yamakami, K., Yoshizawa, N., Wakabayashi, K., Takeuchi, A., Tadakuma, T., and Boyle, M.D. (2000). The potential role for nephritis-associated plasmin receptor in acute poststreptococcal glomerulonephritis. Methods *21*, 185-197.

Yoshizawa, N., Oshima, S., Sagel, I., Shimizu, J., and Treser, G. (1992). Role of a streptococcal antigen in the pathogenesis of acute poststreptococcal glomerulonephritis. Characterization of the antigen and a proposed mechanism for the disease. J Immunol *148*, 3110-3116.

Yoshizawa, N., Yamakami, K., Fujino, M., Oda, T., Tamura, K., Matsumoto, K., Sugisaki, T., and Boyle, M.D. (2004). Nephritis-associated plasmin receptor and acute poststreptococcal glomerulonephritis: characterization of the antigen and associated immune response. J Am Soc Nephrol *15*, 1785-1793.

12

Glomerular Pathology in Patients with HIV Infection

Enrique Morales, Elena Gutierrez-Solis,
Eduardo Gutierrez and Manuel Praga
Nephrology Department, Hospital 12 Octubre, Madrid
Spain

1. Introduction

The course and prognosis of patients infected with the human immunodeficiency virus (HIV) is changing dramatically following the introduction of highly active antiretroviral therapy (HAART), with increased patient survival and decreased morbidity (Mocroft et al, 1998).

Current therapy offers patients increased survival by making it more susceptible to certain comorbidities (Fang et al, 2007). Cardiovascular and renal diseases are the prototype of diseases whose prevalence increases progressively with the prolonged survival and aging (Braithwaite et al, 2005). On the other hand, besides specifically associated nephropathy or HIV coinfection with hepatitis C virus (HCV) with prolonged survival of the HIV-infected population, the spectrum of kidney disease in patients with HIV also reflects the growing burden of comorbid diabetes and hypertension and development chronic renal disease (Wyatt et al, 2007; Mocroft et al 2007; Szczech, 2004).

The prevalence of chronic kidney disease in HIV patients may be between 5 to 15% depending on the series. However, it has been manifested as albuminuria or proteinuria may be present up to 30% in some cohorts of HIV-infected patients (Szczech et al, 2002). The prevalence of renal histological involvement has ranged from 1-15% depending on the different autopsy series (Shahinian et al, 2000). Patients with HIV infection may develop different types of glomerular diseases, vascular lesions and tubulointerstitial nephritis related in some cases with the virus itself or other co-infections (Williams et al, 1998).

In this chapter we will review at different types of glomerular diseases found in patients with HIV infection, highlighting its etipopatogenia, clinical presentation, diagnosis and therapeutic alternatives.

2. Glomerular diseases in patients with HIV infection

Association between HIV infection and renal disease was first described in 1984, shortly after isolation of the virus (Rao et al, 1984). The glomerular diseases are relatively common complication in patients infected with HIV, with a wide range of clinical presentations and with a poor prognosis in most cases. Although HIV-associated nephropathy (HIVAN) has been considered the most frequent and most representative glomerular disease, after the generalized treatment of HIV-infected patients with HAART therapy has allowed the emergence of other glomerular diseases with a higher incidence than the general population, see Table 1.

- HIVAN
- HIV-Associated glomerulonephritis. Immune complex glomerulonephritis
  - Membranoproliferative glomerulonephritis
  - Membranous nephropathy
  - Mesangial glomerulonephritis (IgA)
  - Focal segmental glomerulosclerosis non-collapsing
  - Lupus-like glomerulonephritis
  - Postinfectious glomerulonephritis
- Other nephropathies
  - Thrombotic Microangiopathy
  - Malignant hypertension
  - Amyloidosis

Table 1. Glomerular diseases in patients with HIV infection

2.1 HIV-associated nephropathy

This type of glomerular disease is HIV-associated nephropathy best described (Rao et al, 1987). The disease affects mostly males, intravenous drugs users and black patients (D'Agati & Appel, 1997). U.S. is the third leading cause of end-stage renal disease (ESRD) in African Americans between 20 and 64 years of age and the most common cause of ESRD in HIV-1 seropositive patients (Eggers & Kimmel, 2004; Shahinian et al, 2000). Prevalence is variable, ranging from 4% in clinical studies and 10% in autopsy (Mazbar et al, 1989). Although these renal findings can be seen in patients with asymptomatic or primary HIV infection, most of patients have low CD4 cells count and advanced disease.

Among the specific mechanisms involved, in addition to genetic susceptibility (several polymorphisms that influence susceptibility to HIV infection), the virus can be seen in glomerular epithelial cells (Kimmel et al, 1993; Röling et al, 2006). Transgenic mice were crated with HIV-DNA construct inserted into the genome and developed a histological picture and clinical presentation very similar to that of humans (Bruggeman et al, 1997). The viral genome is detected in different renal structures (tubular cells, podocytes, glomerular parietal epithelial cells), even in cases without renal involvement, indicating that the presence in the renal tissue is not sufficient to cause nephropathy (Lu & Ross, 2005; Mikulak & Singhal, 2010). There are many mediators and the expression of nonstructural viral proteins, cytokines and growth factors can modulate and amplify renal injury. The mechanism of viral entry into renal epithelial cell is still unknown. CCR5 and CXCR4 are coreceptors to CD4 that mediate HIV-1 entry into lymphocytes. These receptors have not been demonstrated on renal epithelial cells in vivo (Eitner et al, 2000). Recently, have been described the DEC-205 receptor, which facilitates the entry of the virus in renal tubular cells (Hatsukari et al 2007).

HIVAN is a characterized by a constellation of pathologic findings involving glomerular, tubular and interstitial compartments. Glomerular pathologic findings include a collapsing focal segmental glomerulonephritis, with a marked retraction of glomerular capillary loops, and occlusion of the lumen (D'Agati & Appel, 1998). Podocytes show intense hypertrophy and hyperplasia, which is associated with decrease expression of podocyte maturity markers and accumulations of protein in their cytoplasm. On the other hand, there is a characteristic intense tubulointerstitial involvement, which gives it a matter of some exclusivity over other nephrotic syndromes. These changes consist of dilatation of the renal tubules, which sometimes are proliferative microcyst, and large proteinaceous cylinders in light, cell infiltrates and areas of fibrosis (D'Agati & Appel, 1998; Klotman, 1999). Immunofluorescence usually shows mesangial deposits of IgM and C3 and electron microscopy, are frequently observed tuboreticular inclusions in the cytoplasm of endothelial cells. These structures are synthesized by the stimulation of alpha-interferon, as in the cases of patients with lupus nephritis. The histological differential diagnoses of focal segmental glomerulosclerosis are the collapsing nephropathy heroin abuse, caused by bisphosphonates, interferon or parvovirus (Klotman, 1999).

Main manifestation of HIV-associated nephropathy is a nephrotic syndrome (Herman & Klotman, 1998). However, although the proteinuric can be massive in many cases (more than 8-10 g/24 h), most patients with HIVAN do not have significant peripheral edema. Moreover, patients with HIVAN are usually not hypertensive, a remarkable finding considering that more than 90% of black patients with renal insufficiency of other causes exhibit hypertension. The kidneys are usually normal in size or larger. Most patients also have advanced renal failure at the time of diagnosis.

Evolution without HAART is poor, with rapid development of renal failure requiring dialysis within the first year of diagnosis, and with a high mortality (Winston et al, 1998). The beneficial effects of HAART on HIVAN have been shown in individual clinical observations. There are reports of resolution of renal disease with the administration of HAART, with a recurrence of renal disease after stopping treatment (Scialla et al, 2007).

Although no controlled clinical trials have demonstrated the effectiveness of any therapeutic measure in the HIVAN, it is recognized that HAART prevents or reduces the risk of developing HIVAN and if this occurs, the patients may have a slower course and lower mortality than in untreated patients (Lucas et al, 2004). Another treatment option is recommended in these patients using drugs that blocker renin-angiotensin-aldosterone system (BRAAS). These drugs are a part like any other chronic proteinuric nephropathy (Wei et al, 2003). Some studies have shown a decrease in proteinuria and a trend towards stabilization of renal damage in patients with HIVAN treated with corticosteroids. However, this treatment was not without significant side effects (Smith et al, 1994), so it should be limited to cases in which treatment with HAART have not produced any improvement and if we rule out opportunistic infections. Finally, we can find some curious case of spontaneous improvement of the glomerular pathology (Morales et al, 2002). The indications for renal replacement therapy with dialysis or transplantation in patients with HIVAN are similar to those followed in other chronic renal disease in the general population.

2.2 Immune-mediated glomerulonephritis

Patients with HIV infection have a higher incidence of other glomerulonephritis whose pathogenesis is generally attributed to glomerular deposition of immune complexes (Balow, 2005; Nochy et al, 1993), see **Table 2.**

	City/Country	Number of patients	Gender (M/F)	HCV (+)%	Race	Types of Glomerular diseases	Ref
Williams DI et al	London	17	13 M, 4 F		47% blacks 53% caucasians	HIVAN 41%, MN 23%, HUS 12%, others 24 %	9
Rao TKS et al.	Nueva York	55	49 M, 6 F		100% blacks	HIVAN 90%, Mesangial GN 10%	11
Mazbar SA et al.	San Francisco	27	26 M, 1 F		63% blacks 37% caucasians	HIVAN 27%, MPGN 27%, Interstitial nephritis 9%, immune complex GN with IgG-IgM 9%, 28 % others	15
NocheD et al.	Paris	60	51 M, 9 F		48% blacks 52% caucasians	43 % HIVAN, Immune complex GN 37%, lupus like nephritis 16%, HUS 11.5%	33
Casanova S et al.	Italy	26	21 M, 5 F		100% caucasians	Immune complex GN 65.5%, MPGN 15.5%, lupus like nephritis 11.5%, minimal change 7.5%	34
Connolly JO et al.	London	34	25 M, 9 F		55.8% blacks 41.1%caucasians	50 % HIVAN, 14.5 % MN, 6% MPGN, 12 % HUS, 3% Immune complex GN, 14.5 % others	53
Shahinian V et al.	Texas	389	362 M, 27 F		54 % blacks 35% caucasians	26% unknown, 7 % HIVAN, 7% immune complex GN, 17 % ATN, 25% crystal induced nephropathy	14
Szczech La et al.	EEUU	89	73 M, 16 F		88% blacks 12% others	47% HIVAN, 53 % non-HIVAN	6
Cheng JT et al.	EEUU	14	8 M, 6 F	100	93% blacks 7% caucasians	79% MPGN, 21% MN	36
Stokes MB et al.	EEUU	12	11 M, 1 F	100	58% blacks 42% caucasians	41% MPGN, 41 % mesangial GN, 8% MN, 8 % HIVAN	37
Gutiérrez et al.	Madrid, Spain	27	23 M, 4 F	77.8	11% blacks 89% caucasians	29.6% MPGN, 25.9% Non-collapsing FSGS, 22.2% mesangial GN, 14.8% HIVAN.	45

Table 2. Different studies with renal disease in HIV patients

In Europe, especially in Caucasians, glomerular immune complex glomerular diseases are more common than HIVAN and may take several forms. The immune-mediated glomerulonephritis would be the counterpart among the white population to what is represented by the HIVAN in the black (Casanova et al, 1995).

The pathogenesis of these types of glomerulonephritis remains largely unknown; there is a local formation or glomerular deposition of circulating immune complexes that may contain HIV antigens and polyclonal antibodies. We can not rule out the involvement of an immune response against associated viral infections. The clinical features are very striking (gross hematuria, edema, acute renal failure, and hypertension), although cases of more subtle presentation and are diagnosed incidentally, see **Table 3.** Hypergammaglobulinemia is common, reflecting a polyclonal B cell activation. However, the role of some viral co-infections very frequent among HIV patients, such hepatitis C (HCV) and hepatitis B virus (HBV), appears to be decisive, particularly in MPGN and NM.

Very limited information is presently available regarding treatment and clinical outcomes in patients with immune-mediated GN in patients with HIV infection. Until now we have not information about the therapeutic interventions used in patients without HIV infection (steroids, immunosuppressants, calcineurin inhibitors) can change the course of immune-complex glomerulonephritis.

	HIVAN	MPGN	IgAN	FSGS-NC	MN	PIGN	Lupus-like	Amyloidosis	MAT
Nephrotic syndrome	4	3	0	3	4	1	4	4	1
Macroscopic hematuria	0	2	4	0	0	3	2	0	2
Acute renal failure	1	1	2	1	1	3	1	1	4
Hypertension/ Malignant hypertension	1	1	3	1	1	1	1	0	3
Hypo-complementemia	0	3	0	0	0	4	1	0	0
Cryglobulins (+)	0	3	0	0	0	1	1	0	0
Coinfection HCV/HBV	0	4	1	1	2	0	2	1	0
Treatment	HAART BSRAA S	BSRAA VHC (+) (INF+RBV) (S+PF+RTX)	BSRAA	BSRAA	BSRAA Several clinical (S+IMS)	BSRAA Several clinical (S)	HAART S	HAART Secondary aetiology	Plasma P

HIVAN: HIV-associated nephropathy; MPGN: membranoproliferative GN; IgAN: IgA nephropathy; FSGS-NC: Not collapsing forms of FSG; MN: membranous nephropathy; PIGN: Postinfectious GN; MAT: Thrombotic microangiopathy; HAART: Highly active antiretroviral therapy; BSRAA: Blockers of the system renin-angiotensin-aldosterone; S: steroids; INF: interferon; RBV: ribavirin; RTX: rituximab; P:Plasmapheresis. Degrees: (0-4): (Never-Always)

Table 3. Most common presentations and laboratory markers in glomerular diseases in patients with HIV infection

2.2.1 Membranoproliferative glomerulonephritis

The most common clinical presentation is nephrotic syndrome with macroscopic hematuria or microhematuria and normal renal function or mild renal function impairment. Up to 90% of cases there are co-infected with HCV (Morales et al, 1997; Cheng et al, 1999). Cryoglobulins are detected in most cases with elevated rheumatoid factor and decrease of complement, especially C4. The clinical and serological profile is very similar to the membranoproliferative GN associated with HCV patients without HIV infection. For all these reasons it is considered that this is a pathogenetically GN induced by HCV, without the concomitant presence of HIV play a prominent role (Stokes et al, 1997).

In some cases the extrarenal manifestations of cryoglobulinemia include clinical presentation, with vasculitis cutaneous, and even gastrointestinal manifestations alveolar hemorrhage. In these cases we can find an acute renal failure with hematuria and proteinuria, and characteristic histological finding of membranoproliferative GN with deposits of cryoglobulins in glomerular capillary lumens. Cryoglobulins are usually of a mixed IgG-IgM.

The safety and efficacy of HCV treatment with interferon and ribavirin in patients coinfected with HIV has been evaluated in numerous series in the literature (Kadan & Talal, 2007). There are series of cases in which an effective antiviral treatment correlated with improvement in renal manifestations (Kamar et al, 2006). However, we find cases in which there is no negativity of cryoglobulins despite the negativity of HCV-RNA, and can even clinical manifestations (Morales et al, 2007). There are cases in which clinical aggressiveness may be amenable to immunosuppressive treatment. High-dose steroids and plasmapheresis may improve the clinical course, although has increased HCV replication and risk of worsening liver disease. Rituximab is an anti-CD20 monoclonal antibody that has produced a prolonged improvement of renal manifestations in cases that can not be eradicated HCV (Kamar et al, 2006).

In cases of membranoproliferative GN is not associated with HCV; the experience is limited and can recommend the use of drugs that block the RAAS, since its effect antiproteinuric, renoprotective and antihypertensive.

2.2.2 IgA nephropathy

Series have described several cases of IgA nephropathy in patients infected with HIV. The actual incidence is unknown, but in a study of 116 autopsies in patients with HIV infection were detected IgA glomerular deposits by 7.7% (Beaufils et al, 1995).

Patients infected with HIV develop IgA antibodies against specific HIV antigens and this seems to be the pathogenic basis of this nephropathy. On the other hand, can produce idiotype IgA antibodies against other antibodies IgG and IgM directed against viral antigens. Renal lesions may result from HIV antigen-specific immune complexes that are derived from the circulation and from in situ complex formation (Kimmel et al, 1992).

Clinical presentation is similar to that of idiopathic IgA nephropathy: microhematuria with occasional episode of gross hematuria after infection mainly located in the upper respiratory tract and different proteinuria degrees. The long-term prognosis depends mainly on the amount of the proteinuria. In addition to these developments chronic, slowly progressive, characteristic of IgA nephropathy, patients may also develop acute complications similar to those of the IgA idiopathic acute renal failure that is associated with macroscopic hematuria is a widely known complication (Gutierrez et al, 2007) and development of hypertension malignant (MHT) (Chen et al, 2005). In episodes of gross hematuria may develop acute tubular necrosis, tubular abnormalities consist in a high proportion of tubules that are filled by red blood cells (RBC) casts and signs of tubular necrosis that are more evident in tubules that are occupied by RBC casts, see **Figure 1**.

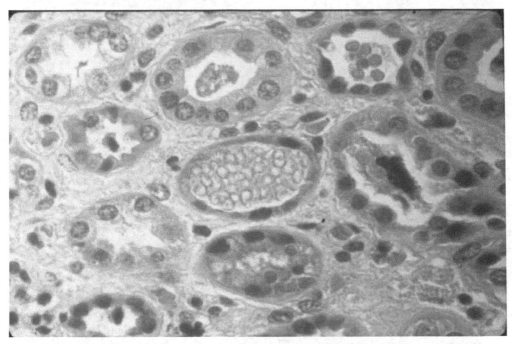

Fig. 1. Tubules filled by red blood cells, showing diminished number of lining epithelial cells and nuclear pyknosis.

Regarding the MHT, is observed in a significant percentage (5% -7%) of cases of idiopathic IgA, but some series indicate that its incidence may be even higher in HIV-associated IgA nephropathy. In our experience, most of the cases with HIV-infection and IgA nephropathy presented malignant hypertension (Gutierrez et al, 2007). The prognosis is poor and many cases progress to irreversible end-stage renal failure, see **Figure 2**. However, in some patients the effective control of blood pressure drug type inhibitors of angiotensin converting enzyme (ACE) inhibitors and / or antagonists of the angiotensin receptor (ARB) manages to partially reverse renal failure.

In some patients with HIV infection, as also in Idiopathic IgA renal manifestations may be associated with systemic manifestations of the type of vasculitis cutaneous, arthritis and various digestive disorders, all components of the Schönlein-Henoch syndrome.

At the present there is a little information about the treatment and outcomes of patients with HIV infection. Therefore, according to the recommendations in idiopathic IgA, it is recommended to treat all patients who develop significant proteinuria (>0.5-1 g / day) or hypertension, with ACE inhibitors or ARB, since the antiproteinuric and renoprotective effect of these drugs, also tested with IgA nephropathy (Praga et al, 2003).

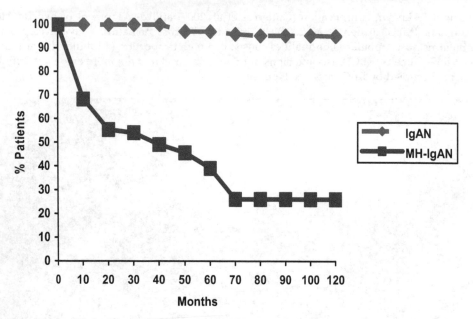

Fig. 2. Renal survival of patients with mesangial IgA nephropathy and MHT and mesangial nephropathy patients without MHT.

2.2.3 Focal segmental glomerulosclerosis non-collapsing

Among the different histological forms of focal glomerulosclerosis, have also been reported not collapsing glomerulosclerosis in patients with HIV (Haas et al, 2005). The pathogenesis and the exact relationship of these GN may have HIV or other pathogens have not been investigated.

Very limited information is available about the real incidence, clinical and developmental characteristics and therapeutic possibilities of this entity. In our experience, this type of glomerular disease is the second most common presentation in our HIV-infected patients (Gutierrez et al, 2007). The most common clinical presentation was proteinuria, and nephrotic syndrome was observed in 72% of cases. All patients were treated with HAART and BSRAA; at the end of treatment no patient need dialysis and 60% had renal insufficiency (Gutierrez et al, 2007).

In idiopathic forms, not associated with HIV, proteinuria and nephrotic syndrome are common manifestations. Some cases progress rapidly to ESRD. Corticosteroids administered for a long time for months and calcineurin inhibitors drugs are treatment options supported by experience. However, given the absence of data on HIV-infected patients and the susceptibility of these patients to infections, careful observational studies are needed before recommending these options. The optimization of antihypertensive and antiproteinuric drugs (ACEI/ARB) can exert a favorable effect, as in idiopathic less aggressive forms.

2.2.4 Membranous nephropathy

Membranous nephropathy (MN) is a typical example of glomerular disease mediated by deposition of immune complexes. MN is a recognized complication of renal malignancies and infections. Among these, HBV and HCV have been associated with the development of MN and syphilis, and various parasitic diseases.

In this context, the frequent presence of HBV and HCV co-infection and the increasing incidence of syphilis and other infectious processes suggests that there may be a predisposition of patients with HIV infection to the development of MN, although not known actual incidence and its outcome.

The characteristic clinical presentation is nephrotic syndrome, although minorities of cases show no nephrotic range proteinuria. In forms idiopathic, there are two therapeutic strategies that have proven effective in controlled prospective studies, immunosuppression with steroids plus cyclophosphamide or chlorambucil, and calcineurin inhibitors drugs (cyclosporine, tacrolimus) (Praga, 2008). However, consider that a high percentage (up to 50% in some series) have spontaneous remission within the first years of the disease (Polanco et al, 2010) for this reason may be preferable initially attitude conservative in patients with HIV-infection. All chronic proteinuric nephropathies may be beneficial to use renin-angiotensin-aldosterone system blockers (ACEI/ARB). If we can identify an infectious agent as pathogenic factor, the treatment could potentially resolve the kidney problem.

2.2.5 Postinfectious glomerulonephritis

Although the descriptions are limited (Enriquez et al, 2004), patients with HIV infection could be theoretically exposed to the development of postinfectious GN due to its higher rate of infection. The clinical picture is generally abrupt, with hypertension difficult to control, often gross hematuria and mild and transient impairment of renal function frequently. There are typical red blood cell casts present in urinary sediment and hypocomplementemia. Renal biopsy shows a diffuse endocapillary GN with proliferation of mesangial and endothelial cells, Glomerular and interstitial infiltration of monocytes and lymphocytes is present. Glomerular accumulation of neutrophils is common and is termed "exudative". Ultrastructural studies demonstrate the subepithelial "humps" which are typical although not pathognomonic of postinfectious GN.

The history of an infection, usually 1-2 weeks, followed by a short asymptomatic period and the typical abrupt onset of nephritic syndrome for the diagnosis in many cases, along with the study of the sediment and the detection of hypocomplementemia. The majority of cases have benign course with conservative treatment of the infectious process and complications (hypertension, edema). The descriptions of acute postinfectious GN in patients with endocarditis or localized infections are characteristic, although they have published very few cases among HIV-infected patients.

2.2.6 Lupus-like glomerulonephritis

Lupus-like glomerulonephritis, defined by the presence of a "full house" of glomerular immunoglobulin and complement deposits on immunofluorescence in the absence of serologic evidence of systemic lupus erythematosus (SLE). There is presently little information known about the etiology, its treatment, or its long-term outcome.

Its main histological features are cell proliferation and mesangial matrix, the presence of hyaline thrombi and massive deposit of immune complexes in capillary walls, which reach mimic the "wire loops" typical of lupus nephritis and are the origin of name ("lupus-like") that has been proposed for these cases. In immunofluorescence, as occurs in lupus nephritis, deposit detects all types of immunoglobulins (IgG, IgA, IgM) and various fractions of complement (Haas et al, 2005; Weiner et al, 2003). However, the term may be misleading, because the similarities end with lupus in the histological aspects of renal biopsy. There are no systemic symptoms similar to lupus flares and serology (ANA and anti-DNA, hypocomplementemia) is negative.

Most reported cases present with nephrotic syndrome and progressive deterioration of renal function. No information about the natural history of this process and whether or not modify therapeutic interventions. Regarding the pathogenesis, there are only speculations. It is proposed that, in addition to frequent infections with HBV, HCV and other infectious agents, HIV itself through several of its proteins (p24, gp41, gp120) can induce a systemic response of immunoglobulin, causing a large amount of circulating immune complexes that would be trapped nonspecifically in the glomerulus, alternatively, the HIV proteins could be initially deposited in the glomerulus (planted antigens) and subsequently be detected by the antibody in situ formation of immune complexes (Weiner et al, 2003).

Although we can be exceptionally patient with HIV infection and the coexistence of lupus with renal involvement, and it would be important to make a diagnosis difference between the two entities. In patients with both HIV infection and a diagnosis of SLE, three patterns of disease occurrence have been described: HIV following SLE diagnosis, SLE following HIV infection, and simultaneous diagnosis of HIV and SLE. Since the appearance of an autoimmune disorder in patients with a pre-existing immunodeficiency would not be expected, at least from a mechanistic standpoint, we will focus our review on patients with existing HIV who developed signs and symptoms consistent with a new diagnosis of lupus. SLE and HIV infection are two diseases whose clinical and serologic presentations may occasionally mimic one another, but with pathogenic mechanisms that theoretically are mutually exclusive. The seemingly paradoxical coexistence of these two immune disorders offers intriguing insights into the complex cellular and humoral immune networks that govern autoimmune phenomena and self tolerance.

Finally, the clinical management of the HIV positive lupus patient represents a therapeutic challenge for the physician due to the delicate equilibrium that needs to be achieved between SLE remission and HIV control (Gindea et al, 2010).

2.3 Other nephropathies in patients with HIV infection
2.3.1 Thrombotic microangiopathy

Thrombotic microangiopathy (TMA) is a known complication of HIV infection (Connolly et al, 1995; Alpers, 2003). Published reports of the incidence of TMA evaluated during the pre-HAART era vary considerably, depending on the type of study performed, diagnostic criteria used to evaluate patients, and stage of HIV disease (Connolly et al, 1995). It is likely that this under-diagnosed entity, as shown in autopsy studies (Gadallah et al, 1996) and patients with progressive deterioration of renal function, the presence of MAT in renal biopsy exceeded the incidence of HIVAN (Peraldi et al, 1999).

Endothelial cell injury appears to be the primary event causing platelet activation and deposition in the microvasculature. On these microthrombi mechanical destruction would occur, anemia, schistocytes, elevated LDH and Coombs test negative. Direct cytopathic roles of HIV as well as other factors such as malignancy, drugs, and infectious agents have been implicated in the pathogenesis of HIV-TMA. It is known that various HIV proteins can directly damage endothelial cells, inducing apoptosis therein (Alpers, 2003).

In experimental animals infected with HIV often develops MAT, so it is suspected that HIV itself plays a key role in endothelial damage (Eitner et al, 1999). It is also the possibility that anticardiolipin antibodies/antiphospholipid frequently detected in HIV patients (Boue et al, 1990) have pathogenic importance. In the primary antiphospholipid syndrome or lupus erythematosus associated with MAT may be triggered. Although not able to demonstrate that HIV-infected patients with anticardiolipin antibodies are at higher risk for MAT, it is an intriguing association. In idiopathic MAT has been achieved in many cases to elucidate the molecular basis of the disorder, especially those with family history: gaps ADAMS-13 and other enzymes that degrade the von Willebrand factor in type forms PTT and alterations of the complement system in the SHU. There is no evidence that these disorders occur in the MAT of patients infected with HIV. Although the majority of patients present in a more advanced stage of HIV disease, TMA can be the initial presenting symptom of HIV infection.

Clinical features are those of idiopathic TMA (Eitner et al, 1999), and the diagnosis should be suspected in any patient with new onset thrombocytopenia and microangiopathic haemolytic anaemia. Most patients are male and young and progressive deterioration of renal function is associated with the typical hematological findings MAT: schistocytes anemia with peripheral blood, thrombocytopenia, elevated LDH. Although most cases present a clear and rapidly progressive deterioration of renal function, similar to pictures of hemolytic uremic syndrome (HUS), others can have predominant neurologic manifestations, as in thrombotic thrombocytopenic purpura (TTP).

Kidney biopsy shows changes similar to idiopathic MAT: platelet-fibrin thrombi in preglomerular arterioles and the glomerular capillaries, arterioles with endothelial edema imaging in "onion skin" and mesangiolysis with widening of subendothelial space. When there are extrarenal manifestations (neurological, cardiac) vascular lesions are similar in the vessels of the affected organs.

Therapy with plasma exchange or infusion appears to be efficacious. A rapid diagnosis and institution of plasmapheresis is crucial for a favorable outcome. The long term prognosis of HIV-TMA is unfavorable and may depend on the stage of HIV infection. The recent data after the use of highly active retroviral treatment, however, are unavailable and current prognosis is therefore uncertain.

2.3.2 Malignant hypertension

Malignant hypertension is defined by the presence of unacceptably high blood pressure with grade III hypertensive retinopathy (hemorrhages and exudates) or IV (papilledema more vascular lesions). As we noted earlier, is a casual presentation of idiopathic IgA nephropathy, but its impact on the rest of idiopathic GN is rare. By contrast, preliminary studies indicate incidence of MHT special not only in IgA nephropathy patients with HIV, in which may be the most frequent presentation of this entity, but in other glomerular diseases associated with HIV (Morales et al, 2008). On the other hand, entities such as membranoproliferative GN, membranous and focal glomerulosclerosis, in which the MHT is a rare complication, there are a significant number of cases when associated with HIV infection. In our experience, malignant nephrosclerosis (arteriolar fibrinoid necrosis with intimal thickening and luminal narrowing; see **Figure 3**) was detected in six cases (three of them with IgAN, one with C-FSG, one with NC-FSG and one with MGN).

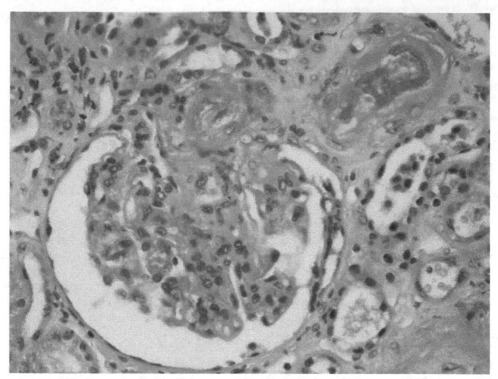

Fig. 3. Renal biopsy of patient 1 (Table 1), showing a glomerulus with mesangial proliferation (the immunofluorescence showed predominant deposits of IgA) and vascular lesions of malignant nephrosclerosis (fibrinoid necrosis) in the afferent arteriole. (hematoxylin;eosin; x400).

The typical symptoms of MHT (markedly increased BP, blurred vision due to retinal haemorrhages and severe headache). To interpret this catastrophic prognosis in HIV patients with GN and MHT, we speculate that the development of MHT has an irreversible detrimental influence on glomerular diseases already having a rather poor prognosis by themselves, see **Figure 4**.

On the other hand, the development of chronic renal failure could likely exacerbate the appearance of infectious and cardiovascular complications in these HIV-infected patients because both patients with chronic renal failure and HIV infection are particularly prone to the appearance of such complications (Grinspoon & Carr, 2005; Kamin & Grinspoon, 2005; Gupta et al, 2005). Other possible pathogenic pathways to explain this particular propensity of HIV patients with glomerular diseases to MHT could rely on the already known higher incidence of thrombotic microangiopathy (TMA) among HIV patients (Alpers, 2003). Both TMA and MHT could be interpreted as clinical manifestations of a systemic endothelial injury, due to a direct toxic effect of HIV, other infectious agents (particularly HCV and HBV) or other factors (such as drug addictions) linked to the environment of HIV infection. On the other hand, the presence of antiphospholipid antibodies is also more common among HIV patients, and these autoantibodies could play a role in endothelial vascular damage (Alpers, 2003; Galrao et al, 2007).

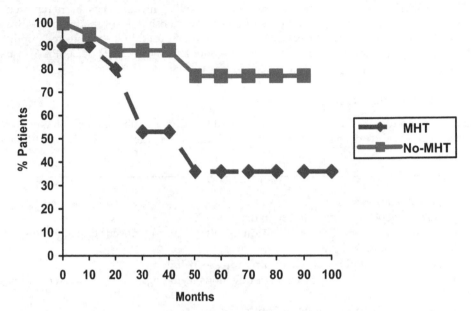

Fig. 4. Probability of renal survival (absence of chronic dialysis) in HIV patients with or without malignant hypertension.

In addition, considering the dismal prognosis of our patients in spite of HAART treatment and a satisfactory control of blood pressure, early detection and treatment of hypertension in HIV patients with glomerular diseases are mandatory.

2.3.3 Amyloidosis

In autopsy series of patients infected with HIV, as well as reviews of renal biopsies, amyloidosis is a relatively common finding (Lanjewar et al, 1999; Joseph et al, 2000). This is a secondary amyloidosis, type AA. Many studies have been suggested that frequent chronic infections may be responsible for this complication. However, it is possible that HIV infection itself plays a pathogenic role. Described a high level of SAA, acute phase reactant which is the precursor of AA amyloid in patients infected with HIV (Husebekk et al, 1986) and experimental models have shown that a significant proportion of animals infected develop amyloidosis (King et al, 1983).

As is common in amyloidosis, massive proteinuria and nephrotic syndrome were the most common renal manifestations in the cases described. There are no studies about specific therapeutic options in these patients, apart from trying to eradicate the underlying infectious process.

2.3.4 Hypertensive and diabetic nephropathy

Metabolic complications of HAART (dyslipidemia, changes in body fat, insulin resistance, diabetes mellitus) and the aging of the infected population suggest that kidney damage secondary to diabetes and hypertension may have increasing importance in patients infected HIV (Masia-Canuto et al, 2006).

In some series of renal biopsies of patients with HIV infection has been reported the presence of diabetic nephropathy in 6% of cases, hypertensive nephropathy in 4% (Szczech et al, 2004).The recommended treatment is similar to that used in the uninfected population and should include strict control of blood pressure and the early use of BSRAA to try to reduce proteinuria.

3. Tubular and interstitial renal disease

Patients infected with HIV can present a wide variety of tubular and interstitial renal disease secondary to drugs, infections and/or tumors; see Table 4 (GESIDA, 2010; Blok & Weening, 1999).

- Acute tubular necrosis
- Interstitial nephritis associated with drugs
  - Renal failure and Fanconi syndrome (certain reverse transcriptase inhibitors)
- Allergic interstitial nephritis
- Cristal-induced nephropathy (certain protease inhibitors)
- Interstitial nephritis associated with infections (cytomegalovirus, tuberculosis, hongos, Salmonella, Legionella, etc)
- Kaposi sarcoma and Lymphoma infiltrative
- Rhabdomyolysis

Table 4. Tubular and interstitial renal disease

The recommendations for the treatment of these nephropathies consist of drug withdrawal or correction of the precipitating cause, corrections, electrolyte, and in interstitial nephritis immunoallergic the administration of a short course of corticosteroids.

4. Conclusion

In conclusion, due to the wide range of kidney damage in people with HIV infection, it is difficult to predict the renal histology according to clinical criteria, so renal biopsy is mandatory for histologic diagnosis. In addition, the course and prognosis of these patients has changed radically since the introduction of antiretroviral therapy, with higher survival, so early diagnosis is essential and the establishment of an alternative therapy to prevent progression of renal disease.

5. References

Alpers CE (2003). Light at the end of the TUNEL. HIV-associated thrombotic microangiopathy. *Kidney Int* 2003; 63:385-396.

Alpers CE (2003). Light at the end of the TUNEL. HIV-associated thrombotic microangiopathy. *Kidney Int* 2003; 63:385-396.

Balow JE (2005). Nephropathy in the context of HIV infection. *Kidney Int* 2005; 67(4):1632-3.

Beaufils H, Jouanneau C, Katlama C, Sazdovith V & Hauw JJ (1995). HIV-associated IgA nephropathy -A postmorten study. *Nephrol Dial Transplant* 1995; 10:35-38.

Blok K & Weening JJ (1999). Interstitial nephritis and nephritic syndrome in patient from Zambia. *Nephrol Dial Transplant* 1999; 14:1016-1017.

Boue F, Dreyfus M & Bridey F (1990). Lupus anticoagulant and HIV infection: a prospective study. *AIDS* 1990; 4:467-471.

Braithwaite RS, Justice AC, Chang CC, Fusco JS, Raffanti SR & Wong JB et al (2005). Estimating the proportion of patients infected with HIV who will die of comorbid diseases. *Am J Med* 2005; 118: 890-898.

Bruggeman LA, Dikman S, Meng C, Quaqqin SE, Coffman TM & Klotman PE (1997). Nephropathy in human immunodeficiency virus-1 transgenic mice is due to renal transgene expression. *J Clin Invest* 1997; 100:84-92.

Casanova S, Mazzucco G, Barbiano di Belgiojoso G, Motta M, Boldorini R & Genderini A, et al (1995). Pattern of glomerular involvement in human immunodeficiency virus-infected patients: an Italian study. *Am J Kidney Dis* 1995; 26:446-453.

Connolly JO, Weston CE & Hendry BM (1995). HIV associated renal disease in London hospitals. *Q J Med* 88: 627-34, 1995.

Cheng JT, Anderson HL, Markowitz GS, Appel GB, Poque VA & D'Agati V (1999). Hepatitis C virus-associated glomerular disease in patients with human immunodeficiency virus coinfection. *J Am Soc Nephrol* 1999; 10:1566-1574.

Chen Y, Tang Z, Yang G, Shen S, Yu Y & Zeng C et al (2005). Malignant hypertension in patients with IgA nephropathy. *Kidney Blood Press Res* 2005; 28:251-258.

D'Agati V & Appel GB (1997). HIV infection and the kidney. *J Am Soc Nephrol* 1997; 8:138-152.

D'Agati V & Appel GB (1998). Renal pathology of human immunodeficiency virus infection. *Semin Nephrol* 1998; 18: 406-421.

Eitner F, Cui Y, Hudkins KL, Schmidt A, Birkebak T & Aqv MV et al (1999). Thrombotic microangiopathy in the HIV-2-infected macaque. *Am J Pathol* 1999; 155:649-661.

Eitner F, Cui Y, Hudkins KL, Stokes MB, Segerer S & Mack M, et al (2000).Chemokine receptor CCR5 and CXCR4 expression in HIV-associated kidney disease. *J Am Soc Nephrol* 2000; May;11(5):856-67.

Eggers PW & Kimmel PL (2004). Is there and epidemic of HIV infection in the US ESRD Program?. *J Am Soc Nephrol* 2004; 15:2477-2485.

Enríquez R, Cabezuelo JB, Escolano C, Pérez M, Amorós F & Gutiérrez-Rodero F, et al (2004). Postinfectious diffuse proliferative glomerulonephritis and acute renal failure in an HIV patient. *Clin Nephrol* 2004; 61:278-281.

Fang CT, Chang YY, Hsu HM, Twu SJ, Chen KT & Lin CC, et al (2007). Life expectancy of patients with newly-diagnosed HIV infection in the era of highly active antiretroviral therapy. *QJM* 2007; 100:97-105.

Gadallah MF, El-Shahawy MA, Campese VM, Todd JR & King JW (1996). Disparate prognosis of thrombotic microangiopathy in HIV-infected patients with and without AIDS. *Am J Nephrol* 1996; 16:446-450.

Galrão L, Brites C, Atta ML, Atta A, Lima I & Gonzalez F et al (2007). Antiphospholipid antibodies in HIV-positive patients. *Clin Rheumatol* 2007; 26: 1825–1830.

Gindea S, Schwartzman J, Herlitz LC, Rosenberg M, Abadi J & Putterman C (2010). Proliferative Glomerulonephritis in Lupus Patients with Human Immunodeficiency Virus Infection: A Difficult Clinical Challenge. *Semin Arthritis Rheum* 2010 Dec; 40(3):201-9.

Grinspoon S & Carr A (2005). Cardiovascular risk and body-fat abnormalities in HIV-infected adults. *N Engl J Med* 2005; 352: 1721–1722.

Gupta SK, Eustace JA, Winston JA, Boydstun II, Ahuja TS & Rodriguez RA et al (2005). Guidelines for the management of chronic kidney disease in HIV-infected patients: recommendations of the HIV Medicine Association of the Infectious Diseases Society of America. *Clin Infect Dis* 2005; 40: 1559–1585.

Gutiérrez E, González E, Hernández E, Morales E, Martínez MA & Usera G, et al (2007). Factors that determine an incomplete recovery of renal function in macrohematuria-induced acute renal failure of IgA nephropathy. *Clin J Am Soc Nephrol* 2007; 2:51-57.

Gutiérrez E, Morales E, Gutiérrez Martínez E, Manzanares MJ, Rosello G & Mérida E et al (2007). Glomerulopatías asociadas a la infección por VIH: Una perspectiva española. *Nefrología* 2007; 27: 439-447.

Haas M, Kaul S & Eustace JA (2005). HIV-associated immune complex glomerulonephritis with «lupus-like» features: a clinicopathologic study of 14 cases. *Kidney Int* 2005 67:1381-1390.

Hatsukari I, Singh P, Hitosugi N, Messmer D, Valderrama E & Teichberg et al (2007). DEC-205-mediated internalization of HIV-1 results in the establishment of silent infection in renal tubular cells. J Am Soc Nephrol 2007; 18(3):780-787.

Herman ES & Klotman PE (2003). HIV-associated nephropathy: Epidemiology, pathogenesis and treatment. *Semin Nephrol* 2003; 23:200-208.

Husebekk A, Permin H & Husby G (1986). Serum amyloid protein (SAA): an indicator of inflammation in AIDS and AIDS-related complex. *Scand J Infect Dis* 1986; 18:389-394.

Joseph A, Wali RK & Weinman EJ (2000). Renal Amyloidosis in AIDS. *Ann Intern Med* 2000;133(1):75

Kadan JS & Talal AH (2007). Changing treatment paradigms: hepatitis C virus in HIV-infected patients. *AIDS* 2007; 21:154-168.

Kamar N, Rostaing L, Alric L (2006). Treatment of hepatitis C-virusrelated glomerulonephritis. *Kidney Int* 2006; 69:436-439.

Kamin DS & Grinspoon SK (2005). Cardiovascular disease in HIV-positive patients. *AIDS* 2005; 19: 641–652.

Kimmel PL, Phillips TM, Ferreira-Centeno A, Farkas-Szallasi T, Abraham AA, Garret CT (1992). Idiotypic IgA nephropathy in patients with human immunodeficiency virus infection. *N Engl J Med* 1992; 327:729-730.

Kimmel PL, Ferreira-Centeno A, Farkas-Szallasi T, Abraham AA & Garret CT (1993). Viral DNA in microdissected renal biopsy tissue from HIV infected patients with nephrotic sybdrome. *Kidney Int* 1993; 43:1347-1352.

King NW, Hunt RD & Letvin NL (1993). Histopathologic changes in macaques with an acquired immunodeficiency syndrome (AIDS). *Am J Pathol* 1983; 113:382-388.

Klotman PE (1999). HIV-associated nephropathy. *Kidney Int* 1999; 56:1161-1176.

Lanjewar DN, Ansari MA, Shetty CR, Maheshwari MB & Jain P (1999). Renal lesions associated with AIDS -an autopsy study. *Indian J Pathol Microbiol* 1999; 42:63-68.

Lu TC & Ross M (2005). HIV-associated nephropathy. *Mt Sinai J Med* 2005; 72(3):193-9.

Lucas GM, Eustace JA, Sozio S, Mentari EK, Appiah KA & Moore RD (2004). Highly active antiretroviral therapy and the incidence of HIV-1-associated nephropathy: a 12-year cohort study. *AIDS* 2004; 18:541-546.

Masia-Canuto M, Bernal-Morell E & Gutierrez-Rodero F (2006). Lipid alterations and cardiovascular risk associated with antiretroviral therapy. *Enferm Infecc Microbiol Clin* 2006; 24:637–48.

Mazbar SA, Schoenfeld PY & Humphreys MH (1989). Renal involvement in patients infected with HIV: Experience at San Francisco General Hospital. *Kidney Int* 37:1358-1370, 1989.

Mikulak J & Singhal PC (2010). HIV-1 and kidney cells: better understanding of viral interaction. *Proc Natl Acad Sci U S A* 2010; 107(9):4281-6.

Mocroft A, Vella S, Benfield TL, Chiesi A, Miller V & Gargalianos, P, et al (1998). Changing patterns of mortality across Europe in patients infected with HIV-1. EuroSIDA Study Group. *Lancet* 1998; 352:1725-1730.

Mocroft A, Kirk O, Gatell J, Reiss P, Gargalinos P & Zilmer K, et al (2007). Chronic renal failure among HIV-1-infected patients. *AIDS* 2007; 21:1119-1127.

Morales E, Alegre R, Herrero JC, Morales JM, Ortuño T & Praga M (1997). Hepatitis-C-Virus associated cryoglobulinaemic membranoproliferative glomerulonephritis in patients infected by HIV. *Nephrol Dial Transplant* 1997; 12:1980-1984.

Morales E, Martinez A, Sánchez-Ayuso J, Gutierrez E, Mateo S, Martínez MA, Herrero JC & Praga M (2002). Spontaneous improvement of the renal function in a patient with HIV-associated focal glomerulosclerosis. *Am J Nephrol* 2002; 22(4):369-71.

Morales E, Rosello G, Hernández E, Gutierrez E, González E & Praga M (2007). Persistence of symptomatic cryoglobulinemia after disappearance of HCV-RNA in patients with cryoglobulinemic membranoproliferative glomerulonephritis treated with interferon and ribavirin. *J Am Soc Nephrol* 2007, 18:787A.

Morales E, Gutierrez-Solis E, Gutierrez E, González R, Martínez MA & Praga M (2008). Malignant hypertension in HIV-associated glomerulonephritis. *Nephrol Dial Transplant* 2008; 23(12):3901-7.

Nochy D, Glotz D, Dosquet P, Pruna A, Guettier C & Weiss L et al (1993). Renal disease associated with HIV infection: A multicentric study of 60 patients from Paris Hospitals. *Nephrol Dial Transplant* 1993; 8:11-19.

Panel de expertos del Grupo de Estudio de Sida (GESIDA) y del Plan Nacional sobre el Sida (PNS) (2010). Diagnosis, treatment and prevention of renal diseases in HIV infected patients. Recommendations of the Spanish AIDS Study Group/National AIDS Plan]. *Enferm Infecc Microbiol Clin* 2010; 28(8):520.e1-22.

Peraldi MN, Maslo C, Akposso K, Mougenot B, Rondeau E & Sraer JD (1999). Acute renal failure in the course of HIV infection: A single-institution retrospective study of ninety-two patients and sixty renal biopsies. *Nephrol Dial Transplant* 1999; 14: 1578-1585.

Polanco N, Gutiérrez E, Covarsí A, Ariza F, Carreño A & Vigil A, et al (2010). Grupo de Estudio de las Enfermedades Glomerulares de la Sociedad Española de Nefrología. Spontaneous remission of nephrotic syndrome in idiopathic membranous nephropathy. *J Am Soc Nephrol* 2010; 21(4):697-704.

Praga M, Gutiérrez E, González E, Morales E & Hernández E (2003). Treatment of IgA nephropathy with ACE inhibitors: A randomized and controlled trial. *J Am Soc Nephrol* 2003; 14:1578-1583.

Praga M (2008). Response to 'Tacrolimus in membranous nephropathy'. *Kidney Int* 2008; 74(6):824.

Rao TK, Filippone FJ, Nicastrti AD, Landesman SH, Frank E & Chen CK et al (1984). Associated focal and segmental glomerulosclerosis in the acquired inmunodeficency syndrome. *N Engl J Med* 310 (11):669-73, 1984.

Rao TK, Friedman EA & Nicastri AD (1987). The types of renal disease in the acquired immunodeficiency syndrome. *N Engl J Med* 1987; 316:1062-1068.

Röling J, Schmid H, Fischereder M, Draenert R & Goebel FD (2006). HIV-associated renal disease and highly active antiretroviral therapy-induced nephropathy. *Clin Infect Dis* 2006; 42:1488-1495.

Scialla JJ, Atta MG & Fine DM (2007). Relapse of HIV-associated nephropathy after discontinuing highly active antiretroviral therapy. *AIDS* 2007; 21:263-264.

Shahinian V, Rajaraman S, Borucki M, Grady J, Hollander M & Ahuja TS (2000). Prevalence of HIV-associated Nephropathy in Autopsies of HIV-Infected Patients. *Am J Kidney Dis* 35(5):884-888, 2000.

Smith MC, Pawar R, Carey JT, Graham RC, Jacobs GH & Menon A, et al (1994). Effect of corticosteroid therapy on human-immunodeficiency virus-associated nephropathy. *Am J Med* 1994; 97:145-151.

Stokes MB, Chawla H, Brody RI, Kumar A, Gertner R, Goldfarb DS & Gallo G (1997). Inmune Complex Glomerulonephritis in Patients Coinfected With Human Inmunodeficiency Virus and Hepatitis C Virus. *Am J Kidney Dis* 1997; Apr 29 (4):514-525.

Szczech LA, Gange SJ, Van der Horst C, Bartlett JA, Young M & Cohen MH, et al (2002). Predictors of proteinuria and renal failure among women with HIV infection. *Kidney Int* 2002; 61: 195-202.

Szczech LA, Gupta SK, Habash R, Guasch A, KalayjianR & Appel R, et al (2004). The clinical epidemiology and course of the spectrum of renal diseases associated with HIV infection. *Kidney Int* 66:1145-1152, 2004.

Wei A, Burns GC, Williams BA & Mohammed NB (2003). Long-term renal survival in HIV-associated nephropathy with angiotensin-converting enzyme inhibition. *Kidney Int* 2003; 64:1462-1471.

Weiner NJ, Goodman JW & Kimmel PL (2003). The HIV-associated renal disease: Current insight into pathogenesis and treatment. *Kidney Int* 2003; 63:1618-1631.

Williams DI, Williams DJ, Williams IG, Unwin RJ, Griffiths MH & Miller RF (1998). Presentation, pathology and outcome of HIV associated renal disease in a specialist centre for HIV/AIDS. *Sex Transm Inf* 1998; 74:179-184.

Winston JA, Burns GC & Klotman PE (1998). The human immunodeficiency virus (HIV) epidemic and HIV-associated nephropathy. *Semin Nephrol* 1998; 18:373-377.

Wyatt CM, Winston JA, Malvestutto CD, Fishbein DA, Barash I & Cohen AJ, et al (2007). Chronic kidney disease in HIV infection: an urban epidemic. *AIDS* 2007; 21:2101-2110.

Permissions

The contributors of this book come from diverse backgrounds, making this book a truly international effort. This book will bring forth new frontiers with its revolutionizing research information and detailed analysis of the nascent developments around the world.

We would like to thank Richard J. Glassock, MD, MACP, for lending his expertise to make the book truly unique. He has played a crucial role in the development of this book. Without his invaluable contribution this book wouldn't have been possible. He has made vital efforts to compile up to date information on the varied aspects of this subject to make this book a valuable addition to the collection of many professionals and students.

This book was conceptualized with the vision of imparting up-to-date information and advanced data in this field. To ensure the same, a matchless editorial board was set up. Every individual on the board went through rigorous rounds of assessment to prove their worth. After which they invested a large part of their time researching and compiling the most relevant data for our readers. Conferences and sessions were held from time to time between the editorial board and the contributing authors to present the data in the most comprehensible form. The editorial team has worked tirelessly to provide valuable and valid information to help people across the globe.

Every chapter published in this book has been scrutinized by our experts. Their significance has been extensively debated. The topics covered herein carry significant findings which will fuel the growth of the discipline. They may even be implemented as practical applications or may be referred to as a beginning point for another development. Chapters in this book were first published by InTech; hereby published with permission under the Creative Commons Attribution License or equivalent.

The editorial board has been involved in producing this book since its inception. They have spent rigorous hours researching and exploring the diverse topics which have resulted in the successful publishing of this book. They have passed on their knowledge of decades through this book. To expedite this challenging task, the publisher supported the team at every step. A small team of assistant editors was also appointed to further simplify the editing procedure and attain best results for the readers.

Our editorial team has been hand-picked from every corner of the world. Their multi-ethnicity adds dynamic inputs to the discussions which result in innovative outcomes. These outcomes are then further discussed with the researchers and contributors who give their valuable feedback and opinion regarding the same. The feedback is then collaborated with the researches and they are edited in a comprehensive manner to aid the understanding of the subject.

Apart from the editorial board, the designing team has also invested a significant amount of their time in understanding the subject and creating the most relevant covers. They scrutinized every image to scout for the most suitable representation of the subject and create an appropriate cover for the book.

The publishing team has been involved in this book since its early stages. They were actively engaged in every process, be it collecting the data, connecting with the contributors or procuring relevant information. The team has been an ardent support to the editorial, designing and production team. Their endless efforts to recruit the best for this project, has resulted in the accomplishment of this book. They are a veteran in the field of academics and their pool of knowledge is as vast as their experience in printing. Their expertise and guidance has proved useful at every step. Their uncompromising quality standards have made this book an exceptional effort. Their encouragement from time to time has been an inspiration for everyone.

The publisher and the editorial board hope that this book will prove to be a valuable piece of knowledge for researchers, students, practitioners and scholars across the globe.

List of Contributors

Abdelaziz Elsanjak and Sharma S. Prabhakar
Department of Medicine, Texas Tech University Health Sciences Center, USA

Matthew C. Pickering
Centre for Complement & Inflammation Research (CCIR), Imperial College, London, United Kingdom

Joshua M. Thurman
Division of Nephrology and Hypertension, University of Colorado Denver School of Medicine, Colorado United States of America

Dawinder S. Sohal and Sharma S. Prabhakar
Department of Medicine, Texas Tech University Health Sciences Center, USA

Francois Berthoux
Dialysis and Renal Transplantation Department, University Hospital of Saint-Etienne, Medical Faculty of Saint-Etienne, Saint-Etienne Cedex 2, France

Amir Kamal Aziz
Nephrology and Dialysis Department, Louis Pasteur Hospital, Dole, France Dimitrios Kirmizis and Aikaterini Papagianni Aristotle University, Thessaloniki, Greece

Francesco Paolo Schena
Renal Unit, University of Bari, Bari, Italy

Maria Pia Rastaldi
Renal Research Laboratory, Fondazione IRCCS Ca' Granda Ospedale Maggiore, Policlinico & Fondazione D'Amico per la Ricerca sulle Malattie Renali Milano, Italy

L. Guilherme, S. Freschi de Barros, A.C. Tanaka and J. Kalil
Heart Institute (InCor), School of Medicine, University of São Paulo, São Paulo, Brazil

J. Kalil
Clinical Immunology and Allergy Division, School of Medicine, University of São Paulo, São Paulo, Brazil

L. Guilherme, S. Freschi de Barros and J. Kalil
Immunology Investigation Institute, National Institute for Science and Technology, University of São Paulo, São Paulo, Brazil

...eiro Castro
...logy Division, School of Medicine, University of São Paulo, São Paulo, Brazil

...neet Singh
...nzies School of Health Research, Cahrles Darwin University, Darwin, NT, Northern ...rritory Medical Program, Flinders University, SA, Australia

Toru Watanabe
Department of Pediatrics, Niigata City General Hospital, Japan

Vincent Ho
Department of Medicine, Campbelltown Hospital and School of Medicine, University of Western Sydney, Sydney, Australia

Jason Chen
Department of Anatomical Pathology, Royal North Shore Hospital, Sydney, Australia

W. Michael McShan and Roya Toloui
Department of Pharmaceutical Sciences, University of Oklahoma Health Sciences Center, Oklahoma City, USA

Enrique Morales, Elena Gutierrez-Solis, Eduardo Gutierrez and Manuel Praga
Nephrology Department, Hospital 12 Octubre, Madrid, Spain